MODULAR COGNITIVE-BEHAVIORAL THERAPY FOR CHILDHOOD ANXIETY DISORDERS

Guides to Individualized Evidence-Based Treatment

Jacqueline B. Persons, *Series Editor*

Providing evidence-based roadmaps for managing real-world cases, volumes in this series help the clinician develop treatment plans using interventions of proven effectiveness. With an emphasis on systematic yet flexible case formulation, these hands-on guides provide powerful alternatives to one-size-fits-all approaches. Each book addresses a particular disorder or presents cutting-edge intervention strategies that can be used across a range of clinical problems.

Cognitive Therapy of Schizophrenia
David G. Kingdon and Douglas Turkington

Treating Bipolar Disorder: A Clinician's Guide to Interpersonal and Social Rhythm Therapy
Ellen Frank

Modular Cognitive-Behavioral Therapy for Childhood Anxiety Disorders
Bruce F. Chorpita

Cognitive-Behavioral Therapy for PTSD: A Case Formulation Approach
Claudia Zayfert and Carolyn Black Becker

Modular Cognitive-Behavioral Therapy for Childhood Anxiety Disorders

Bruce F. Chorpita

Series Editor's Note by Jacqueline B. Persons

THE GUILFORD PRESS
New York   London

© 2007 The Guilford Press
A Division of Guilford Publications, Inc.
72 Spring Street, New York, NY 10012
www.guilford.com

Printed in Canada

This book is printed on acid-free paper.

Last digit is print number: 9 8 7 6 5 4 3 2 1

Library of Congress Cataloging-in-Publication Data

Chorpita, Bruce F.
    Modular cognitive-behavioral therapy for childhood anxiety disorders / Bruce F. Chorpita.
      p. cm. — (Guides to individualized evidence-based treatment)
    Includes bibliographical references and index.
    ISBN-13: 978-1-59385-363-1 ISBN-10: 1-59385-363-7 (pbk. : alk. paper)
    1. Anxiety in children—Treatment.   2. Cognitive therapy for children.   I. Title.   II. Series.
    [DNLM: 1. Anxiety Disorders—therapy.   2. Cognitive Therapy—methods.   3. Child.
WM 172 C551m 2006]
    RJ506.A58C53 2006
    618.92′8522—dc22

                                                                    2006024796

About the Author

Bruce F. Chorpita, PhD, is Professor of Clinical Psychology, Clinical Adjunct Professor of Psychiatry, and Codirector of the Center for Cognitive Behavior Therapy at the University of Hawaii. He is an internationally recognized expert on childhood anxiety disorders and on innovations in treatment design and dissemination. Dr. Chorpita has generated more than 75 publications on anxiety disorders and children's mental health and has received many awards and honors for his work, including a commendation from the governor of Hawaii for his teamwork with the Hawaii Department of Health in 2004 and the Hawaii Regents' Medal for Excellence in Research in 2005.

Locally, Dr. Chorpita has chaired Hawaii's Evidence Based Services Committee since 1999. The committee is composed of psychologists, psychiatrists, psychiatric nurses, clinical social workers, family members, and other professionals who regularly review the scientific literature to inform state clinical practice guidelines on treatment and prevention of child mental health problems. From 2001 to 2003 Dr. Chorpita also served as the Clinical Director of the Hawaii Department of Health's Child and Adolescent Mental Health Division, providing leadership and oversight to statewide practice development activities in public mental health.

Dr. Chorpita has served on the editorial boards of numerous professional journals and since 2005 has been Associate Editor of the *Journal of Abnormal Child Psychology*. He also worked nationally on practice policy as a member of both the American Psychological Association Division 53 Committee on Evidence-Based Treatment and the Division 12 Committee for Science and Practice. Since 2002 he has been a member of the Research Network on Youth Mental Health, a national collaborative group of experts working to identify, test, and implement promising mental health practices for children. Dr. Chorpita has also received research and training grants from the National Institute of Mental Health, the Hawaii Departments of Education and Health, and the John D. and Catherine T. MacArthur Foundation.

Series Editor's Note

Every anxious child is different. Some have separation anxiety, some have obsessive–compulsive disorder, and some worry. Some have families who encourage the child to confront his or her fears and overcome them, and others do not. And although, as Bruce F. Chorpita, the author of this volume, points out, "nobody likes exposure," some move smoothly through it, whereas others have depressive symptoms or oppositional behaviors or other problems that interfere with the treatment. This volume provides the busy clinician with a single guide to the effective treatment of all these children.

This book, which is part of the series Guides to Individualized Evidence-Based Treatment, aims to facilitate the transportation of evidence-based therapies from the ivory tower to the front lines of clinical settings. The series presents strategies clinicians can use to individualize treatment to meet the needs of each unique case while remaining evidence based. In this case, the evidence base is particularly strong; the treatment presented in this volume has been shown to be effective for treating childhood anxiety in a controlled study (Chorpita, Taylor, Francis, Moffitt, & Austin, 2004).

The book begins with a clear presentation of the cognitive-behavioral conceptualization of clinical anxiety in children and its treatment. The goal here is to teach clinicians the fundamentals of cognitive-behavioral conceptualizations of anxiety and its treatment in a way that will allow them to develop a cognitive-behavioral conceptualization of each child's anxiety and carry out a principle-driven treatment of it. Thus, treatment is guided by principles rather than by a list of interventions. Whereas some approaches provide only a step-by-step protocol that lists a series of interventions to be carried out for every patient (cf. Wilson, 1998), this book strives for more by providing clinicians with guidance to improve clinical judgment rather than to minimize it.

To meet the needs of each child and family, the treatment is organized in modules (Wilson, 2000). All anxious children receive some modules (e.g., learning to make a fear ladder to rate anxiety severity), but only some receive others (e.g., the module that teaches parents to ignore avoidance or other countertherapeutic behaviors by the child). An algorithm guides the clinician's selection of modules for each case. All the modules have the same format; this consistency allows the clinician to quickly learn a module and pull it into a treatment plan. Because Chorpita views exposure as the heart and soul of an effective treatment of anxiety, exposure, both imaginal and *in vivo,* is described in careful detail. Some modules address noncompliance, oppositional behaviors, avoidance, and other problems that interfere with the exposure and other fundamental components of the treatment. The treatment is also highly idiographic in that it is guided by data collected from each patient as treatment proceeds. The clinician uses the fear ladder at the beginning of each session to monitor the child's progress in treatment, and the results of this assessment feed directly into the agenda for that session.

Bruce Chorpita's clinical experience, judgment, and wisdom provide invaluable guidance. A key concept is "Back to fundamentals." That is, if the child is not responding to the treatment, Chorpita recommends taking a close look at fundamentals to be sure they are being delivered before reworking the treatment plan. His scholarship, clinical experience, teaching skills, and sparkle, energy, and sense of humor shine through every page. The racial, ethnic, and cultural diversity of Hawaii, where this treatment was developed, also adds a special richness to the material.

I am delighted to include this book in the Guides to Individualized Evidence-Based Treatment series. I'm certain it will make an important contribution to the treatment of children who suffer from anxiety disorders and to the development of idiographic, principle-driven, cognitive-behavioral therapies more generally.

JACQUELINE B. PERSONS, PhD
San Francisco Bay Area Center for Cognitive Therapy

Acknowledgments

This book is dedicated to my wife, Catherine Sustana, for her constant support in all my endeavors, and to our two children, Marie and Nicholas, who have taught me so much about working with children and yet regularly remind me how much I still don't know.

Thanks are due to Eric Daleiden, who as a friend and a colleague participated in dozens of conversations with me about these ideas. Lucky for me, he has the special skill of taking ordinary concepts and making them into great ones. In the end, this book is as full of his ideas as it is of my own.

I extend thanks to my mentors and teachers who taught me how to think about human behavior and the technology to alleviate human suffering. In graduate school, David Barlow taught me practically everything that was then known about anxiety and its treatment, ultimately making it possible for me to develop new ideas of my own. At the same time, Tim Brown taught me assessment and diagnostics with Cartesian precision.

Anne Marie Albano literally taught me how to be a cognitive-behavioral therapist, first using a manual, and then flexibly addressing cases whenever the manuals did not fit. Later, Ron Drabman's "handout" approach to supervision—together with what I learned from Anne Marie—served as the inspiration for the modular design and flexible application of cognitive-behavioral therapy that are outlined in this book.

I am grateful to my colleagues for their continual encouragement and generosity. Every one of these people supported my efforts on this project or helped improve my thinking about it in some way: Tina Donkervoet, Nancy Gorman, Laurie Garduque, Charles Glisson, Scott Henggeler, Kimberly Hoagwood, Peter Jensen, Christopher Lonigan, Chuck Mueller, Tom Ollendick, Jackie Persons, Paulie Schick, Jason Schiffman, Sonja Schoenwald, Michael Southam-Gerow, John Weisz, and Karen Wells. I feel lucky to know all of them.

I also wish to thank the graduate students who worked on this protocol with me long before it close to becoming a book. Alissa Taylor, Sarah Francis, Aukahi Austin, Catherine Moffitt, Jennifer Gray, Farrah Greene, Charmaine Higa, Brad Nakamura, John Young, Kii Kimhan, and Letty Yim, among others, helped me to develop, test, and refine these procedures over almost 10 years—many of them working as cotherapists with me along the way. Many of the worksheets and handouts, too, are the products of their creativity and initiative. Thanks are due not just to those mentioned but also to all of my graduate and practicum students for giving me the opportunity to teach and to learn about cognitive-behavioral therapy and to help them help children. I couldn't ask for a better job.

I feel fortunate to be able to acknowledge the support from the National Institute of Mental Health, the John D. and Catherine T. MacArthur Foundation, and the Hawaii Departments of Health and Education, which kept our programs running all these years.

Finally, my sincerest gratitude is offered to the children and families of my community whose struggles brought them to our center and gave us all the opportunity to serve, to learn, and to teach. It has been a humbling experience, and one that I will continue to treasure.

Contents

PART IV. TREATMENT MODULES

MODULAR COGNITIVE-BEHAVIORAL THERAPY FOR CHILDHOOD ANXIETY DISORDERS

PART I
GETTING STARTED

ONE

Why This Manual?

The most serious thinking about how to treat the children and families in our program happens mostly on Friday mornings. Within the confines of the University of Hawaii's Center for Cognitive Behavior Therapy, we provide mental health services to children between the ages of 6 and 18, mostly referred from Hawaii public schools and the Department of Health. A handful of those served are self-referred families from around the Pacific region who have sought specialty treatment for complex anxiety problems. The cases are almost always challenging—much harder than I remember seeing when I was receiving my own graduate training (a confession that my current trainees find quite satisfying), and there are nearly 15 therapists who require my regular supervision for their cases. Many of them are graduate students in training, and thus—quite appropriately—tend to request more guidance than the average practitioner. We meet for several hours each Friday morning to discuss cases and make decisions.

Friday is also the only day that we all see each other as a cohesive program—the graduate students, postdoctoral staff, and faculty supervisors. We typically all have lunch together after our morning meeting, giving us an important opportunity to socialize and share ideas, which is then followed by research and training meetings in the afternoon. This schedule means that we have only a small window of opportunity on Friday morning to make important decisions about our ongoing cases. These are some of the most important decisions we make all week, so we have to get them right. No one goes to lunch until we feel confident about the treatment plans.

Over nearly a 10-year period, the level of clinical complexity of this work has served to reform and even threaten many of my beliefs about effective therapy approaches. On the one hand, the children and families we were seeing had so many more challenges than I was first accustomed to that it seemed that many of the manualized approaches with which I had been trained would have limited success. I felt this not because I believed the techniques would not work, but because the family situations were often so complicated, the comorbidity so severe, or the need for treatment gains so rushed that the delivery of the appropriate techniques might never occur or would not occur quickly

enough to keep a family from giving up on us. For example, a child referred to us by a
school social worker in October, and who has been out of school for more than a month,
would not have time to cover all the requisite steps in a typical anxiety treatment manual before getting back into the classroom. It had to happen "yesterday." Similarly, an
anxious child with challenging oppositional behaviors might not be inclined to participate and cooperate with cognitive-behavioral therapy (CBT), and perhaps would
require some strategies for managing disruptive behavior. Other times, a case would go
longer than 12–16 weeks, with clear evidence of the need to continue treatment, yet most
manualized treatments for anxiety would have ended by then. Finally, children very
often had more than one anxiety problem, which could mean that different manuals
might be needed (e.g., one for obsessive–compulsive disorder, one for social anxiety).
My training told me it was important to use treatments backed by scientific evidence,
but how could treatment manuals be followed in such cases?

At the same time, I was often training new therapists to perform in these challenging circumstances without the luxury of time to go over every detail of every technique
every Friday. Even if we didn't want to use a manual for the reasons described above,
time constraints meant we would have to somehow. Without some structured way to
teach the key strategies that work for childhood anxiety, there simply would not be
enough time to train clinicians properly or to accept many of the referrals that seemed
likely to benefit from our program. Training materials had to be written down and structured, so how could we *not* use a manual?

I eventually realized that solving this dilemma would require a new kind of manual.

THREE CRITICAL ISSUES

That manual would come to be organized around three main issues. First, to state the
obvious, the best treatment plan in the world has little chance if the child and family are
unwilling or unable to participate in the protocol. Thus *engagement* is always one of the
first issues to address. A minimum level is necessary for the protocol to work, and given
the fact that anxiety treatments can sometimes be uncomfortable for children and even
parents, more engagement is probably better. That said, there is more to treating anxiety
than a good therapeutic relationship, and indeed there is no evidence to suggest that
engagement alone is sufficient for success. There are other things to think about as well.

With childhood anxiety, those other things involve specific procedures that are well
documented but not always easy to implement. Properly exposing a child to a feared situation or appropriately constructing a list of feared situations takes special skills. In relatively straightforward circumstances, implementing the techniques can predominate
clinical thinking, and without a doubt, it is important for us to get the techniques right.
For that, it seemed, a manual would be ideal—all the techniques could be written down
with their steps laid out neatly for therapists to follow. So the second issue is about the
basic component strategies of CBT, or what I call the *fundamentals*.

There is, however, still one other critical issue that arises, particularly as cases present more complex circumstances with their family, schools, or community. This issue

concerns the pace, the timing, or selection of techniques themselves, not simply their proper execution. Should we start practicing feared situations with a child? How soon? Does this child need to practice some cognitive therapy skills first? Are social skills going to be important? How should we deal with a child's inability to perform therapy "homework"? This aspect of therapy is not about execution of techniques but rather about their selection, order, pace, intensity, and so forth—how they work together.

To take an example, consider an anxious 8-year-old girl who has trouble learning cognitive restructuring skills for some reason or another. On the one hand, the therapist might be wasting time going over cognitive material if it will ultimately be grasped only partially and hence offer little strategic value. So perhaps it makes sense to skip the cognitive exercises and move forward with other parts of the protocol. On the other hand, maybe taking the time to master a cognitive technique early in treatment would pay off richly later in treatment. Spend more time on cognitive skills? Skip cognitive skills? This kind of thinking came up all the time with our cases and required some time and effort to evaluate.

My experience with practicing clinicians, and indeed even my own training in university-based research clinics, suggested that these decisions were made in a way that did not always fit with a predetermined selection, order, or length of therapy sessions as dictated by many treatment manuals. Thus this third issue involves *case formulation*. By developing a working idea of why problems are the way they are, therapists have a guide for determining how to select, sequence, and pace known clinical strategies. In addition to addressing *engagement* and therapy *fundamentals*, this new manual would have to provide a framework for *case formulation*, too.

NO MORE SUPERVISION AS USUAL

In research the term "treatment as usual" refers to the actual care that is delivered under typical clinical circumstances. Although I have not seen the term "supervision as usual" used anywhere, it seems this concept applies equally well in that context. Given the lack of evidence on what content characterizes "supervision as usual," I can only write anecdotally about it. Supervision is the time when the deepest critical thinking about a case is meant to occur. In my opinion, "supervision as usual" seems to be characterized, at worst, by narrative descriptions of the therapy sessions themselves (e.g., "he said this, and then I said that") and, at best, by therapist-nominated problems that might warrant attention (e.g., "I don't know why she's not doing her homework again"), that is, if supervision happens at all. In many community practice settings, it simply does not happen, or it involves a checklist review of caseloads and current crises.

Wading through these issues and getting to the heart of the matter—the formulation—can take lots of time for any one case, and there may not always be sufficient time. But that is not the only problem. What has always made me uneasy is the well-known literature on confidence and clinical decision making: the idea that more discussion and details often add little to the accuracy of decisions, but merely increase therapist confidence (e.g., Oskamp, 1962). Perhaps our discussions were going nowhere clinically and simply ending when everyone's confidence level rose enough to inspire a collective urge to move to the next case. Or to lunch. Even in our luxurious university setting, supervision as usual was definitely a problem.

Outside the university setting, the problem could only be worse: Such time to discuss and reflect on cases is generally unavailable or very limited. Thus, over the same 10-year period, these issues regarding clinical supervision were the subject of much discussion in our state mental health system as well. In my work with the state Departments of Health and Education, I learned just how much more time we have at our university center to conduct supervision. Not surprisingly, most practitioners in the field participated in clinical supervision approximately once a month. The time and resources for thinking about cases were meager, and given our beliefs about the importance of quality review and case formulation, something needed to be fixed.

As part of a university and state mental health partnership in practice development, several of us quietly plotted the death of "supervision as usual." A model eventually emerged to help restructure supervision (i.e., the process of making decisions about cases) so as to improve efficiency and effectiveness (e.g., Chorpita & Donkervoet, 2005; Daleiden & Chorpita, 2005). In essence, this model was an attempt to codify strategies addressing this third issue—case formulation—and to make it work for clinicians who did not have the luxury of time to regularly review every case in detail. In an attempt to address concerns about supervision, we made some important discoveries about how to innovate our own clinical decision making. Whether one participates in supervision or not, these ideas are highly relevant to the routine decisions and considerations of clinical work.

FUNDAMENTALS MEET CASE FORMULATION

So how do we incorporate these new ideas about flexible case formulation and clinical decision making into a treatment manual? Treatment manuals are supposed to be static and linear, right? Well, not necessarily. Over time, my colleagues and I came to see how *case formulation* could be combined with detailed instructions for clinical strategies drawn from well-tested evidence-based approaches (i.e., the *fundamentals*), and this combination would provide the basis for how best to proceed with a given client. This manual is therefore organized on those principles. On the one hand, clear and discrete descriptions of how to execute important clinical techniques are needed. These are provided in Part IV of this book, where each technique is described in its own self-contained unit or *module* so it can be easily performed by following the steps as outlined. The outlines of these techniques are relatively straightforward, for the most part, and may already be part of some therapists' repertoires. The challenge, however, is that the fundamentals are easy to do poorly and difficult to do well. Making them seem natural and fitting to each individual child's problem can take some practice and time. Once mastered, though, they are like reliable tools in one's toolkit.

Much of the rest of this book is really about case formulation—figuring out what to do when, for which reasons. This first chapter provides the overall framework for these decisions and points to how to use other parts of the book for different decisions under various circumstances. As with the fundamentals, mastery of case formulation takes some practice, too.

THE FRAMEWORK FOR CASE FORMULATION

Back to Friday morning. If we accept the notion that not every child will receive the same exact course of strategies in the same order for the same period of time, then we also must acknowledge the likelihood that clinicians will be faced with a seemingly overwhelming number of choices at various decision points. Ideally, each of these decisions should be as informed as possible, yet there are so many sources of information that it can quickly become difficult to know what information to use at any given moment. More often than not, the key decisions are not quite in focus, or when they are, the information relevant to those decisions is either overlooked or unavailable.

The case formulation model that drives our decision process for this protocol is outlined in Figure 1.1. Note that decisions are represented by diamonds and proceed in a structured order. Each decision is also informed by one or more pieces of information, which can come from a variety of sources (represented by stacked documents with a curved lower edge). One key principle is that decisions are not made in the absence of the appropriate information; the information sources for the key decisions are shown in the first column. Finally, decisions can lead to actions, which are denoted by labeled rectangles, and each of these actions can be further supported by sources of information, which appear in the fourth column of the figure.

Beginning in the upper-left hand corner, the figure shows that the first decision a clinician faces is treatment selection. In the context of this manual, one must therefore decide whether the child's problem is primarily anxiety and therefore appropriate for the methods and techniques described. To make this decision, the clinician performs a comprehensive assessment and uses the results of the assessment to decide whether the primary problem area for the child is anxiety (with or without comorbidity—more on that later). Chapter 3 of this book provides information about how that assessment is performed and how that decision is made.

If treatment for anxiety is appropriate, the clinician must then address the question of whether treatment is actually possible. In other words, in order to benefit from the strategies and skills outlined in the manual, a child and family must be able to engage in treatment—that is, to meet regularly, and in most cases, be willing to rehearse skills outside of meetings with the therapist. Information about whether engagement exists often involves scheduling (e.g., days to get the first appointment scheduled). If therapy is already ongoing, this information can involve other sources of information, such as the frequency of missed sessions, amount of incomplete homework, or the frequency and promptness with which phone calls are returned. If the level of engagement threatens the ability to administer the protocol altogether, then engagement must be addressed. Although common, these circumstances do not typically characterize the majority of cases; thus the strategies for working on engagement appear later in the book (Chapters 6 and 11).

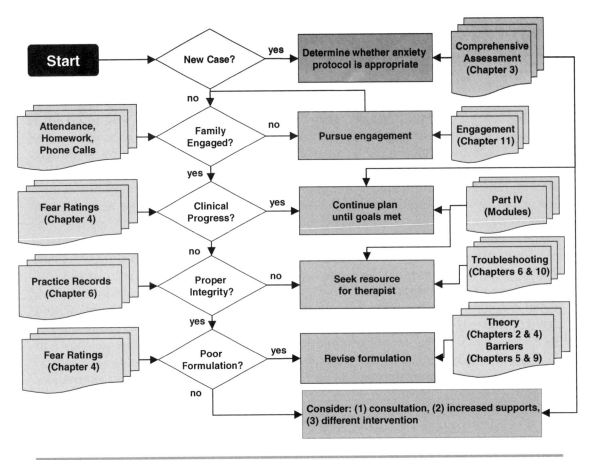

FIGURE 1.1. Case formulation: how to think with a manual. Adapted from Daleiden and Chorpita (2005). Copyright 2005 by W. B. Saunders. Adapted by permission.

Once engagement is observed or established, the decision making will then focus heavily on clinical progress. For a new case, this means getting a strategy in place that allows progress to be measured repeatedly over time. Repeated measurement of anxiety for this purpose is discussed in Chapter 4 and involves a list of feared situations for the child. This aspect of treatment allows one continually to reassess the success of the case formulation and adjust as necessary.

Once measurement is in place, ratings are obtained on a weekly basis, and these ratings inform a recurring review of clinical progress, as suggested by Figure 1.1. By this time, the therapist will be working from a treatment plan that suggests which techniques to use in what order (all treatment begins with a core plan that gets revised as needed). The details of the basic treatment plan and how it works are presented in Chapter 4. If the child is making progress, continuation of that treatment plan is recommended. Note that the action ("continue plan until goals met") is informed by the *fundamentals*, that is, the steps outlined in the treatment modules, as well as by information from the initial assessment, which spells out some of the goals for treatment.

If a child is not improving according to quantifiable ratings of progress, one must again consider the *fundamentals* (i.e., the proper execution of specific manualized techniques). In other words, clinicians should ask themselves whether they are performing the intervention properly. Because most of the treatment is organized around exposure, I have devoted three chapters to this single technique, covering the basics as well as how to troubleshoot its implementation. Troubleshooting involves the review of several records and information sources taken directly from treatment sessions (covered in Chapter 5). The same review of integrity is made not just for exposure but for all other clinical strategies as well, and Chapter 10 outlines methods to troubleshoot those. If there are problems with the implementation of specific techniques, Chapters 5 and 10 can to be used to identify possible solutions; more generally, additional therapist review of the modules could be needed.

Considering fundamentals should always precede jumping to case formulation decisions. In our supervision group, for example, before concluding that the basics are not working, a therapist must first demonstrate that these techniques were actually implemented properly. If not, then the tactic should be to fix the fundamentals rather than shifting to another direction. In my experience in training graduate students and community practitioners alike, there appears to be a strong bias toward jumping to a new plan. Who wants to believe he or she is not good at something? I certainly don't, and it is this rather normal reaction that often pushes a therapist prematurely onto a new plan when the old plan might have been fine—just poorly executed. Given the ubiquity of this error, the notion of "sticking to the plan" is given some serious attention in Chapter 4, which introduces the idea of the core treatment plan—in essence, every therapist's basic approach. That said, sometimes sticking to the plan simply does not work, and evidence mounts to justify a new approach. For example, comorbid oppositional behavior may interfere with even the best-designed exposure exercises. At this point, the appropriateness of the plan itself (here, to continue exposure) should be reconsidered. Given the complexity of revising a treatment plan, this decision should typically be informed by multiple sources of information. Important sources include clinical theory about childhood anxiety (Chapter 2), information about how treatment works under ideal circumstances (Chapter 4), information about how treatment works under less than ideal circumstances (Chapter 8), and strategies for selecting a new treatment plan consistent with a revised formulation (Chapter 9). In the context of a core theory about anxiety, the therapist is encouraged to hypothesize a new treatment plan and take appropriate action. The flowchart begins again in the upper left ("Start"), and the therapist continues to review engagement, clinical progress, and technical integrity, in turn. Although this method may sound complicated, in practice such reformulation often takes the form of "adding in" a reward program or a time-out program to address interference or obstacles with the ongoing treatment plan.

If the child is not improving despite what appears to be proper engagement, solid fundamentals, and an appropriate treatment plan, the therapist encounters the least desirable set of circumstances: being clinically "stuck" (see bottom rectangle in Figure 1.1). One should arrive at this stage only after reviewing all the prerequisite decisions and exhausting all other options. In this difficult set of circumstances, one may have to consider getting outside consultation, increasing the intensity of the intervention (e.g., considering a structured placement, adding other therapeutic supports), or whether another intervention altogether would be appropriate. Note that this action is informed by the initial assessment as well, which can be revisited to determine whether an entirely different approach would have been warranted (e.g., treating something other than anxiety). Fortunately, in our experience, this set of circumstances is rather rare. Most problems with clinical progress seem to be due to the earlier considerations outlined in Figure 1.1. Nevertheless, everyone can get "stuck" now and then, so this outcome is included in the figure for completeness.

HOW TO USE THIS MANUAL

Addis and Krasnow (2000) conducted a survey of practicing psychologists regarding their attitudes toward treatment manuals. One key finding is that practitioners for the most part do not use them. Here is the good news: The mere fact that you are reading a section called "How to Use This Manual" means you are exceptional. Keep up the good work (there is a lot more yet to read).

The bad news is that manuals may have some properties that make them unpopular or difficult to use. Two main themes presented by clinicians were that manuals do not emphasize (1) the importance of the therapeutic relationship or (2) individual case conceptualization. Let's briefly consider each of these in turn, because they speak directly to how to use this manual.

I have already said it, and I will say it again: The therapeutic relationship is important. One need not refer to the substantial and sometimes controversial literature on general versus specific factors in psychotherapy to be aware of this point. If an anxious child refuses to meet with you, you cannot get the job done. Thus a primary consideration in an ongoing case involves level of engagement (Figure 1.1). As mentioned earlier, this notion is covered generally in Chapter 11 and given special consideration regarding its most central procedures in Chapter 6.

That said, trying to teach someone how to manage the therapeutic relationship is a bit like trying to teach someone to be funny. This manual will give you plenty of things to consider regarding engagement, but chances are these are skills you already possess. Most of the therapists I have trained have shown remarkable ability to charm, delight, challenge, confront, and amuse the children they serve. It is an incredibly important skill and for many, perhaps, a gift. The book offers some illustrations, but if you are a practicing clinician, chances are your repertoire in this area is already an established part of your success. Go with what works for you and build off the suggestions and ideas in this book only when it seems appropriate.

Regarding the second theme, individual case conceptualization, this manual is a direct attempt to be different. The protocol is built around a case formulation framework, as outlined in Figure 1.1, and a flexible treatment planning algorithm covered in detail in Chapter 4. The case formulation and treatment planning processes are a major part of the protocol. Therapists should always know where they are with respect to the information in Figure 1.1 and should further know how the specific clinical strategies being used are tied to the formulation. It is best to read the main chapters of the book to get a solid idea of how the case formulation and treatment planning process work. Once these are well understood, the vast majority of the "reading" of the protocol will involve selective use of the modules in Part IV. They do not need to be read front to back. They should be selected and implemented only as needed, in the order fitting the treatment plan that makes the most sense.

And finally, let us not forget what manuals may do best: detail the procedures for how to perform specific strategies. One of these strategies is so important, so central, so incredibly essential to learn, that three entire chapters and two treatment modules are devoted to it: exposure. Therapists in our program are taught to be masters of exposure. It is the most important tool in the anxiety treatment arsenal, and everything else a therapist does is designed to support it. So, read those parts and get good at exposure. If you are already good, then get better. It makes all the difference.

In summary, this protocol balances three areas: (1) engagement and the therapeutic relationship, (2) fundamentals (especially exposure), and (3) case formulation. All are important, and just like the figure shows, all are considered in that order. At least, that's how we do it every Friday.

TWO

About Anxiety

Throughout this manual the topics of engagement, technical integrity, and case formulation are revisited. Skill in any of these areas, however, must first build on a basic understanding of the phenomenology and clinical theory of anxiety in children. For example, it far is easier for a therapist to engage a shy child knowing something about the effects of novelty or escape contingencies on anxiety. Likewise, regarding technical integrity, it is very possible to follow the steps of exposure in a manner that is quite wrong—even harmful—without a solid understanding of the concepts of extinction and habituation. Finally, case formulation is also likely to suffer when one cannot easily draw on theory to prioritize one strategy over another at any point in time. So this second chapter is principally about how anxiety works. Let us first begin with some examples of what anxiety looks like.

KRISTI

Kristi was 14 years old and one of four children in a single-parent family of Asian and Pacific Island descent. Kristi's mother had not finished high school, worked part time while raising her four children, and earned less than $15,000 a year. The mother stated that Kristi was "a really good kid" and that she was both bright and sensitive. She was an excellent swimmer and liked to spend time in the ocean or collecting things on the beach.

When she came to our program, Kristi said she had stopped attending school for the preceding 5 months because her classmates often teased her. Even aside from the teasing, Kristi expressed having feelings of constant distress and discomfort when around her peers, as well as fears of speaking or reading in class, working with a group of other children, or eating and drinking in front of others. She was quite worried that others would think she was "a loser."

In addition to her social fears, Kristi also had concerns about separation from her mother and home, stating that she feared something bad would happen to her while she was at school, such as getting sick or being kidnapped by a stranger. If she had to leave home, Kristi often complained of physical symptoms, such as headaches, stomachaches, and nausea. For the preceding 6 months, Kristi would sometimes vomit when anticipating the possibility of going to school. This reaction was complicated further by Kristi's persistent feeling that she was at risk of becoming seriously ill and that she needed to avoid all sources of germs as well as certain foods. Given her mother's limited resources and numerous life demands, Kristi's mother was understandably exhausted by the situation and had become somewhat overwhelmed and hopeless about Kristi's returning to school.

Upon visiting our program, Kristi showed elevated anxiety and depressed mood on a variety of psychological measures. For example, on a standardized clinical rating scale, the clinical interviewer rated the distress and interference associated with Kristi's anxiety problems as being "moderate to severe," meaning her normal life was pretty much on hold. An independent measure of functioning confirmed that Kristi's most severe areas of impairment were school functioning, moods, and emotions. That same measure also confirmed her impairment regarding interacting with her peers. Finally, in conjunction with a diagnostic interview, Kristi was assigned a primary diagnosis of separation anxiety disorder, with additional diagnoses of social phobia and a specific phobia of contracting an illness or disease.

DOUG

Doug was almost 11 years old and an only child of Japanese ethnicity living at home with his mother, father, and maternal grandmother. His mother had completed college, and his father had received a general equivalency diploma (GED). Their annual family income was approximately $70,000. Doug was described by his teachers as polite and smart but also very serious. Prior to his initial evaluation with our program, Doug had been prescribed antidepressants and antianxiety medication. Doug and his mother reported an extensive treatment history, including two separate inpatient hospitalizations for anxiety and depressive concerns—rather uncommon for children at Doug's age.

Doug reported having frequent panic attacks—the primary concern—that led him to avoid such situations as school, crowded places, and riding in the car. These attacks appeared to come "out of nowhere" and were very frightening, although Doug preferred to describe them to us as "feeling sick" rather than as "feeling afraid." The attacks would reach a high level of intensity within only a minute or two, and involved increased heart rate, dizziness, difficulty breathing, and a sick feeling in his stomach. The feelings usually persisted until Doug was able to escape the situation. For example, his parents would pull over the car and let him out to get fresh air, or his teacher would send him to the nurse's office at school. Although Doug was attending school at the time of the assessment, Doug's mother reported that it was a struggle each morning to get him to go to school and that he often came home early, causing disruptions with her part-time job, which she was now considering quitting.

In addition to his panic, Doug also had experienced feelings of depressed mood for the preceding 2 months. He said that nothing had seemed fun lately and that he no longer wanted to see his friends or go out with family on the weekends. He also reported the presence of persistent and excessive worries about his grandmother, his grades at school, and any new things that were planned. These worries were often accompanied by severe restlessness, muscle tension, and irritability.

From an objective standpoint, Doug's anxiety was quite severe. His score on a self-report measure of anxiety placed him in the 99th percentile on separate scales for separation anxiety, panic, and generalized anxiety, and in the 98th percentile on yet another scale for depression. Furthermore, his score on an anxiety and depression scale completed by his mother placed him in the 99th percentile for these problems as well. On a standardized measure of life functioning, Doug's greatest areas of impairment involved his moods and emotions, but he also demonstrated impairment on scales measuring performance at school, performance at home, behavior toward others, and ability to think clearly. In a diagnostic interview at our program, Doug received a primary diagnosis of panic disorder with agoraphobia and additional diagnoses of major depressive disorder, recurrent, severe, and generalized anxiety disorder.

MARY

Mary was a 7-year-old girl with four siblings in a two-parent European American family. Mary's mother had a 2-year college degree, and her father had a graduate degree. Their family income was $42,000. Mary was a charming girl, albeit shy, and she was very bright and cooperative. She excelled in the role of caretaker, getting along quite well with her younger siblings. She also loved to talk about her pet mouse, which, as she proudly stated, she took care of all by herself, giving him water and food and playing with him every day.

During an initial assessment in our program, Mary and her mother reported that Mary was afraid of the dark to the extent that she would wake up her parents approximately three times per week. Mary also reported that she found it difficult to spend the night at friends' houses, enter dark rooms, or be in dark rooms of the house alone. Her younger brother often teased her by threatening to turn off the lights or telling her about monsters in her closet. Her parents also reported that Mary frequently pulled out her hair while in bed at night, which they believed was due to the anxiety.

On a standardized measure of childhood psychopathology completed by her mother, Mary ranked in the 96th percentile for anxiety and mood problems. Mary's score on a standardized measure of life functioning indicated impairment in moods, emotions, and school performance, the latter due mainly to her being sleepy at school much of the time. On a structured diagnostic interview, Mary was diagnosed with specific phobia of the dark and trichotillomania.

IMPACT OF ANXIETY

Despite the differences in diagnoses and specific focus of their worries, what Kristi, Doug, and Mary have in common are problems related to excessive anxiety and avoidance of situations that are an important part of their daily functioning (e.g., interacting with peers, going to school, or sleeping in bed at night). These problems qualify for the label of anxiety disorder in that these children demonstrate anxiety that goes above and beyond a developmentally appropriate level and causes great distress or interference with life functioning. These problems do not normally go away on their own, unlike separation anxiety in toddlers or fear of the dark in preschoolers. Whether a diagnosis is assigned or not, the critical issue for these three children is that the anxiety is excessive to the point of interfering with daily functioning. This is perhaps one of the best criteria by which to evaluate the clinical nature of an anxiety concern; that is, the anxiety creates sufficient interference that a family feels they cannot get by without professional assistance.

As a general class, anxiety represents the most common category of psychiatric disorders in children (see Albano, Chorpita, & Barlow, 2003; Bernstein & Borchardt, 1991; Costello et al., 1996), constituting the primary reason children and their families seek specialty mental health services (Beidel, 1991). Anxiety can be as troubling as it is common. For example, research has shown that childhood anxiety disorders negatively impact a broad range of factors, including academic performance (e.g., Dweck & Wortman, 1982) and social functioning (e.g., Strauss, Frame & Forehand, 1987; Turner, Beidel, & Costello, 1987). Furthermore, children with anxiety disorders often have more than one disorder at the same time, which can include additional anxiety disorders or other disorders such as depression or attention-deficit/hyperactivity disorder (ADHD; e.g., Albano, Chorpita, & Barlow, 1996; Keller et al., 1992). For example, Last, Strauss, and Francis (1987) found that 80% of children with a principal diagnosis of an anxiety disorder had at least one additional Axis I disorder. In this regard, Kristi, Doug, and Mary are fairly typical—all experienced impairment in multiple life circumstances, and all demonstrated multiple diagnoses.

The natural course of anxiety disorders is not encouraging either. Accumulating evidence supports the idea that anxiety disorders having an early onset in childhood can continue well into adulthood (Albano et al., 2003). It is therefore safe to say that the impairment associated with anxiety in children has important long-term implications for adult functioning (Kendall, 1992; Ollendick & King, 1994b), with studies showing that anxiety symptoms worsen over time (Kendall, 1994) and may eventually lead to depression (e.g., Alloy, Kelly, Mineka, & Clements, 1990; Barlow, Chorpita, & Turovsky, 1996; Chorpita & Barlow, 1998). For Doug, this unfortunate outcome had already manifested by the age of 10.

Anxiety has implications for legal and educational classification as well. For example, a high proportion of children with anxiety disorders can be considered "seriously emotionally disturbed." Costello and colleagues (1996) defined serious emotional disturbance (SED) as the conjunction of a clinical diagnosis plus "functional impairment that substantially interferes with or limits the child's role of functioning in family, school, or community activities" (cf. Substance Abuse and Mental Health Services Administration, 1993). In a study surveying children with a wide range of clinical diagnoses, Costello and colleagues found that 45.8% of those with anxiety disorders were classified as SED, using a conjunction of three measures of impaired functioning (Costello et al., 1996).

This SED classification has immediate implications for service funding at the individual level (e.g., whether a child may be eligible for Medicaid funding) and has broader policy implications as well, regarding the development and support of service programs targeting disorders with high community impact. Thus the overall picture is that anxiety disorders in children are relatively common, often run a chronic course, and frequently produce substantial functional impairment in addition to their inherent distress.

ANXIETY SYNDROMES

Unlike some other areas of childhood problems (e.g., attention-deficit disorders), anxiety formally manifests itself in many different ways, and the diversity of anxiety syndromes makes for some apparent challenges regarding treatment. The most recent *Diagnostic and Statistical Manual of Mental Disorders* (DSM-IV-TR; American Psychiatric Association, 2000) outlines 13 different anxiety disorders. What's more, many of these diagnoses have multiple subtypes; for example, specific phobia has five subtypes (i.e., animal type, natural environment type, blood–injection–injury type, situational type, or other type). Fortunately for the practitioner, only a few of these disorders comprise the majority of referrals for treatment of anxiety in children: namely, separation anxiety, generalized anxiety, and social phobia (e.g., Kendall, 1994). Table 2.1 provides a rough sketch of the epidemiological characteristics of these major syndromes, and their individual clinical descriptions follow.

TABLE 2.1. Patterns in the Distribution of Anxiety Disorders among Children and Adolescents

Syndrome	Prevalence estimates	Gender	Age
Separation anxiety disorder	3.5–12.9%	Slightly more common in girls	More common in children
Generalized anxiety disorder	2.9–12.4%	Mixed findings	More common in adolescents
Social phobia	1.1–6.3%	Mixed findings	More common in adolescents
Specific phobia	3.5–9.2%	Evenly distributed	Evenly distributed
Obsessive–compulsive disorder	0.8–4%	Slightly more common in boys, although only in adolescence	Slightly more common in adolescents
Panic disorder	4.7%	Slightly more common in girls	More common in adolescents
Posttraumatic stress disorder	1–3%	More common in girls	Mixed findings

Note. Estimates are based on the collective studies by Anderson, Williams, McGee, and Silva (1987), Cuffe et al. (1998), Essau, Conradt, and Petermann (2000), Flament et al. (1988), Kashani and Orvaschel (1988), Kashani, Orvaschel, Rosenbderg, and Reid (1989), Last, Perrin, Hersen, and Kazdin (1992), Maggini et al. (2001), McGee et al. (1990), Pine (1994), Rutter, Tizard, and Whitmore (1970), Verhulst, van der Ende, Ferdinand, and Kasius (1997), Warren and Zgourides (1988), and Zohar et al. (1992).

Separation Anxiety Disorder

As demonstrated in the example of Kristi, separation anxiety disorder is characterized by age-inappropriate anxiety about being separated from a caregiver. Its core feature involves a fear of something threatening happening to self or caretaker during separation, for example getting hurt, murdered, kidnapped, or lost. Other symptoms can include refusal to go to school, refusal to be alone at home, difficulty going to sleep without a caretaker present, inability to sleep away from home, nightmares about separation, and complaints of physical symptoms during separation, such as stomachaches or headaches. In order to warrant a clinical diagnosis, separation anxiety must occur prior to age 18, must last for at least 4 weeks, and must cause significant distress or significantly interfere with life functioning (American Psychiatric Association, 2000). When defined in this way, separation anxiety disorder is more common among younger children (Albano et al., 2003), although it can also occur in adolescents, as in Kristi's example. It should be distinguished from developmentally normal separation anxiety, which can commonly manifest in infants starting at about 6 months and peaking, on average, around 18 months.

Generalized Anxiety Disorder

Generalized anxiety disorder is characterized by excessive and uncontrollable worry and associated feelings of tension or restlessness. Generalized anxiety disorder is slightly more common in adolescents and can involve concerns about family, friends, grades, or even just minor things. A child with generalized anxiety disorder will find it difficult to stop the worrying once it begins, and the worry will occur most days for at least 6 months (American Psychiatric Association, 2000). In addition to the worry, a child may experience one or more symptoms of central nervous system arousal, such as restlessness, fatigue, poor concentration, irritability, tension, or impaired sleep. In discriminating normal from pathological worry, it is important to verify that the anxiety and worry exhibited by the child are, in fact, excessive and out of proportion to the situation. For example, a child with an abusive father who worries constantly about his mother's and his own safety is probably demonstrating an appropriate level of anxiety and should not be diagnosed with generalized anxiety disorder. Also, the focus of the worry should not be entirely attributable to another anxiety disorder, such as separation anxiety or social anxiety.

Social Phobia

Social phobia is characterized by excessive and disabling fear of social or evaluative situations. These situations must include peers, and the anxiety response can express itself as panic, tantrums, crying, freezing, or shrinking from view (American Psychiatric Association, 2000). To warrant a diagnosis, the social anxiety needs to present for at least 6 months. Although social phobia usually involves a small assortment of social fears, at the extremes it can be "discrete," meaning it involves only a single feared situation (e.g., giving a speech) or "generalized," involving almost all aspects of social functioning. Social phobia is more common among adolescents than among children.

Specific Phobia

Specific phobia is characterized by excessive and disabling fear of a specific object or situation. As mentioned, phobias are organized into a number of basic areas: animal (e.g., dogs), natural/environmental (e.g., swimming), situational (e.g., crowds), blood–injury–injection (e.g., getting a shot), and other (e.g., fear of choking on food, fear of clowns) (American Psychiatric Association, 2000). The fear response typically takes the form of panic or extreme distress and must be present for at least 6 months to warrant a diagnosis. Phobias must produce symptoms that lead to impairment or significant and recurrent distress. For example, a child living in Hawaii might not be diagnosed with a phobia of snakes, given that snakes do not exist in this state and hence offer limited circumstances for distress or interference. Likewise, phobias must be excessive in nature. For example, a child who would not approach an unleashed, barking dog would not be considered phobic, but a child who could not walk to school for fear of the fenced dog across the street probably would be. Although developmentally normal fears (e.g., preschool fears of monsters or animals) are more common in children, phobia diagnoses are equally common in children and adolescents.

Obsessive–Compulsive Disorder

Obsessive–compulsive disorder is typically characterized by repetitive, unwanted thoughts or images (obsessions), often accompanied by rituals performed to reduce or neutralize the anxious thoughts (compulsions). The obsessions go beyond excessive worry, in that they are repetitive and highly intrusive in nature, and the child attempts to suppress or eliminate them. Compulsions—specific ritualized behaviors—are often rigidly performed in response to the obsession and need not be logically or rationally linked with elimination of risk associated with the fear. For example, one might count to 10 to avoid getting germs on one's pillow, or brush one's teeth in a highly symmetrical pattern in order to avoid a cavity. Although obsessive–compulsive disorder can occur with obsessions only or compulsions only, its most common form includes both. The disorder is slightly more common in older children and in all cases can involve a great diversity of fears and obsessions. Obsessions can include thoughts about accidentally hurting others, getting things arranged properly, contacting germs, changing one's appearance, losing loved ones, losing cherished objects, or getting a disease. Compulsions can include such things as counting, washing, checking things repeatedly, rewriting homework or tests, highly repetitive questioning or reassurance seeking, hoarding, or arranging things.

Panic Disorder

Panic disorder is characterized by sudden feelings of intense fear that can seem to come from out of the blue. These are the defining feature, known as panic attacks, and in panic disorder these attacks involve a cycle whereby a sensation of anxiety (e.g., fast heartbeat) leads the child to feel that an attack might begin, which is followed by an escalation of anxiety, which intensifies the sensations, further escalating the anxiety, and so forth, until the anxiety spirals out of control. This panic attack typically includes multiple symptoms of physiological arousal, such as rapid heartbeat, difficulty breathing, shakiness, chest pain, sweating, and dizziness (American Psychiatric Association, 2000). It can also include anxious thoughts such as the fear of dying or losing control. To warrant a diagnosis, the attacks must have occurred more than once and should be accompanied by at least 1 month of persistent apprehension about further attacks, a change in behavior as a result of the attacks, or persistent worry about the consequences of the attacks (e.g., that something is wrong with one's heart). Panic disorder is sometimes accompanied by agoraphobia, the avoidance of places that might trigger feelings of anxiety. The collective evidence on the prevalence of panic disorder in children suggests that it is quite rare (e.g., Anderson et al., 1987; Last et al., 1987; Nelles & Barlow, 1988), although researchers confirmed that prepubertal cases of panic disorder do exist (e.g., Moreau & Weissman, 1992), as was the case with Doug.

Posttraumatic Stress Disorder

Posttraumatic stress disorder is characterized by frightening thoughts, emotional disturbance, and persistent increased arousal resulting from exposure to a traumatic event or events. Such events typically include real or perceived threat of death or serious injury to self or others, such as being in a car accident or witnessing domestic violence. The resulting disturbance lasts at least 1 month and includes features from three domains: (1) a sense of reexperiencing the event, such as through nightmares, flashbacks, or repetitive play with a traumatic theme, and distress or arousal when exposed to cues from the event; (2) emotional or behavioral avoidance of objects or cues related to the event, such as refusing to talk about the event, refusal to go places or do things that remind one of the event, and feelings of emotional numbness, detachment, or hopelessness about the future; and (3) persistent feelings of heightened arousal, such as being easily startled, short-tempered, or having difficulty concentrating or sleeping. When exposed to a traumatic event, girls and younger children are more likely to develop symptoms of PTSD as compared with boys and adolescents, respectively.

GETTING TO THE CORE OF ANXIETY

This manual is less about treating anxiety disorders than it is about treating their core underlying features. This claim is not made in the psychodynamic sense—CBT is not at all about uncovering or interpreting latent conflicts or hidden meaning. Rather, it is meant to emphasize the fact that, despite the heterogeneity of childhood anxiety disorders, the underlying pathological processes are essentially the same.

Kristi, Doug, and Mary each had different diagnoses. Kristi primarily worried about her mother leaving her or getting sick or hurt (i.e., separation anxiety disorder); Doug was concerned about having a panic attack and losing control in front of others (i.e., panic disorder with agoraphobia); and Mary was afraid of what unseen threats might confront her in her dark bedroom (specific phobia, situational type). Nevertheless, all three children shared fundamental characteristics in their reaction to new information, their interpretation of the world around them, their behavior in the face of challenges, and their tendency to experience distress more easily than others. From a treatment perspective, understanding these core features is essential. Fortunately, recent research has begun to shed considerable light on this topic, and it is there that we now turn.

Negative Affectivity

Any discussion of common threads must begin with the construct of negative affectivity (NA; Watson & Clark, 1984), a general temperamental risk factor related to anxiety (Barlow, 2000; Chorpita, 2001; Lonigan & Phillips, 2001; Ollendick, King, & Yule, 1994). High NA in children involves an increased sensitivity to negative events or threatening objects and information (cf. Gray & McNaughton, 1996). In other words, children with high NA are those who get upset, worried, frightened, or sad more easily than others. This temperament—or early personality factor—puts a child at risk to experience a variety of negative emotions throughout life and can lead to anxiety disorders and eventually depression.

Accumulating research has recently outlined the relation between the constructs of NA and specific anxiety syndromes in some detail. Figure 2.1 shows the basic relations identified in children between anxiety dimensions as outlined in DSM-IV-TR (American Psychiatric Association, 2000) and NA, as well as another dimension, physiological hyperarousal, which involves high levels of autonomic responding (e.g., rapid heartbeat, shakiness, dry mouth; Clark & Watson, 1991). In general, findings from a number of studies support the idea that NA is a common influence across many or all anxiety syndromes, whereas physiological hyperarousal is mainly specific to panic disorder (see Figure 2.1). This finding sometimes comes as a surprise: the notion that rapid heartbeat or dry mouth or butterflies in the stomach are not the universal features of anxiety. Rather, NA, or oversensitivity to negative events, objects, and situations, is the hallmark of clinical anxiety (Barlow, 2002).

Variations of this general set of relationships have been confirmed in multiple studies in children and adolescents in both clinical and nonclinical samples (Chorpita, Albano, & Barlow, 1998; Chorpita, 2001; Chorpita & Daleiden, 2002; Chorpita, Plummer, & Moffitt, 2000; Joiner, Catanzaro, & Laurent, 1996; Lonigan, Hooe, David, & Kistner, 1999; Lonigan, Carey, & Finch, 1994) and support the notion that a common process is fundamental to all anxiety disorders. One might ask at this point, why then not treat NA? This is an excellent question, but first it is important to examine some of the other factors that contribute to the development of clinical anxiety in children.

Perception of Control

By itself, this risk factor of high NA might not be enough to trigger the onset of clinical anxiety. However, NA can be further intensified through a variety of experiences in a child's development. One rather central developmental influence appears to be related to a child's sense of control over things that happen in life (Chorpita, 2001). Some research suggests that children who feel they cannot control things (e.g., the behavior of their caretakers, their access to toys or food, the behavior of their peers) are likely to

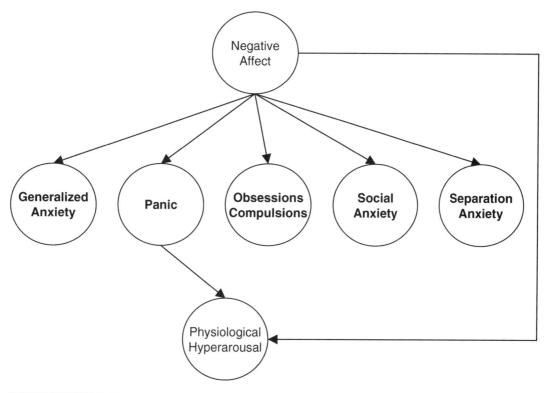

FIGURE 2.1. Relations among dimensions of anxiety, negative affect, and physiological hyperarousal.

react more negatively to threatening events. This sense of things being out of one's control can be intensified through early experiences that limit a child's opportunity to experience the world, to master challenges, and to elicit help at the appropriate times. To overcome anxiety, a child needs to develop a sense that he or she can make bad things less bad by making them go away or by learning how to cope with them (Chorpita & Barlow, 1998; Kendall & Treadwell, 1996).

Specific Life Experiences

In addition to these important experiences with control, specific life experiences can also occur that are believed to lead to the expression of a child's NA in a specific domain (Barlow, 2002; Ollendick, Vasey, & King, 2001; Phillips, Hammen, Brennan, Najman, & Bor, 2005). For example, a child with temperamentally high NA who is bitten by a dog may develop a phobia of dogs; if the child is excessively teased, social phobia might develop; if the child has a bad experience with a stranger, separation anxiety disorder may develop, and so forth. Thus the expression of an anxiety disorder is seen as the cumulative effects of temperament (negative affectivity), early experience that shapes one's view of the world (e.g., experience with control), and specific life events (Barlow, 2000).

The children in all three of our case examples likely demonstrated shy or fearful temperaments (i.e., high NA) early in life, had early experiences that intensified their anxiety in general, and finally had specific negative experiences that contributed to their respective areas of fear or anxiety. For example, Kristi was someone who (as will be seen below) had a strongly negative temperament. Her tendency to "see the glass half empty" was pervasive and had been present for as long as she and her mother could remember. Although we must rely on retrospective report, Kristi's early childhood appeared to be characterized by instability within her family and a lack of encouragement or opportunity to master challenges, especially those involving attending preschool and making friends early on. Her mother was separated from her father already and found it challenging to provide the extra support that Kristi needed at the time she started school. Thus Kristi never learned to feel in control of events, particularly those involving other people and their reactions to her. Finally, a series of stops and starts with preschool and kindergarten presented multiple conditioning experiences that reinforced the development of Kristi's anxiety. Each time she was "pulled" from school, she felt relief, and her strategies to avoid school were inadvertently supported.

These three elements—temperament, early experience, and life events—are believed to play a role in the development of anxiety over time. Understanding the development of anxiety can lead to important and helpful insights about eliminating or managing future risk. For example, with Kristi, we know that given her temperament, care should be taken when introducing her to novel situations and extra support and monitoring of her emotions provided when she encounters big social milestones (e.g., going to high school, dating, starting a job or college). However, in and of itself, understanding the origins of anxiety is by no means the goal of treatment. Regardless of how anxiety develops, it is critical to focus on what features are present now and how those features can be addressed—just as the treatment for a broken leg is the same regardless of how the leg was broken. The three common features of anxiety that are present-focused and traditionally have provided a good therapeutic "handle" to grab onto are the thoughts, feelings, and actions associated with the anxiety itself. Let us next consider these.

ANXIOUS THINKING

One process related to NA that clearly cuts across all anxiety disorders involves cognition—that is, the way children think—and children with anxiety problems think differently from other children in this regard (e.g., Chorpita, Albano, & Barlow, 1996; Treadwell & Kendall, 1996; Vasey & Daleiden, 1994). In general, anxious children are more likely to elaborate on negative information. In other words, relative to other children, they can think of lots of ways that things can go wrong. This tendency shows up in a number of specific ways, including biases in attention, interpretation, and self-talk. For example, in one study, Vasey, Daleiden, Williams, and Brown (1995) presented children with pairs of words on a computer screen and found evidence that anxious children were more likely than nonanxious children to look at the words that were threatening (e.g., "accident"). In a different series of studies, several investigators observed that anxious children are more likely to interpret ambiguous situations as dangerous (Barrett,

Rapee, Dadds, & Ryan, 1996; Bell-Dolan, 1995; Chorpita, Albano, & Barlow, 1996). That is, when asked a question such as "You hear a noise in the middle of the night—what do you think it is?" anxious children come up with a larger number of threatening possibilities (e.g., "a burglar") than do nonanxious children. In yet another line of research, Treadwell and Kendall (1996) observed that anxious children also engage in more negative self-talk than do nonanxious children, telling themselves such things as "I won't be able to handle this situation." Because of the ubiquity of this kind of thinking among the anxiety disorders, it lends itself well to therapeutic intervention.

TWO STAGES: ANXIETY AND PANIC

When the world is viewed in this scary way, the effects on the child are pervasive, and the associated emotions often activate a number of systems in the brain and body. Barlow (1988) initially detailed these events in a comprehensive two-stage model of anxiety and panic, highlighting the notion that anxiety is an emotion whose purpose is to prepare one for confrontation with danger. Initially, when a threat is still somewhat distant, the feelings manifest as worry and tension, and the reactions involve inhibition of gross motor behavior (e.g., children might stop running or playing), narrowing of attention, increased stimulus analysis, increased exploration of environment (e.g., scanning for danger), and priming of hypothalamic motor systems for possible rapid action that may be required. Barlow (1988) and Gray (1987) stated that this response is itself "pure" anxiety. Gray (1987) aptly characterized this reaction as a "stop, look, and listen" response. With children, I often refer to this as "Stage 1" of a two-stage process.

When our 10-year-old Doug is on his way to school, he is probably in Stage 1. He might stop to analyze his surroundings cautiously, imagine the things that might trigger a panic attack, and think about how to avoid them. This apprehensive response is nearly universal in all higher animals: recall how when you first approach a bird, it will typically stop feeding or walking so that it can study you to see what you will do next. This pattern is similar to how a child or adult might react to something novel or potentially threatening. As noted by Barlow et al. (1996), the emotion of anxiety in Stage I often serves a useful purpose in facilitating anticipation and analysis of danger and therefore helping to avoid it.

If the threat intensifies or gets closer, the processing of information escalates, and other parts of the body prepare to confront the danger; we are now in Stage 2. Again, this reaction is typically part of a natural and purposeful response to survive a threatening experience, such as an attack from an angry dog. In this situation, the body is wired to activate additional emotions, often called "fear" or "panic" (Barlow et al., 1996; Gray & McNaughton, 1996), more widely known as the classic "fight-or-flight" response (Cannon, 1929). This response involves increased heartbeat, change in blood pressure, faster breathing, and a cascade of chemicals throughout the body to increase speed, strength, and alertness. Some of these chemicals, such as adrenaline, can have side effects such as shakiness or nausea.

As Doug walks to school, if he detects the first signs of an impending attack, he moves rapidly and fully from Stage 1 (worry and scanning) to Stage 2 (dry mouth, shaky hands, intense breathing, and pounding heart). Similarly, if you charge the bird, it will fly away in a burst of energy—or if that is not possible, it will try to defend itself. All of this is part of the organism's design to handle danger. Again, the problem is that children with anxiety disorders often experience these emotions when there is no real danger, such as when children who always get good grades worry about their next test.

Importantly, both Stage 1 and Stage 2 can be helpful and are often necessary for survival (an idea that is typically very foreign to someone with anxiety problems). It is only when individuals begin to experience anxiety at inappropriate times—when there is no real threat or danger, or when the response intensity is out of proportion to the danger—that the emotion becomes a problem. Barlow (1988) termed this reaction a "false alarm." It is this kind of anxiety—the false alarm—that sometimes requires treatment.

IMPLICATIONS FOR TREATMENT

It makes sense that addressing a core, underlying process should be the key to any successful treatment approach. That premise is, in fact, one basis for the organization of this manual. By focusing on the core features across all anxiety disorders, it is possible to consider a single set of treatment strategies that can address all of them.

This idea is so old in some ways, it has become new again. That is, although there has recently been an increasing specialization of treatment programs for specific anxiety disorders, much of the early work on the treatment of fear and anxiety in children conceptualized anxiety as a unitary syndrome, with a common set of intervention strategies designed to address it as one entity (Barrios & O'Dell, 1998). This is not to say that some variations are not needed to account for individual clinical presentations that, for example, might differentiate obsessive–compulsive disorder from separation anxiety. The proliferation of effective protocols for childhood anxiety disorders does suggest that special considerations are likely helpful in dealing with each separate clinical presentation (Cohen, Deblinger, Mannarino, & Steer, 2004; Ollendick, 1995; March, Amaya-Jackson, Murray, & Schulte, 1998; Kendall, 2002). However, the current approach addresses a variety of those considerations through flexible treatment planning, emphasizing a core set of strategies to address the underlying cognitive, emotional, and behavioral tendencies common to all anxiety disorders. Just how this treatment planning is accomplished is covered in more detail in Chapter 4.

More generally, CBT protocols such as this one are based on the idea that it is important to teach children the skills to identify when the danger is not real (Barlow's "false alarm") and, therefore, when their anxiety is unnecessary. Giving children the ability to identify more accurately when situations are safe helps reduce or even eliminate the accompanying responses of tension, worry, as well as the feelings of fear and panic (Kendall, 1992). This manual, in particular, emphasizes an approach to treatment that attempts to tap and resolve these core anxiety responses that underlie the diversity of anxiety syndromes. The strategies are designed to eliminate the "false alarms" that children experience, helping them distinguish the real threat from the imagined threat. Thus, although Kristi is separation anxious, Doug has panic attacks, and Mary is afraid of the dark, all three need to learn that they perceive danger when danger is not really present.

The therapeutic corrective learning needed to distinguish real from perceived danger is acquired best through direct experience (Foa & Kozak, 1986), and thus all aspects of treatment are designed to support these kinds of learning exercises. Unlike approaches that might seek to impart a large number of skills to a child, this protocol focuses primarily on getting the child to experience situations perceived as threatening and to learn that they are safe. For this reason, exposure—systematic experience with the feared situation—is the central intervention of the treatment and the one that receives the most attention in the protocol. For efficiency, other skills are taught only as needed in order to serve this primary aim of corrective learning. The specific manner in which this protocol is accomplished is described in more detail below, as we find out more about what happens with Kristi, Doug, and Mary.

Of course, any treatment planning rests on the assumption that anxiety is the actual target in question or that there is even some anxiety worth treating. So before we go further, let us first review more closely how to determine what the child's problem is and whether it requires treatment.

THREE

Who Needs This Treatment?

The first step in the treatment process involves determining whether the child has an anxiety disorder that requires treatment. Recall from Figure 1.1 (now adapted in Figure 3.1) that making this decision begins with the comprehensive assessment. Figure 3.1 shows that the comprehensive assessment is used to inform not only the treatment selection decision ("determine whether anxiety protocol is appropriate"), but also decisions about termination of, or major adjustments to, the treatment. In that sense, the comprehensive assessments tend to "bookend" the treatment procedures and principally serve to inform the big question of whether the child has an anxiety problem and hence would benefit from this protocol.

This chapter offers a basic description of the approaches that are most useful to assess anxiety and related difficulties in children and that we have used most often in our own research and training program. Readers seeking a thorough and scholarly review of the assessment of fears and anxieties in childhood are referred to Southam-Gerow & Chorpita (in press). It is also important to keep in mind that decisions about ongoing progress and case formulation generally are not derived from the comprehensive assessment. Those decisions—in light gray in the figure—are discussed in more detail in Chapter 4.

ASSESSMENT DOMAINS

Anxiety in children is best understood through a multifaceted assessment approach that evaluates multiple domains. These domains can be roughly organized into the following six areas, which (if your memory is like mine) are best remembered by their first letters, A–F: Affect, Behaviors and symptoms, Client perspectives, Diagnosis, Environment, and Functioning. In this chapter, a select group of measures within each of the six domains (A–F) is reviewed for their suitability, with tabular summaries of when and how to use each measure. Remember that the overall goal of the comprehensive assessment is to determine whether there is a problem that would require an anxiety treatment.

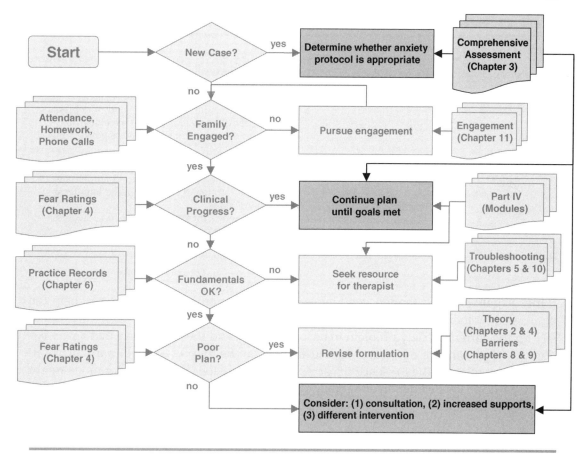

FIGURE 3.1. Comprehensive assessment.

AFFECT

As mentioned in Chapter 2, anxiety disorders appear to be connected by the underlying influence of NA. Understanding this tendency to react to situations with negative emotions is at the core of this protocol, and thus the assessment of NA is of considerable importance. Another affective dimension related to emotional problems is that of positive affectivity (PA; Clark, Watson, & Mineka, 1994). PA is the tendency to react to things with energy or enthusiasm; it has demonstrated an important association with depression, such that low PA (along with high NA) co-occurs with higher depression scores (e.g., Chorpita, 2001). In that sense, PA is one of the dimensions that best discriminates children with anxiety from those with depression (e.g., Chorpita & Daleiden, 2002; Lonigan et al., 1994). At present, the two best-evaluated measures of these dimensions in children are the Affect and Arousal Scale (AFARS; Chorpita, Daleiden, Moffitt, Yim, & Umemoto, 2000) and the Positive and Negative Affect Schedule for Children (PANAS-C; Laurent et al., 1999), which are summarized below (see also Table 3.1).

Measuring NA in children seeking services for anxiety disorders can be rather helpful, in that it provides information about the general tendency to interpret and react to

TABLE 3.1. **Measuring Affect**

When	Recommended measures	Interpretation
Pretreatment	AFARS or PANAS-C	1. High NA suggests increased likelihood of chronicity or comorbidity; therapist should emphasize how CBT strategies can generalize to other areas of fear. 2. Low PA suggests increased likelihood of depression; therapist should consider careful screening for depression or monitoring for depression over the course of treatment.
Posttreatment or reformulation	AFARS or PANAS-C	1. High NA suggests increased likelihood of reemerging anxiety; therapist should emphasize maintenance strategies and encourage long-term rehearsal of skills. 2. Low PA suggests increased likelihood of depression; therapist should consider careful screening and possible treatment for depression.

things negatively. This tendency, which is at the core of anxiety problems, can help the clinician infer the likelihood of, for example, co-occurring anxiety disorders, the propensity for the current anxiety problem to be long-lasting, and the probability that new anxiety foci might emerge over time. Measuring PA can be helpful as well, particularly in terms of identifying the presence of, or risk for, depression. Such considerations might lead a clinician to consider an altogether different intervention than CBT for anxiety disorders, for example.

Affect and Arousal Scale

The AFARS is a 27-item self-report questionnaire for children designed to measure positive and negative affect, along with the nonaffective dimension physiological hyperarousal. The physiological hyperarousal scale measures the presence of autonomic symptoms such as breathlessness, rapid heartbeat, and sweating. As mentioned in Chapter 2, physiological hyperarousal has been found to be associated with some anxiety disorders in children, most notably, panic disorder (Chorpita, Plummer, et al., 2000; Chorpita, 2001). The AFARS asks respondents to endorse how true items are (e.g., "I get upset easily," "I have fun at school," "My mouth gets dry"). The psychometric properties of the AFARS have been found to be favorable in several studies (Chorpita & Daleiden, 2002; Chorpita, Daleiden, et al., 2000; Daleiden, Chorpita, & Lu, 2000).

Positive and Negative Affect Schedule for Children

Another well-researched measure of affect in children is the PANAS-C. This measure is a 27-item self-report scale designed to measure PA and NA in children. Unlike the AFARS, the PANAS-C asks children to rate individual adjectives (e.g., "sad," "blue") with respect to how often they felt that way in the past few weeks. Laurent et al. (1999) reported favorable psychometrics for this measure. In a series of comparative analyses in clinical sample, Chorpita and Daleiden (2002) found that the NA scales of the PANAS-C and AFARS were both associated with measures of anxiety, with the PANAS-C NA scale showing slightly higher validity coefficients. In that same study, the PANAS-C PA scale demonstrated a clear advantage in its association with depression, although it showed some problems with discriminant validity by yielding significant correlations with other measures of NA, worry, and panic. Although the AFARS may have the potential to better predict future anxiety due to its high content validity for temperament, the confirmation of any advantage or lack thereof awaits additional research. Given these findings, we generally prefer to use the PANAS-C as part of the comprehensive assessments in our program.

BEHAVIOR AND SYMPTOMS

Measuring anxious behaviors and symptoms yields direct and interpretable information about the disturbance. Measurement of behavior and symptoms can involve a number of different modalities, the most common of which are self-report, parent-report, and direct observation measures (see Table 3.2). Although self- and parent-report measures are two of the easiest and most efficient strategies, a notable challenge involves balancing different information based on informant perspectives. For example, there is a preponderance of evidence that parents and children do not often agree in their reports of the child's negative emotions (Handwerk, Larzelere, Soper, & Friman, 1999; Klein, 1991; Stavrakaki, Vargo, Roberts, & Boodoosingh, 1987). Thus, the assessment of behaviors and symptoms related to anxiety is arguably best captured through the use of multiple informants, and when self-report and parent-report fail to yield a clear picture of the problem, clinicians might consider observational methods as well.

Self-Report

Obtaining scores on a self-report measure is one of the easiest ways to gauge the nature and intensity of a child's anxiety. One clear advantage provided by self-report measures is that they provide a quantified baseline against which the progress of an intervention can be measured. Contemporary measures of child anxiety can be thought of in terms of two categories: multidimensional and single-syndrome measures. Not surprisingly, multidimensional measures index more than one anxiety syndrome (e.g., separation anxiety, social anxiety). Their advantage is that they provide information regarding different aspects of anxiety across a broad range of dimensions. Their disadvantages are that (1) they can provide comparatively less information about each specific dimension than might be found using single-syndrome measures, and (2) they might involve more items and thereby increase administration time.

Single-syndrome measures, on the other hand, focus the assessment on a particular dimension within the anxiety domain. For example, such a measure might index social anxiety, worry, or separation anxiety only. Such scales can still have multiple dimensions or subscales, but these all load on the single dimension of interest (e.g., multiple aspects of separation anxiety). These measures can be useful for getting lots of information about a specific area but are less useful when there is interest in multiple areas of anxi-

TABLE 3.2. **Measuring Behavior and Symptoms**

When	Recommended measure	Interpretation
Pretreatment	RCADS or MASC	Higher scores reflect increased severity of problem; *T* scores can yield normative reference information about degree of severity.
Pretreatment, if more detailed measurement is needed regarding a specific syndrome	SASC-R, LOI-CV, or PSWQ-C	Higher scores reflect increased severity of problem; some measures will give more detailed information of feared objects or situations, which can be incorporated into treatment.
Pretreatment, if self-report measures do not provide clear picture	Behavioral observation (e.g., behavior avoidance test)	If the design of the behavior avoidance test or observational situation is a good approximation of the natural situation, the child's response is one of the best sources of data regarding intensity of the anxiety. If discrepant from self-report measures, it is generally better to give stronger consideration to this approach.
Posttreatment	MASC or RCADS	Higher scores reflect increased severity of problem; *T* scores can yield normative reference information about degree of severity and should be below 65 for target syndromes.
Posttreatment, if syndrome specific measures were given at pretreatment	SASC-R, LOI-CV, or PSWQ-C	Higher scores reflect increased severity of problem; some measures will give more detailed information of feared objects or situations that can be evaluated to determine specific effects of treatment.
Posttreatment, if self-report measures do not provide clear picture of results	Behavioral observation (e.g., behavior avoidance test)	If the design of the behavior avoidance test or observational situation is a good approximation of the natural situation, the child's response is one of the best sources of data regarding intensity of the anxiety. If discrepant from self-report measures, it is generally better to give stronger consideration to this approach.

ety. An alternative to the use of multidimensional measures is to administer many different single-syndrome measures, although administration time can be prohibitive.

★ In our program, we typically administer a single multidimensional measure as part of the comprehensive assessment. Single-syndrome measures may subsequently be administered for special purposes, such as getting a detailed understanding of social anxiety or obsessions and compulsions that is not otherwise clear from the comprehensive assessment.

Multidimensional Measures

Multidimensional Anxiety Scale for Children. The Multidimensional Anxiety Scale for Children (MASC; March, Parker, Sullivan, & Stallings, & Conners, 1997) is a 39-item multidimensional measure for children ages 8–19. It has the following scales (and subscales): (1) physical symptoms (tense/restless and somatic/autonomic), (2) harm avoidance (anxious coping and perfectionism), (3) social anxiety (humiliation/rejection and public performance fears), and (4) separation anxiety. The measure has demonstrated favorable psychometric properties in its original publication and has shown good test–retest reliability estimates in subsequent research (March et al., 1997; March, Sullivan, & Parker, 1999).

Revised Child Anxiety and Depression Scale. Another multidimensional measure, the Revised Child Anxiety and Depression Scale (RCADS; Chorpita, Yim, Moffitt, Umemoto, & Francis, 2000), is a 47-item self-report questionnaire for children and adolescents ages 8–18, with six scales corresponding to separation anxiety disorder, social phobia, generalized anxiety disorder, panic disorder, obsessive–compulsive disorder, and major depression. The RCADS requires respondents to rate how true each item is with respect to their usual feelings. In a series of studies in both clinical and community samples, the RCADS has demonstrated favorable psychometric properties (Chorpita, Yim, et al., 2000; Chorpita, Moffitt, & Gray, 2005; deRoss, Chorpita, & Gullone, 2002). Two particular strengths of this measure are that (1) it contains scales corresponding to a large number of anxiety diagnostic syndromes, which can be helpful for determining the focus of intervention, and (2) it contains a brief depression scale to assess the presence of depression. Extensive normative data are also available.

Single-Syndrome Measures

Leyton Obsessional Inventory—Child Version. The Leyton Obsessional Inventory—Child Version (LOI-CV; Berg, Rappoport, & Flament, 1986) is single-syndrome measure indexing obsessive–compulsive disorder and consists of a 44-item card sort for children ages 10–18. It requires children to identify the presence of different obsessions or compulsions by placing them into a "yes" or "no" pile. For each endorsed item, separate ratings are also taken for resistance (i.e., the degree to which the respondent resists the obsession or compulsion) and interference (i.e., the degree to which the obsession or compulsion interferes with daily life). For the resistance score, the respondent places each endorsed card into a pile corresponding to "sensible," "habit," "not necessary," "try to stop," or "try very hard to stop" (scored 0, 1, 1, 2, 3, respectively). For the interference score, the respondent places each endorsed card into a pile corresponding to "no interference," "interferes a little," "interferes moderately," or "interferes a lot" (scored 0, 1, 2, 3, respectively). Normative data exist for the three scales, and the psychometric properties are adequate. This measure can be particularly useful for getting a detailed inventory of the types of obsessions and compulsions present in a child who might otherwise not volunteer such information in a clinical interview.

Penn State Worry Questionnaire for Children. The Penn State Worry Questionnaire for Children (PSWQ-C; Chorpita, Tracey, Brown, Collica, & Barlow, 1997) is a single-syndrome measure of worry in children ages 7–17, most commonly used to assess the dimension of generalized anxiety. It is a 14-item self-report questionnaire that measures both the frequency and controllability of worry (e.g., "Many things make me worry"). The PSWQ-C has shown good psychometric properties with respect to clinical worry and generalized anxiety disorder in children. For example, the PSWQ-C has discriminated children with GAD from children with other anxiety disorders and from nonclinical controls (Chorpita, Tracey, et al., 1997).

Social Anxiety Scale for Children—Revised. The Social Anxiety Scale for Children—Revised (SASC-R; La Greca & Stone, 1993) is a 22-item self-report questionnaire consisting of 18 descriptive self-statements and 4 filler items. It is another narrowband measure, tapping the dimension of social anxiety. Each item is rated on a 5-point Likert scale ranging from 1 (*not at all*) to 5 (*all the time*). The factor structure and psychometric properties of this scale are well-supported among both clinical and nonclinical samples of children (Ginsburg, La Greca, & Silverman, 1998; La Greca & Stone, 1993). There is also good evidence of discriminant validity, such that this measure has successfully discriminated socially anxious and nonsocially anxious children (Ginsburg et al., 1998).

Behavioral Observation

Behavioral observation of children in clinic, home, or classroom settings can be quite helpful, particularly when there is discrepancy among sources of information (e.g., in our case example, Doug said he was not afraid to go to school, but his parents disagreed). Because observation procedures are typically more costly and demanding than self-report methods, observation is best used when it is expected to provide important new information about the child's problem that is not available by other means.

Behavior Avoidance Test

A classic procedure for behavioral observation of fear or anxiety is the behavior avoidance test, in which a child is observed encountering a feared stimulus (e.g., Melamed & Siegel, 1975). With such a procedure, the child is gradually brought into increasingly closer contact with a feared object or situation and is usually asked to provide subjective ratings of fear. For example, a child might be asked to rate his or her level of fear on a scale from 1 to 10 every minute or so during the test. Other variables obtained can include the length of time to approach the object, the distance traveled toward the object, or time in contact with object or time spent in the feared situation (Strauss, 1993). Behavior avoidance tests can be done in laboratory or naturalistic settings and have been used to assess a variety of fears, including fear of heights (Van Hasselt, Hersen, Bellack, Rosenblum, & Lamparski, 1979), social concerns (Eisen & Silverman, 1991), fear of blood (Van Hasselt et al., 1979), fear of animals (Evans & Harmon, 1981), and fear of darkness (Kelley, 1976).

The benefits of such procedures include their ability to be customized for a specific child (e.g., a highly specific stimulus can be arranged that best approximates the child's unique anxiety problem) and the fact that they allow for assessment of multiple responses, such as physiological reactivity, avoidance strategies, or social skills. For example, in a social anxiety behavior test, a child could be asked to give a brief speech to three audience members. The assessor can not only take fear ratings but also observe the social performance of the child (e.g., eye contact, tone of voice, pace of speaking), using these results to provide feedback for improvement. Overall, the behavioral avoidance test is one of the best methods for determining frequency and severity of behaviors and symptoms—but again, its use must always be weighed against its cost and inconvenience.

CLIENT PERSPECTIVES

Assessment of client perspectives (e.g., satisfaction with therapy, if it was completed; goals for therapy, if it is beginning) is often an important addition to the assessment of purely clinical syndromes and symptoms (see Table 3.3). These perspectives help put the problem into a larger context. For example, in the case with Mary, although specific phobia was the clinical focus, her declining academic performance was the main reason that her family sought services. Improvement on the phobia was therefore just a step toward a larger goal.

Obtaining information about client perspectives can take many forms. For example, a wide variety of measures exist to assess such constructs as therapy satisfaction (e.g., Doucette & Bickman, 2001), therapeutic alliance (e.g., Shirk & Saiz, 1992), and expected success of the intervention (e.g., Nock & Kazdin, 2001). When established measures are not available to assess some aspect of the client perspective that might be of interest, it is nevertheless a good idea to interview the family to obtain such perspectives. In our program, this information is most often obtained through independent dialogue with child and parents to determine goals (before treatment) and satisfaction with progress (after treatment) in an informal manner.

Getting this kind of information from families is especially important when treating anxiety, because as mentioned earlier, some aspects of the treatment may be uncomfortable for the child, parents, or other family members. For example, exposure exercises can frequently provoke high levels of distress in children, even including crying or yelling for parents' help. It can therefore be important to assess, formally or informally, whether the family feels that the treatment strategy fits the child's problem. Otherwise, there is the potential for premature termination of therapy (e.g., Kazdin, Holland, & Crowley, 1997) based on a misperception that CBT is "making the problem worse."

TABLE 3.3. **Measuring Client Perspectives**

When	Recommended measure	Interpretation
Pretreatment	Clinical interview or selected measures	Therapists should seek to identify possible goals, attitudes, and perceptions of the child and family that might impact the success of the intervention. Challenges identified early can be addressed by the selection of appropriate strategies or modules.
Posttreatment	Clinical interview or selected measures	Concerns identified at posttreatment should be addressed in a debriefing, and reformulation of the case and possible extension of treatment to target new goals should be considered.

DIAGNOSIS

The current "gold standard" for clinical diagnosis involves the structured diagnostic interview (Edelbrock & Costello, 1990; Matarazzo, 1983). As compared with unstructured interviews, structured diagnostic interviews offer superior reliability by standardizing the diagnostic areas to be assessed and use of a controlled question format to reduce interviewer bias (DiNardo, O'Brien, Barlow, Waddell, & Blanchard, 1983; Edelbrock & Costello, 1990). These properties are important, given the particularly differentiated nature of anxiety disorders and the increasingly explicit diagnostic criteria in recent revisions of the *Diagnostic and Statistical Manual of Mental Disorders* (e.g., DSM-IV-TR; American Psychiatric Association, 2000).

Anxiety Disorders Interview Schedule for DSM-IV— Child and Parent Versions

One of the most commonly used structured interviews for childhood anxiety disorders is the Anxiety Disorders Interview Schedule for DSM-IV—Child and Parent Versions (ADIS-IV-C/P; Silverman & Albano, 1996). The ADIS-IV-C/P is a structured clinical interview for parents and children that is specifically designed for DSM-IV diagnosis of childhood anxiety disorders, mood disorders, and selected behavior disorders. A particular strength of the ADIS-IV-C/P is its detail regarding multiple parameters of anxiety disorders. For example, it often directs the interviewer to inquire about such areas as the severity, intensity, interference, avoidance, or uncontrollability of fear and anxiety at both the symptom and syndrome levels with each diagnosis. Separate diagnostic profiles are derived from separate parent and child interviews, which are combined to form a consensus diagnosis (Silverman & Albano, 1996). Good-to-excellent interrater reliability has been demonstrated for the ADIS-IV-C/P (Silverman, Saavedra, & Pina, 2001). Some guidelines for interpretation of diagnostic information appear in Table 3.4.

One of the main limitations to the use of the ADIS-IV-C/P is its lengthy administration time. Assessment of children in our clinical research program routinely takes between 4 and 5 hours, not including scoring, interpretation, or report writing. Given this virtual impossibility for practitioners, some might choose to administer only the portions of the structured interview that seem relevant. Such an approach could base the selection of interview sections on those disorders that appear to be likely candidates, given the other information gathered, and it is the approach we advise for clinicians in practice.*

Another strategy to increase efficiency involves fitting the different assessment measures into the structured interview time. Thus, in our program we routinely administer parent report measures while performing a diagnostic interview with the child, and then administer child self-report measures while performing a diagnostic interview with the parent or caretaker. Finally, another approach to minimize administration cost

---

*Few studies, if any, support this strategy of partial administration; however, this general approach to structured interviewing was outlined in some detail by Chorpita, Yim, and Tracey (2002) and showed considerable promise in modeling simulations. Subsequent tests in a clinical sample by Chorpita and Nakamura (2006) also look promising but are preliminary.

TABLE 3.4. **Considerations for Interpretation of Diagnostic Information: Differential Diagnosis and Co-Occurring Conditions**

Diagnosis	Issue
Differential diagnosis	
Pervasive developmental disorders and psychotic disorders	Commonly associated with impaired social functioning or excessive fears and preclude the diagnosis of separation anxiety, specific phobias, and social phobia.
Generalized anxiety disorder	Often difficult to distinguish from obsessive–compulsive disorder, social phobia, posttraumatic stress disorder, and depression. The worries associated with generalized anxiety disorder are usually not as specific as those with obsessive–compulsive disorder, and they are not accompanied by rituals. Generalized anxiety disorder involves more domains of worrying than just social events. Worrying that occurs exclusively during the course of posttraumatic stress disorder or depression should not be diagnosed as generalized anxiety disorder.
Oppositional defiant disorder	Can involve avoidance of school, crying, and tantrums similar to those seen with anxiety disorders. However, episodes characteristic of oppositional defiant disorder are more pervasive, angry, controlled, or purposeful than those associated with anxiety disorders.
Attention-deficit/ hyperactivity disorder	Can appear similar to anxiety, in that these children have difficulty with concentration and tend to avoid things. However, attention-deficit/ hyperactivity disorder, by itself, usually does not involve the distress, agitation, or inhibition associated with anxiety disorders.
Normal anxiety	Distinguished from anxiety disorders by degree; anxiety disorders involve an excessive amount of what is considered developmentally or situationally appropriate anxiety. For example, a child who is extremely scared of a school in which there is reasonable chance of violence to him or her would not be considered to have an anxiety disorder for that reason alone.
Coexisting/co-occurring conditions	
Other anxiety disorders	Occur in 50–80% of children with an anxiety disorder (Albano et al., 2003). It is not uncommon for children with anxiety disorders to have two or three diagnoses, given the highly differentiated classification of these disorders.
Depression	Occurs in 5–50% of adolescents with anxiety disorders (e.g., Strauss, Last, Hersen, & Kazdin, 1988) but is less common among younger children with anxiety disorders (Strauss, Lease, Last, & Francis, 1988).
Disruptive behavior disorders	Sometimes co-occur with anxiety disorders. In such instances, it is usually necessary to treat the disruptive behavior disorder first, given that successful intervention for anxiety often requires the cooperation of the child in some difficult exercises. Such elements of intervention are often difficult to administer if the child is defiant or uncooperative. Following successful intervention with the behavior problems, a child may be considered an appropriate candidate for an anxiety disorder protocol.
Tic disorders	Occur in 30% of children diagnosed with obsessive–compulsive disorder (Swedo, Rapoport, Leonard, Lenane, & Cheslow, 1989).

TABLE 3.5. **Measuring Diagnosis**

When	Recommended measure	Interpretation
Pretreatment	ADIS-IV-C/P or selected sections	Diagnosis will help yield information to build an intervention strategy tailored to specific anxiety syndromes (see Chapter 7).
Posttreatment or reformulation	ADIS-IV-C/P or selected sections	Diagnosis will help determine whether additional intervention is warranted, but may not be needed.

is to use diagnostic interviewing as a strategy to precede treatment only. Even in a research context, there may be insufficient incremental benefits of administering a full structured diagnostic interview to a child whose diagnostic profile is likely well known from a pretreatment interview and observed during the course of treatment. In such instances, it might make more sense if some other quantified measures of anxiety were taken at posttreatment (e.g., self-report measures). Recommendations for diagnostic assessment appear in Table 3.5.

ENVIRONMENT

It can often be helpful to measure aspects of the child's environment that could be related in some way to the problem or its treatment (see Table 3.6). In most cases, choices of what to measure will be based on the individual features of the presenting case and the specific strategies chosen for intervention. For example, a therapist might choose to assess the parenting practices in a family in which anxiety-related tantrums by the child are frequent. This choice would suggest early on that specific approaches would need to be incorporated to support family members' ability to manage behavioral challenges.

Other possible choices of measures of the environment include a parent diary to track specific responses to the child's anxiety, scales to measure the anxiety of siblings, measures of conflict between parents and child, or tools to assess marital adjustment or satisfaction. For example, in Mary's case, in which she made frequent and unpredictable nighttime visits to her parents' bedroom, it was of interest to us to assess the impact of such behavior on the parents' relationship.

TABLE 3.6. **Measuring Environment**

When	Recommended measure	Interpretation
Pretreatment	Interview, measure, or observation as needed	Therapists should seek to identify intermediate targets for intervention or collateral areas of disturbance that will be reassessed after treatment.
Posttreatment	Interview, measure, or observation as needed	Lack of change from pretreatment might suggest incomplete results from intervention or problem with case formulation.

FUNCTIONING

Measures of child functioning give some indication of the degree of disruption in the day-to-day life and routine of a child. Such measures typically incorporate information about problems with peer functioning, school performance, behavior in the home, and emotional stability and can be used to aid in the classification of children as SED. Table 3.7 summarizes recommendations.

One limitation to these measures is their focus on the outward effects of the syndrome or problem. For example, Costello et al. (1996) pointed out that in the determination of SED, functioning is commonly defined in terms of the overall degree of disruption and does not include a dimension of distress. Because many of the consequences of anxiety are covert and may have subtle, albeit rather grave, effects, many contemporary measures of functioning may be insensitive to some of the more private aspects of interference. For that reason, it is suggested that measures of functioning for children with anxiety not be interpreted in isolation. Rather, they should be supplemented with measures of distress, such as those listed above in the section on behavior and symptoms.

Vanderbilt Functioning Index

The Vanderbilt Functioning Index (VFI; Bickman, Lambert, Karver, & Andrade, 1998) is a 24-item measure tapping dimensions of antisocial behavior, problems at home, problems at school, problems with peers, and self-harm. Psychometric studies support the reliability and validity of the VFI, showing correlations with other established measures, as well as correlations with cost of treatment and use of residential care (Bickman et al., 1998). One of its advantages is that it is a brief scale that can be easily administered to parents.

Child and Adolescent Functional Assessment Scale

The Child and Adolescent Functional Assessment Scale (CAFAS; Hodges, 1998) is a clinician-scored, multidimensional rating scale designed to assess functional impairment as experienced by children and adolescents, ages 5–17, across eight domains of functioning (Hodges & Wong, 1996; Hodges & Wong, 1997). Raters are provided with a list of behavioral descriptors on each of the subscales, from which they must choose

TABLE 3.7. **Measuring Functioning**

When	Recommended measure	Interpretation
Pretreatment	CAFAS or VFI (in conjunction with measures of distress)	Will help yield information on degree of disruption and the focus of impairment.
Posttreatment	CAFAS or VFI (in conjunction with measures of distress)	Should point to remaining areas of concern; if present, specific strategies should be developed to address these remaining problems with functioning.

those items that are most congruent with the child's most severe level of dysfunction during the month preceding the assessment (Hodges & Wong, 1996). Items within each subscale are grouped according to four degrees of impairment—*severe, moderate, mild,* and *minimal or no impairment*—yielding scores of 30, 20, 10, or 0 points, respectively. Data generated from two large-scale evaluation studies indicated that the CAFAS possesses good internal consistency and high interrater reliability (Hodges & Wong, 1996). The CAFAS also correlates significantly and positively with other indicators of impairment, including severity of psychiatric diagnosis and service use (Hodges & Wong, 1996).

EXAMPLE: INITIAL COMPREHENSIVE ASSESSMENT WITH KRISTI

Recall that the first decision informed by a comprehensive assessment is to determine whether a child could benefit from CBT for anxiety (Figure 3.1). The following assessment procedures were conducted with Kristi and her mother at pretreatment, and their interpretation and integration into the decision-making framework are described here in some detail.

Affect

At her pretreatment assessment, Kristi was administered the PANAS-C to evaluate her temperamental affectivity. Her raw scores were 46 for PA and 51 for NA. A PA score of 40 is about 6 points higher than the average for children in our program, so Kristi's score implied that she was more emotionally positive than many of the children we see clinically—a good sign, and one that we interpreted as demonstrating a low risk for depression. Her score of NA, on the other hand, was considerably above average for children seen in our program. With the PANAS-C NA scale, scores above 30 are taken seriously; the average child suffering from anxiety disorders scores about a 34. Depressed children in our program average NA scores in the low 40s, so Kristi's score of 51 was obviously well above average for her negative emotionality. Right away, this score helped inform our first decision: Kristi would likely need treatment. It also suggested to us that we should be looking for comorbidity (i.e., multiple anxiety disorders), and that our treatment approach would have to emphasize generalizability beyond the initial clinical focus, because her tendency to develop new anxiety problems in the future might be higher than average.

Behavior and Symptoms

Krsiti's scores on the RCADS supported our hypotheses regarding appropriateness of treatment and comorbidity. These *T* scores were as follows: separation anxiety disorder (78), social phobia (69), generalized anxiety disorder (56), panic disorder (52), obsessive–compulsive disorder (44), and major depression (56). The elevations on the first two scales placed her in the 99th and 97th percentile for separation anxiety and social anxiety, respectively. Taken together with the PANAS-C scores, these results lent further support to the notion that Kristi would benefit from an anxiety treatment protocol.

Client Perspectives

Kristi's mother was quite clear in our clinical interview that she was overwhelmed by Kristi's refusal to attend school and nearly constant complaints of physical distress. As a single mother raising four children, Kristi's mother felt that she was out of options and that the school would soon give up on Kristi—transferring her either to home schooling or to another school. She needed help quickly, and the goal was obviously to get Kristi into school as soon as possible. From the perspective of deciding whether or not to treat, there was clear evidence that the family wanted help and that the consequences of not getting help could be severe. It also became clear that in addition to addressing the anxiety related to the school refusal, some specialized intervention strategies might be needed to deal with Kristi's frequent complaining to her mother. This information was integrated into the case formulation once the treatment began.

Diagnosis

Kristi and her mother both participated in the full administration of the ADIS-IV-C/P. Based on these interviews, Kristi was assigned a primary diagnosis of separation anxiety disorder, with additional diagnoses of social phobia and a specific phobia of contracting an illness or disease. In this case, child and parent reports were relatively convergent, with both mother and child describing the separation anxiety and social anxiety in some detail. Only Kristi reported her fear of contracting a disease. The interview allowed us to gather a wealth of information about the specific triggers and symptoms associated with Kristi's diagnostic syndromes. For example, it was clear that Kristi's social anxiety was focused on being teased or simply observed by her peers. The fact that she met diagnostic criteria for three disorders lent still more support to the idea that Kristi would require a formal treatment protocol.

Environment

We assessed the environment informally, by gathering interview information about family background, resources available to the mother, and the home setting. Significant details included the fact that mother was separated from Kristi's father and had no one in her own peer group available to provide reasonable social support. She was raising four children on part-time wages and lived in state-subsidized housing. From the mother's report, Kristi's siblings had no discernible behavioral or emotional concerns, but were nevertheless "typical challenging kids." The home environment offered some inducements for Kristi to stay home from school, including unrestricted access to television and food while the mother worked. The collective information about the environment further suggested that Kristi's problem would not likely resolve on its own or merely through additional effort on the part of Kristi's mother.

Functioning

Following the interview, the clinical interviewer completed the CAFAS. Kristi's scores for School Performance and Moods/Emotions scales were each 30, indicating "severe" impairment, and representing the highest score possible (worst possible functioning). Kristi also scored a 20, "moderate," for the Behavior towards Others scale, suggesting that she had impairments in relations with her peers, which we now knew were due to her social anxiety and withdrawal. Summing these scales yielded a CAFAS total score of 80, well into the range considered severe for anxiety cases in our program. In fact, we often provide services for children with "uncomplicated" anxiety, whose total CAFAS scores are as low as 10 or 20. In such cases, the anxiety and distress can be severe, but interference with multiple domains of functioning is less heavily demonstrated. Given her CAFAS score of 80, Kristi's case required little reflection about whether the impairment justified intervention.

SUMMARY

Kristi's comprehensive assessment illustrates how multiple measures and strategies were used to determine the appropriateness of her receiving treatment of any kind and, in particular, treatment for anxiety problems (the first rectangle in Figure 3.1). The collective results painted a picture of significant impairment resulting from a preponderance of anxiety problems. Given the school and home situations, it was clear that a formal intervention would be appropriate to remedy the problem.

The comprehensive assessment approach, such as that used at pretreatment with Kristi, could also be performed prior to termination to document what gains had been made and whether additional services or supports might be needed. Reviewing the posttreatment assessment results with child and parents can also act as a way to summarize accomplishments, consolidate knowledge, and provide positive feedback.

Finally, a comprehensive assessment is sometimes warranted when a case is characterized by big problems that cannot seem to be resolved easily (see Figure 3.1, bottom rectangle). For example, it is sometimes important to step back and thoroughly investigate lack of progress that cannot be accounted for by problems with the case formulation, the therapist's technical integrity using the protocol, or obvious barriers such as poor engagement. Sometimes these assessments reveal new developments or challenges that can serve to substantially alter a treatment approach (e.g., use an entirely different protocol or select a primary treatment target other than anxiety).

The comprehensive assessment in our case example involved the administration of specific instruments or procedures in each domain; however, it is important to keep in mind that the comprehensive assessment is more a process than merely a list of measures. Different circumstances might warrant a different collection of strategies. What defines the comprehensive assessment are the overarching goals of identifying the nature and extent of problems and interference across multiple domains in order to inform decisions about when to start, stop, or abandon the treatment approach. The clinician is advised to assemble the appropriate tools to meet those goals, using the guidelines outlined above to direct decision making.

FOUR

The Core Treatment Plan

Having introduced the basic concepts, briefly reviewed theory, and outlined assessment procedures, we can now turn to the details of treatment itself. The purpose of this chapter is to develop the notion of the "core treatment plan"—the treatment path that represents the most common scenario, and the one best informed by treatment research.

As mentioned in Chapter 1, we can assume for now that most cases will not begin with significant engagement problems. If this assumption is not true in a given setting or context, then perhaps a different plan is warranted, but in our program, even in the context of serving children in the public mental health system, significant problems with engagement emerge in no more than about a third of cases. Thus, most of the time it is safe to assume that we can go forward with the core treatment plan.

This notion of the core treatment plan is central to the proper use of this protocol from beginning to end. The concept draws from the substantial literature on clinical decision making that has repeatedly shown how actuarial information—statistics from prior observations about how common or likely something is—is nearly uniform in its superiority over clinical judgment (Dawes, Faust, & Meehl, 1989; Meehl, 1954). In other words, despite considerable training, clinical experts often perform worse when making specific predictions than do formulas using basic statistics on such things as prevalence or probabilities.

In one illustration, Dawes et al. (1989) reviewed the classic study by Goldberg (1968), in which a simple mathematical decision rule for diagnosing neurosis versus psychosis was created using scales from a well-known personality inventory. This scale-score decision rule was compared with expert judgments from 29 clinicians from seven different service units (e.g., hospitals, clinics). In a head-to-head test, clinicians were correct an average of 62% of the time, with the best judge being correct on 67% of the decisions, whereas the simple mathematical formula was correct for an average of 70% of the decisions. Goldberg found that the clinician judges did no better even when given substantial additional training on this diagnostic decision. Amazingly, even when the judges were given the outcome of the mathematical rule and were free to use it in their decision making, they were not as accurate as the rule itself.

Shocking? This illustration demonstrates the ease with which biases can be introduced into clinical decision making and supports the notion of "sticking to the rule" when a good rule is available. What, then, is the role of the clinician? To that end, Dawes and colleagues noted that there are some circumstances under which actuarial rules are inferior. The most well known is classically referred to as the "broken leg" scenario, based on the anecdote of a successful formula for predicting someone's weekly attendance at a movie theater—which should be discarded if one discovers that the individual in question is wearing a cast on his or her leg. In other words, there will be times when there is obvious evidence that the rule in question is no longer appropriate, and sound clinical judgment should carry the day.

So what does this line of thought have to do with developing a treatment plan? Actually, the case formulation model central to this protocol is no different. Therapists are tempted to see the exceptions to the rule, to see how the treatment could be modified or individualized. Although active case formulation is expected at the appropriate times, individualization of the treatment should be conceptualized as a departure from the core treatment plan and should be occasioned by the metaphorical broken leg. In other words, the therapist should attempt to implement the core plan and make modifications only when observations and evidence indicate significant threats to that approach.

So what is the basic plan of action? The answer is exposure, and lots of it. The entire protocol is organized around getting the anxious child to participate in exposure exercises; all other strategies are designed to support or enhance those effects. The latter part of this chapter covers how that plan is implemented.

Where did the core plan originate? Why is exposure the centerpiece of the treatment? This emphasis on exposure comes from observation and review of the great many studies on the successful treatment of anxiety. The aggregate summary of these procedures must provide the clue, and so we proceed next with a brief review of the literature on CBT for anxiety.

TREATMENTS FOR ANXIETY

The treatment strategies outlined in this protocol are based heavily on the work of Barlow (1988) and Beck and colleagues (Beck, Rush, Shaw, & Emery, 1979) in adults, its extensions for children by Kendall and colleagues (e.g., Kendall, Kane, Howard, & Siqueland, 1990), the behavioral therapy for phobic children developed in the early part of the 20th century (Jones, 1924), and its extensions and elaborations over the past 30 years (e.g., Ollendick & Francis, 1988; Ollendick & King, 1998). Numerous positive findings have emerged with respect to these treatments (see Chorpita & Southam-Gerow, 2006). In over 200 investigations, the protocols that have consistently demonstrated the strongest results in children and adolescents include modeling, exposure, and CBT (see Table 4.1). Let's consider each of these three strategies in turn.

TABLE 4.1. Summary of Best Supported Treatments for Childhood Fears and Anxieties

Intervention	Compliance	Gender	Age	Ethnicity	Therapist	Frequency	Duration	Format	Setting
Exposure and variants	97%	Both	3–17	European American, African American	Undergraduate, BA, MA, PhD	Daily to weekly	1 day to 20 weeks	Group, individual	Clinic, community, school
Cognitive techniques and variants	92%	Both	2–17	European American, African American, Hispanic/ Latino, Asian American, Native American, Pacific Islander	Undergraduate, MA, PhD	Daily to weekly	1 day to 20 weeks	Group, individual, group with parent, individual with parent	Clinic, school, community, dental office
Modeling and variants	100%	Both	2–18	European American, African American	MA, PhD	Twice per day to weekly	1 day to 18 weeks	Group, individual, child with parent	Clinic, community, school, laboratory, dental office, hospital

Note. Compliance refers to the average number of children who completed the study protocol. Ethnicity is listed in order of frequency within protocol type. BA, bachelor's degree; MA, master's degree or enrolled graduate student; PhD, doctoral degree. Adapted from Chorpita and Southam-Gerow (2006). Copyright 2006 by The Guilford Press. Adapted by permission.

Exposure

The strategy of exposure typically involves a child's real or imagined confrontation with a feared stimulus. The different variants of exposure involve modifications of the intensity, duration, or order of stimuli, and may include other clinical strategies as well, such as relaxation or rewards. Two major variations of exposure involve whether the stimulus is confronted directly or whether it is imagined. Direct confrontation is usually termed *in vivo* exposure and requires the child to be in the presence of the actual feared object or situation, such as petting a dog or giving a speech in front of others (e.g., Obler & Terwillinger, 1970). For a variety of reasons, it is sometimes preferable to have the child imagine the feared object or stimulus, a procedure commonly referred to as *imaginal* or *in vitro* exposure. This strategy usually involves a therapist describing a scene that includes the feared stimulus, while the child listens and imagines the details as vividly as possible. Such strategies can be particularly helpful for exposure to stimuli or events that are not easily performed *in vivo*. For example, a child who has a fear of an upcoming surgery might be exposed *in vivo* to the hospital setting or other related stimuli, but confrontation with the event itself (i.e., surgery) is more easily performed through imaginal exposure. Exposure has been shown to be effective in reducing childhood fears and anxieties in more than 35 randomized, controlled tests (Chorpita & Southam-Gerow, 2006) and is applicable across a wide range of contexts and child characteristics (see Table 4.1).

Cognitive-Behavioral Therapy

As its name implies, CBT involves both cognitive and behavioral techniques. Although cognitive procedures are a defining feature of CBT programs, it should come as no surprise that *exposure is still of central importance in CBT*. In fact, CBT for anxiety can best be thought of as exposure *plus* many other techniques, such as the use of thought exercises, rewards, praise, and differential reinforcement strategies—in other words, lots of nice extras to make exposure work better.

Some precursors of formal cognitive techniques were first tested in the 1970s, when they were referred to as self-management or self-talk strategies. For example, in a study on the treatment of fear of darkness, Kanfer, Karoly, and Newman (1975) tested three strategies to address children's fear of the dark: coping self-talk, stimulus self-talk, or neutral self-talk. In the coping self-talk condition, children were instructed to repeat a phrase emphasizing their bravery and ability to cope with the dark (e.g., "I am brave"). In the stimulus self-talk condition, children repeated positive statements about the dark, without reference to coping (e.g., "The dark is a fun place"). Finally, in the neutral self-talk condition, children repeated a nursery rhyme unrelated to the dark. Results pointed to advantages of both the coping self-talk and stimulus self-talk strategies.

More recent protocols have elaborated these procedures with a specific aim toward altering the perception of threat or danger, a process sometimes called "cognitive restructuring." This approach initially involves steps of identifying negative thoughts or perceived threats and challenging them with alternative thoughts or interpretations. Cognitive exercises in this protocol should not be perceived as independent from exposure, however. That is, much of the success of cognitive restructuring is achieved through practice exercises that teach the child, through both experience and reasoning, that his or her anxiety is not necessary—that what he or she perceives as dangerous is really safe. Primarily, this approach provides corrective experiences; that is, children practice what they are afraid of and thereby learn that the bad things they fear do not usually come true. One of the main problems with anxious children is that by avoiding what they are afraid of, they limit the possibility for these corrective learning experiences. The therapist's role is to act as a guide who encourages and supports the child as he or she attempts to engage in these experiences so that things misperceived as threatening can eventually be seen as safe. Collectively, CBT protocols enjoy a substantial amount of empirical support, with over 50 controlled demonstrations of successful performance across a wide variety of child characteristics (see Figure 4.1). In this protocol, the encouragement of corrective learning is most often done informally as part of exposure, such as by asking the child afterward "How did it go?" to help him or her identify success and recognize "safety." Formal cognitive procedures are typically added only when exposure alone appears not to be working well.

Modeling

Modeling involves the child's observation of another person interacting successfully with a feared stimulus. For example, a therapist might pet a dog to demonstrate to a child that the dog is safe and need not be feared. There are many variations of this basic technique, depending primarily on the nature of the model and the type of behaviors expected of the child. For example, with *live* modeling, the model performs the behaviors directly for the child (e.g., Bandura, Grusec, & Menlove, 1967; Murphy & Bootzin, 1973), whereas with *symbolic* modeling, the model is shown interacting with the stimulus on a video or in a photograph (e.g., Lewis, 1974). In *covert* modeling, the child is asked to imagine the model interacting with the feared stimulus, and in *participant* modeling, the child first observes the model interacting with the stimulus and is then asked to perform the same behaviors as the model (i.e., participates in *in vivo* exposure; e.g., Ritter, 1968). In several between-group design investigations, modeling has demonstrated superior treatment effects relative to no-treatment control and wait-list conditions (Bandura, Blanchard, & Ritter, 1969; Blanchard, 1970; Murphy & Bootzin, 1973; Ritter, 1968). In this protocol, modeling is never used alone, given the scarcity of evidence that it works without exposure. Instead, it is often implicitly combined with exposure. For example, when a child has trouble performing a feared task, the therapist might perform it first so that the child can watch and then imitate.

THE IMPORTANCE OF EXPOSURE

Finding Common Elements of Therapy

How can the literature be used to inform the core treatment plan? Well, if one looks at all the successful treatments performed for anxiety, patterns emerge that reveal common strategies across a great many protocols. In a preliminary demonstration of this model, Chorpita, Daleiden, and Weisz (2005a) found one set of strategies for phobias and a sep-

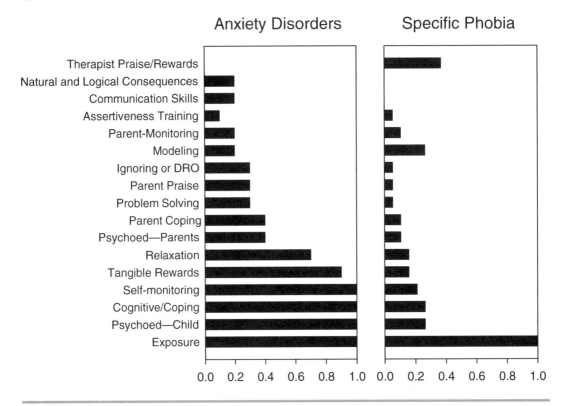

FIGURE 4.1. Frequency of the presence of specific clinical strategies among selected protocols with empirical support. DRO, differentiatial reinforcement of other behaviors. Adapted from Chorpita, Daleiden, and Weisz (2005a). Copyright 2005 by Springer. Adapted by permission.

arate set for the other anxiety disorders. These patterns are shown in Figure 4.1. The results suggested that successful demonstrations of treatment for specific phobia (1) always involved exposure, (2) sometimes involved therapist praise, modeling, psycho-education, and/or cognitive strategies, and (3) rarely used other strategies. The successful empirical demonstrations for the treatment of anxiety disorders other than phobias *always* involved exposure, psychoeducation, cognitive strategies, and self-monitoring, and *often* used rewards, relaxation, parent psychoeducation, and/or parent coping strategies, with *occasional use* of some of the other strategies listed. As is clear from this summary analysis, exposure is the only "universal" component and can be reasonably considered a core ingredient of successful interventions that target fears and anxieties. Particularly noteworthy is that these aggregate profiles represent studies collectively targeting the full spectrum of anxiety disorders.

Other Support for Exposure

Although sufficient dismantling research has not been conducted with CBT for childhood anxiety disorders to confirm that exposure is necessary and not merely common, additional evidence of specific, active effects of exposure can be inferred from two related studies. In an investigation of the additive effects of treatment components implemented with two children exhibiting nighttime fears, Ollendick, Hagopian, and Huntzinger (1991) used a multiple-baseline design across subjects, in which two different treatment components were sequentially applied. Subsequent to the introduction of a combination of cognitive techniques, including self-induced relaxation, self-monitoring, and verbal self-instruction, rewards were implemented for an increase in exposure to the feared situation. Results suggested that reinforced exposure was the critical component in this treatment approach, given that treatment effects were observed only upon the introduction of rewards for heightened levels of exposure (Ollendick, et al., 1991).

An additional source of support for exposure, or the behavioral component of CBT, as the active component of this treatment approach can be ascertained from a randomized clinical trial of CBT for anxiety disordered children (Kendall et al., 1997). In this investigation, children were treated sequentially with two treatment components: a cognitive educational treatment component, followed by an exposure treatment component. Analyses of midtreatment data revealed no significant treatment effects across child or parent indicators, suggesting that the cognitive educational treatment component, in isolation, was not responsible for any observed differences between the treatment and the wait-list control groups. However, comparisons of the second segment of treatment (exposure) with the first and second segments combined suggested that the behavioral treatment component was uniquely associated with the observed outcomes. Although it is possible that these findings suggest the necessity of an initial cognitive procedure to set the stage for exposure, an alternative interpretation of the results is simply that treatment gains are not observed until exposure is enacted, thus suggesting that exposure itself is responsible for observed therapeutic outcomes.

CORE TREATMENT PLAN: THE "CORE FOUR" PROCEDURES

So we have an emerging picture that exposure is the centerpiece of the treatment protocol. It is no coincidence that Part II of this text devotes three chapters to the discussion of exposure. But exposure takes preparation. One must first do the work of figuring out what feared objects should be part of exposure and then prepare the child to engage in it successfully. Also, it makes sense to review how exposure has helped as the treatment comes to a close. We cannot just "jump right in" at the beginning of therapy, nor can we just "jump right out" at the end. Pure exposure by itself would be hard to distinguish from simply scaring someone repeatedly—and obviously would not be successful in achieving therapeutic aims.

Thus, as part of the core treatment plan, it is suggested that all children receive a minimum set of four procedures, the "core four," believed to represent the main ingredients of treatment. These are noted in Figure 4.2: (1) the development of a list of fears (the "Fear Ladder"), (2) education about anxiety ("Learning about Anxiety"), (3) the practice of feared situations ("Practice," which can be *in vivo* or imaginal), and (4) education about maintaining new gains and skills ("Maintenance"). The first two procedures essentially set the stage for exposure (the third procedure) by creating a list of goals and

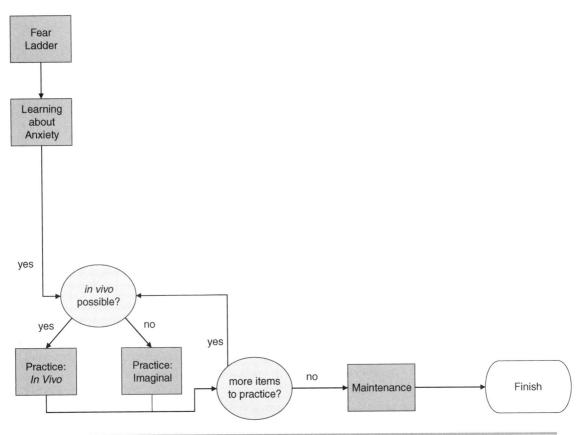

FIGURE 4.2. Flowchart for the core treatment plan.

the processes by which to measure those goals and providing a rationale for exposure. The fourth procedure is essentially designed to encourage the child to continue a life-style that involves habits of approach and exposure whenever anxiety becomes prob-lematic. So that's it—the core treatment plan—the scenario that we first imagine applies to all children receiving the protocol.

PERIODIC ASSESSMENT AND THE CLINICAL "DASHBOARD"

Now back to the case formulation framework. Figure 4.3 shows how the ongoing deci-sions being made are intended to evaluate treatment progress. This decision point is where the periodic assessment comes in, first mentioned briefly in Chapter 3. In our pro-gram, it is an expectation that measures of progress be taken repeatedly for all anxiety cases. These measures are then graphed over time and used to guide decisions about whether the set of core procedures is working.

    In addition to tracking some index of progress, it is advisable to represent the his-tory of therapy strategies as well. These strategies can be plotted together on the same instrument, such that one can view both treatment progress and therapist activities at a

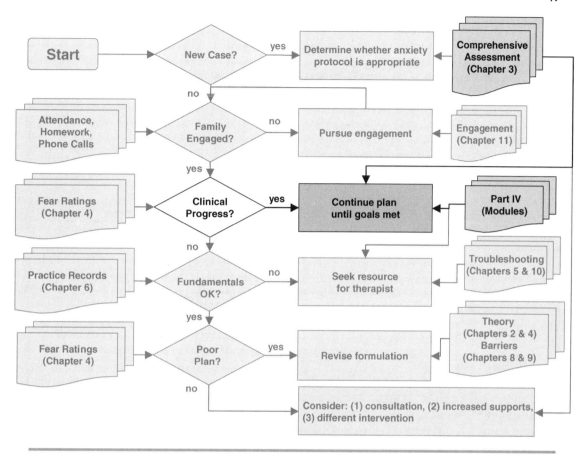

FIGURE 4.3. Progress supports the treatment plan.

glance (see the example of "Susie" in Figure 4.4). These displays or graphs function like a dashboard in a vehicle, summarizing key information in a convenient and rapidly interpretable way (see Daleiden & Chorpita, 2005). The driver—or therapist—is thus able to focus quickly on where he or she has been and ascertain where he or she is going.

My colleague Eric Daleiden—a clinical evaluation wizard—has also referred to this simple dashboard as the "two-chambered heart." Aptly named, it is indeed the heart of the strategy for case formulation and progress review and shows both the inputs (therapy procedures) and outputs (clinical progress measures) that occur with each beat.

In this example, the top panel, referred to as the "progress pane," graphs the child's self-reported and mother-reported fear ratings averaged across a list of fears, such that higher scores represent greater fear level. A downward sloping line thus indicates progress. By both child and mother's report, Susie's average fear ratings decreased from approximately 6 on a 10-point scale to between 1 and 2 over the course of 11 weeks.

The bottom panel, referred to as the "practice pane," is a graph of the history of specific clinical strategies employed over time. The treatment begins in this example with the list of feared items ("Fear Ladder") being constructed on the first day and psychoeducation occurring for both child and parent in a single session about 2 weeks later

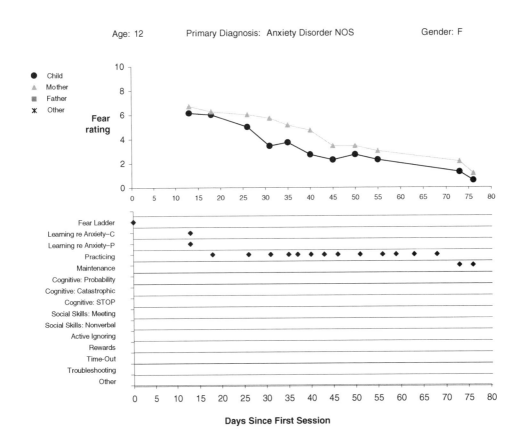

FIGURE 4.4. A clinical "dashboard" for a case using the core four procedures.

("Learning about Anxiety" for child and parent). As shown in the figure, there are then 13 sessions of exposure ("Practicing"), approximately weekly, followed by 2 sessions of wrap-up and review ("Maintenance").

Putting this clinical dashboard back into the context of the case formulation framework, the ratings for Susie's case would lead to the decision "continue plan until goals met" (Figure 4.3), given the regularity with which progress was observed in the progress pane (Figure 4.4). For the most straightforward of cases, then, it is these "core four" procedures, outlined in modules in Part IV, that constitute the treatment plan. When progress is not observed, the framework suggests that one should attend to the quality of the fundamentals. It is to the most important of these—exposure—that we now turn our full attention.

PART II
THE ART OF EXPOSURE

FIVE

How to Conduct Exposure

Chapter 2 served to establish the premise that anxiety disorders may be more alike than different in terms of their developmental, genetic, familial, affective, and temperamental components. Thus the current model conceptualizes the core processes of anxiety—as opposed to the different anxiety disorders—as the optimal targets of intervention. Chapter 3 showed how to determine whether anxiety was the primary problem, and Chapter 4 addressed how exposure appears to be the best candidate for addressing that problem, once identified. It follows that any therapist skilled in the treatment of anxiety must master the art of exposure. This pursuit is where most of the work is won or lost. If a therapist can perform exposure skillfully, he or she can be very effective; if a therapist cannot, he or she runs the risk of being minimally effective.

Like so many therapeutic procedures that can be subtle in their complexity, exposure sounds easy but is not. It is defined as presenting the feared stimulus to the child—which sounds relatively straightforward. However, there are dozens of ways to conduct exposure incorrectly, many of which could even be quite harmful. To make matters more challenging, there is no single way to conduct exposure correctly, either. Such complexity therefore justifies the title of this section as "The *Art* of Exposure."

THEORETICAL BACKGROUND

The object of exposure is to present the feared object or situation to the child (either *in vivo* or *in vitro*) in a way that fosters new learning. A variety of behavioral theories have been proposed to support the notion that presentation of a conditioned stimulus (e.g., feared object) in the absence of the unconditioned stimulus (e.g., feared outcome) should eliminate the conditioned response (i.e., the fear; Eysenck, 1979; Marks, 1969; Pavlov, 1927; Watson & Morgan, 1917; Watson & Rayner, 1920; Wolpe & Rowan, 1988). In other words, presenting the signal for danger (e.g., dog) in the absence of the actual danger (e.g., bite) should weaken their association and hence reduce the fear response to the signal (i.e., dog). Although other behavioral theories have emerged (e.g., Mowrer, 1939;

Rachman, 1977; Seligman, 1970, 1971), all suggest that extinction is the primary mechanism by which anxiety is reduced (see Chorpita & Southam-Gerow, 2006).

One of the other major theories related to the acquisition and reduction of anxiety is social learning theory (Bandura, 1969), which adds observation as an additional pathway for learning and unlearning fears. Bandura's theory is consistent with the notion that exposure to a feared stimulus minus the feared outcome should result in eventual fear reduction, but also offers an additional strategy, modeling, described in Chapter 4. Research has supported both modeling and exposure as methods of fear reduction, although modeling is implemented, almost universally, as a *supplement* to exposure. In other words, a child might observe someone else confront a stimulus first before confronting it him- or herself. With this protocol, it is recommended that modeling be incorporated into the exposure exercises, whenever necessary, to accelerate or enhance the gains.

Somewhat more recent cognitive models have had increasingly important implications for exposure and its successful implementation. For example, Lang's (1977) bioinformational theory posits three important aspects of memory related to fear: (1) information about the feared stimulus, (2) information about the fear-related responses (behavioral, physiological, and verbal), and (3) the individual's interpretations of the stimulus and response. When fear-relevant memories are activated, the person is likely to engage in avoidance behaviors. In many ways, this notion is consistent with Gray's (1987) model, wherein the individual in Stage 1 would analyze the situation and upon accessing stored information related to successful avoidance of a perceived threat, would seek to engage in those same avoidance behaviors again (Chorpita, 2001).

Foa and Kozak (1986) articulated one of the most important extensions of ideas about exposure in what is known as "emotional processing theory." These researchers posited cognitive "fear structures" that contain information related to the threat and the fear response. For example, one might associate being alone in one's bed in the dark with fear and thus escape from the dark with relief. The object of treatment is to provide corrective information that darkness in one's bedroom does not lead to harm and therefore is not a real threat (recall Barlow's notion of the "false alarm"). According to the emotional processing model, modification of these beliefs is highly challenging without activation of the fear structures (i.e., evoking the fear itself). Thus the model explains why simply telling someone not to be afraid of the dark is unlikely to help. According to the model, the corrective information has to be delivered when the fear structure is activated—that is, when someone is experiencing anxiety about the darkness *in the moment*. Hence, even within the context of their cognitive model, exposure therapy remains the critical component. An important corollary is that exposure must occur at a sufficiently intense level for any corrective learning to occur. In short, corrective learning occurs when exposure is (1) fear provoking but (2) lacks the feared consequences.

THE BASICS

The Fear Thermometer

How do we know if exposure is indeed fear provoking? We take ratings. This concept of taking global fear ratings during performance of anxiety-provoking exercises dates back to early assessment strategies (mentioned briefly in Chapter 3) known as behavior avoidance tests (Lang & Lazovic, 1963). These procedures have formal origins dating back as far as Jones (1924).

Wolpe and Lazarus (1966) offered the classic description of how to take such global fear ratings using a metric of subjective units of distress, which has dominated the practice of behavioral assessment of fear and anxiety for the past 40 years.

The fear thermometer is a tool designed to assist in eliciting such ratings from children, with anchors to reflect the range of fear from no fear to maximum fear. Anecdotally, the use of a temperature metaphor has proven particularly useful for children, who have a reasonable amount of experience with thermometers at an early age.* The use of fear thermometers with children has been documented throughout the literature for at least the past 30 years (e.g., Giebenhain & Barrios, 1986; Melamed, Hawes, Heiby, & Glick, 1975).

An example of the fear thermometer used with this protocol appears in Figure 5.1. The scale ranges from 0 to 10, with 0 representing *no fear*, and 10 representing *as much fear as one could imagine*. "Readings" are taken with this thermometer throughout exposure exercises, as is described in more detail below.

Item Selection

The first step of an exposure exercise is to select an item to practice. Naturally, the stimulus should not be so challenging that the child refuses to engage in the exercise, but, as implied by Foa and Kozak's (1986) emotional processing model above, the exercise cannot be too easy either. As a general rule, the more difficult the exposure, the better, provided that the child can be successful and will not refuse to participate. Generally the process of selecting an item to practice involves (1) review of the list of feared items (i.e., fear ladder), created using the first treatment module, and (2) a sensitive and thoughtful discussion with the child. A sample fear ladder from our work with Kristi is shown in Figure 5.2; here the first item selected for exposure is circled (saying "no" to friends),

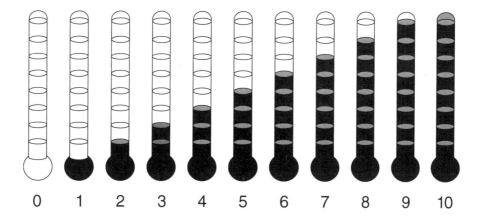

FIGURE 5.1. Fear thermometer.

---

*The increasing use of digital, instant-read thermometers in medical settings and even in homes may portend an end to the utility of this metaphor, as has already happened with other gems such as "broken record."

Date : _____

Please give a rating for how scary each of these things
is today. Remember to use the scale from 0 to 10.

Filled out by: (✔child ( ) parent   ( ) other _____

0 1 2 3 4 5 6 7 8 9 10

Talking in class	9
Working with the teacher	8
Meeting new people	7
Writing on the board	6
Talking on the phone	5
Eating in the cafeteria	5
Saying "no" to my friends	4
Being teased	4

FIGURE 5.2. Sample fear ladder for Kristi.

which might be an appropriate starting point early in treatment. Numbers to the right of items in the figure are their fear thermometer ratings.

Using the Practice Record

Extinction (commonly referred to as "habituation," although see Barlow, 1988, for subtle differences) is tracked in this protocol by using the practice record. Two types of practice records are used: continuous practice records and discrete practice records. Continuous practice records are designed to allow the therapist to take fear thermometer ratings at fixed intervals (e.g., every minute, every 3 minutes) during the performance of an exposure exercise. One might take ratings every minute while a phobic child pets a dog, or every 5 minutes while standing in a high place. Once a child has been taught how to use the fear thermometer, ratings can be taken by simply verbally prompting the child (e.g., "What is your rating now?").

Figure 5.3 shows a continuous practice record completed for Kristi while she performed an exposure exercise for reading aloud. In this exercise, Kristi was provided with a book and asked to read aloud for at least 4 minutes. Before beginning the exercise, the therapist took an initial fear rating, which was 9. Then the therapist kept time with a watch. After Kristi began reading, the therapist prompted her for a fear rating approxi-

Goal: Each time you practice, take ratings every_____ minutes. Stop after_____minutes or when your rating comes down to a _____ .

Start Date: __March 3__

Day __Today's session__

Item __Reading aloud__

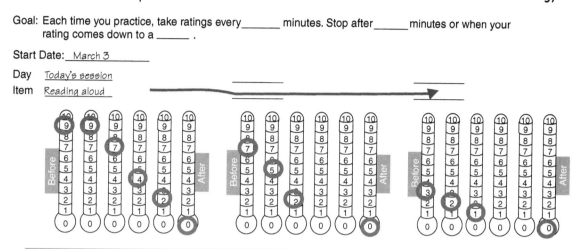

FIGURE 5.3. Kristi's continuous practice record for reading aloud.

mately once each minute. These were recorded on the practice record. After the exercise was complete, the therapist recorded a final rating on the practice record as well. This sequence was repeated twice more, with subsequent trials requiring less time due to Kristi's rapid decrease in anxiety on the second and third trials.

Discrete practice records are used for exposure exercises that cannot be performed continuously. One of Kristi's social fears was that of drinking a beverage while others were watching. Her worries included the possibility that she would spill something on herself or that others would simply stare at her and think she looked foolish while she drank. Because we could not ask Kristi to drink water continuously, we instead performed exercises in which she took a brief sip of water, providing a rating before and after. Her practice record for drinking water appears in Figure 5.4. Note that she took 10 sips of water during the course of the exposure session.

Goal: Each time you practice, repeat_____ times or until your rating comes down to_____. You can do it!

Start Date: __March 19__

Day __Today's session__

Item __Drinking beverage__

FIGURE 5.4. Kristi's continuous practice record for drinking water.

Goals of Exposure

The short-term goals of exposure are twofold: (1) within-trial habituation and (2) between-trial habituation. Habituation is typically detected through a decrease in reported fear level. For example, if a child initially reports a fear level of 8 on the fear thermometer, a subsequent report of 5—keeping the situation constant—would imply habituation. When such decreases occur within the context of a practice episode, they are called within-trial habituation. When such decreases occur across practice episodes (e.g., on a subsequent day or even just a few minutes later), they are called between-trial habituation. On the practice records, within-trial habituation can be detected by connecting the lines from one rating to the next, such that a downward slope implies habituation and a level or increasing slope does not. Between-trial habituation can be detected by connecting the "Before" ratings across multiple trials, with the slopes interpreted in the same way as for within-trial habituation. Figure 5.5 gives examples of both of these types of habituation from a practice session with Mary. The dashed line refers to between-trial habituation, and the solid lines refer to within-trial habituation. With all lines sloping downward, this practice record is evidence of successful exposure.

Therapist Behavior before Exposure

When setting up an exposure practice, the therapist needs to focus the child on the fact that the exercise is a learning experience. It is important to build on information from the earlier psychoeducation (i.e., Learning about Anxiety module, which covers the basic treatment model and background information about anxiety), reminding the child that the anxiety is likely to be a false alarm, and that the best way to find out if the anxiety is appropriate or not is to test the experience and find out if something bad really happens. In setting up an exposure for Kristi, that explanation might sound something like this:

Goal: Each time you practice, take ratings every ___3___ minutes. Stop after ___15___ minutes or when your rating comes down to a _0, 1, or 2_.

Start Date: _August 13_

Day   _Wed_   _Friday_   _Sunday_
Item _Bedroom at night_   _(same)_   _(same)_

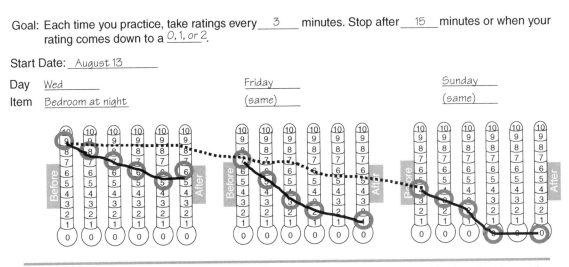

FIGURE 5.5. Mary's continuous practice record showing between-trial (dashed line) and within-trial (solid line) habituation.

"OK, Kristi. Now you talked about how you are most afraid that when you eat in front of other people, they are going to laugh at you. Is that right? As we talked about before, the best way to find out if your fear is just a 'false alarm' is to test out that idea. And we also talked about how, if you do have some anxiety, that if you wait long enough, it will just go away. Are you ready to try a little practice like that with me now? Let's have you eat some of these chips, and I will watch you for a few minutes. While we do that, I am just going sit quietly and take ratings with the fear thermometer so we can see what happens to your anxiety. Do you have any questions before we start?"

Be sure to answer questions and be clear that the purpose of the exercise is to learn whether something is a false alarm—not to be free from anxiety.

Therapist Behavior during Exposure

Many therapists have a difficult time knowing what to do during exposure—particularly because there is very little that the therapist should actually be doing. Sitting in silence while a child bravely or not so bravely tolerates discomfort can feel awkward and unnatural to many therapists. Nevertheless, it is advisable that the therapist does not distract or reassure the child during exposure, otherwise the meaning of the stimulus may be changed. For example, telling Mary "there is nothing scary here with us in the dark" may neutralize that experience of being afraid in the dark for her, and later when she encounters the dark on her own, her anxiety might return because that reassurance (i.e., the therapist's presence) is no longer available.

In most circumstances, the therapist's best choice is to observe quietly and to take ratings. Occasional corrective prompts for approach may be necessary if minor problems arise during the exercise. For example, telling Kristi "remember to keep looking up at me every now and then while you are eating" may be advisable. As a general rule, the choice to speak or intervene should be based on the intention to increase approach, and the therapist should always consider the risk of becoming too distracting or reassuring, both of which are problematic. It can help to keep in mind the notion drawn from emotional processing theory that the fear structure must be activated for corrective information about the lack of real danger to be incorporated during the exercise. Too much distraction or reassurance can "deactivate" the fear structure.

Therapist Behavior after Exposure

Once the exposure is complete, the therapist can then be as warm and reassuring as needed. As can be inferred from the considerable literature on exposure, praise can be a powerful tool at this point. "High-fives," "thumbs up," or other gestures of success are important now. And although generalized praise is always important and effective (e.g., "Wow! You did it!"), even better is specific feedback about the approach behaviors or other positive aspects of performance ("Wow, Kristi, you did the whole exercise without stopping. I really like how you kept making eye contact, too!").

Whether incorporating formal cognitive exercises or not, now is also the time to review and consolidate any learning that occurred as a result of the exercise. These types of questions are typically very helpful:

1. "So what did you notice happened to your anxiety as time went on?" (Here child typically notes that anxiety decreases on its own over time.)
2. "Did the [bad thing, e.g., someone laughing] come true?" (Here the child might observe that the feared consequences did not occur.)
3. "Were you able to handle it better than you thought?" (Here the child might note that it was easier than expected, once begun.)
4. "What was the hardest part?" (Here the child might note that the anticipatory anxiety was the worst part of the whole experience, implying that it is better to just jump in and get started next time than to wait around and deliberate or worry.)
5. "What do you think will happen over time if you keep practicing this one at home?" (Here the child should predict that continued practice will lead to further reductions in anxious responding.)

At this point, it can be very helpful to instill a sense of pride and victory in the child by asking him or her either to repeat or at least describe the success to a parent or some other positive figure. Often when children perform an exposure exercise in front of the parent, it can trigger spontaneous praise and excitement from the parent (who perhaps thought success was unlikely), which, in turn, generate strong feelings of accomplishment in the child. These feelings are important "capital" that the therapist will want to bank on when later exercises are potentially more challenging or difficult to complete.

Basic Troubleshooting of Exposure

As noted at the beginning of this chapter, many things can go wrong with exposure, but two events are of primary therapeutic importance: the absence of either between-trial or within-trial habituation. One of the therapist's primary responsibilities in conducting exposure is to assess for the presence of both types of habituation, and if either is absent, to take immediate corrective actions.

Figure 5.6 shows a continuous practice record for Mary with evidence of a failure to obtain within-trial habituation. If this problem surfaces, the therapist should either extend the length of the exposure until habituation does occur or begin with an easier stimulus in future exercises. It is preferable to choose the former solution if possible, because the fewer "steps backward" taken during exposure, the better. It is usually important to verify the child's ongoing understanding that exposure exercises move forward whenever possible; they do not move backward to easier items. Thus, in this example, the exposure trial should be extended for as long as needed (e.g., 30 additional minutes) for habituation to occur.

It is important not to let the practice record format dictate the length of an exposure; doing so might lead to premature termination of exposure. That is, if the therapist chooses to take ratings every minute and gets to the end of the first grouping of ratings

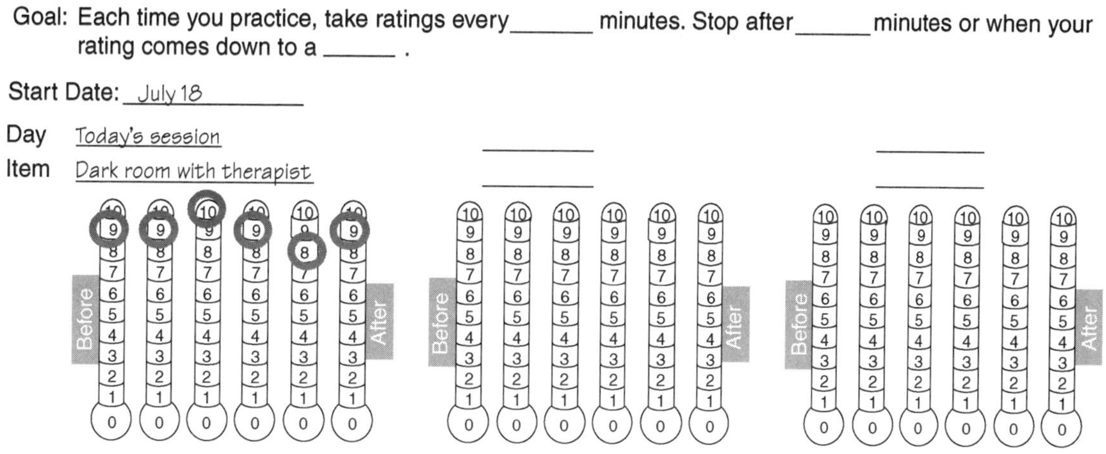

Goal: Each time you practice, take ratings every_____ minutes. Stop after_____minutes or when your rating comes down to a _____ .

Start Date: _July 18_____

Day   _Today's session_   _____   _____

Item   _Dark room with therapist_   _____   _____

FIGURE 5.6. Mary's continuous practice record showing failure to obtain within-trial habituation.

on the practice record without observing habituation, then the therapist should continue the exercise and connect the first cluster of ratings with the second (see Figure 5.7). The decision to stop an exposure exercise should always be based on the child's actual response, not on the format of the measure being used. Remember, the goal is *habituation*, not completing the form perfectly. Some therapists in our program even make their own forms for children who repeatedly "go long" in exposure practices.

Related to the failure to observe within-trial habituation is the pattern of escalating fear ratings. For example, a child might give a fear thermometer rating of 4 to begin, only to have it climb to 7 or 8 over the next few minutes. The first time this escalation happens for a therapist learning exposure, the supervisor might wonder whether the therapist should start taking his or her own ratings! It is not fun, and it takes some trust to believe that the ratings will indeed decrease.

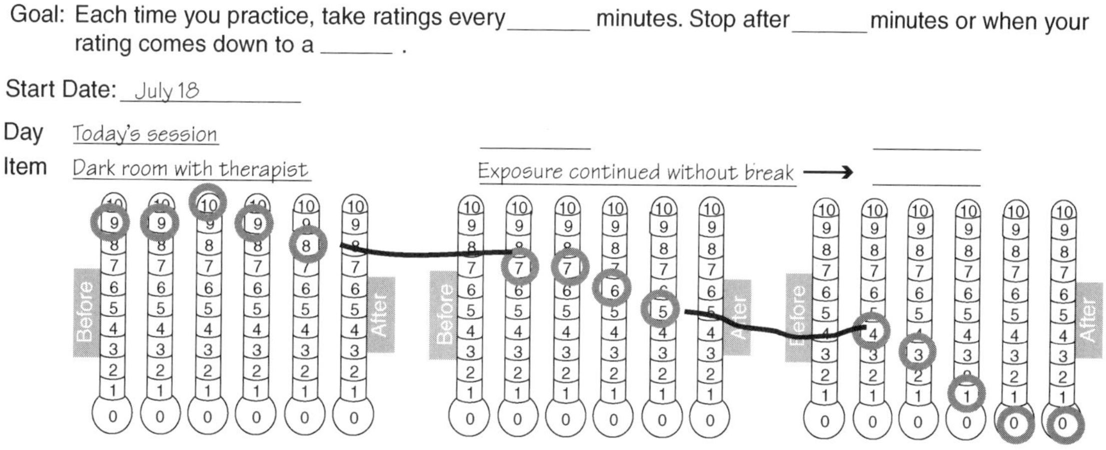

Goal: Each time you practice, take ratings every_____ minutes. Stop after_____minutes or when your rating comes down to a _____ .

Start Date: _July 18_____

Day   _Today's session_   _____   _____

Item   _Dark room with therapist_   Exposure continued without break ⟶   _____

FIGURE 5.7. Sample continuous practice record showing a single extended trial.

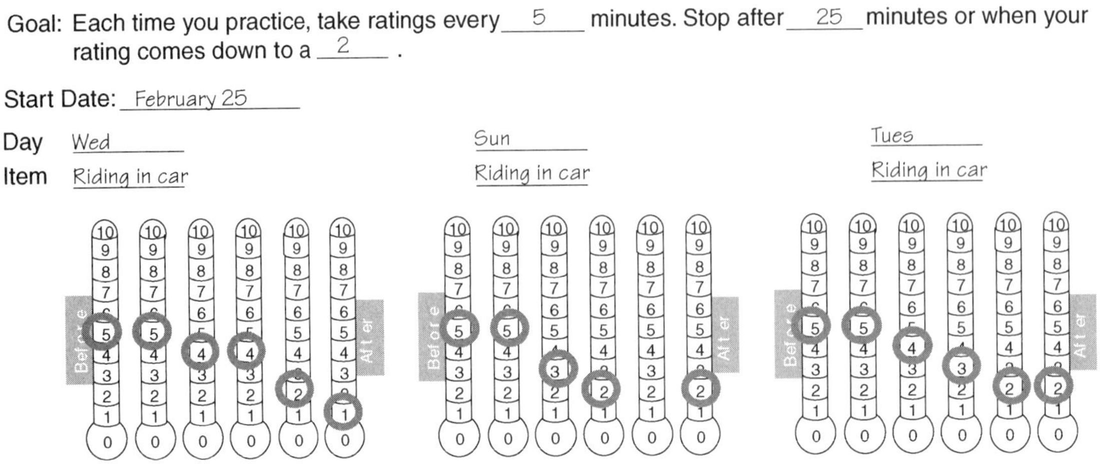

Goal: Each time you practice, take ratings every ___5___ minutes. Stop after ___25___ minutes or when your rating comes down to a ___2___ .

Start Date: _February 25_____

Day   _Wed_____   _Sun_____   _Tues_____
Item _Riding in car_   _Riding in car_   _Riding in car_

FIGURE 5.8. Doug's continuous practice record showing failure to obtain between-trial habituation.

In such circumstances it is best to continue with the exercise, if at all possible. The anxiety should level off and eventually subside. In more extreme circumstances, for which it looks like the level of distress would cause the child to terminate the exercise, it is advisable to reduce the intensity of the exercise, if possible. For example, with a dog exposure, it might mean moving the dog slightly farther away for the moment. In general, therapists are reminded to be patient in waiting for the habituation and to select carefully, from the outset, exercises that are likely to be both challenging *and* successful.

Failure to obtain between-trial habituation is the other common challenge likely to be encountered with exposure. This failure is most often detected when reviewing records from exposure practices performed at home. Figure 5.8 shows a continuous practice record that Doug and his mother completed during the week at home. It shows evidence of a failure to obtain between-trial habituation. If this problem occurs, the therapist should decrease the time between exposure practices, which means scheduling more exposure. In this example, Doug practiced only once every few days, and although there was habituation within each trial, the exercises remained just as difficult to initiate each time. For example, from Wednesday to Sunday his fear had time to return. In this situation, it would therefore be advisable to have Doug repeat the same exposure practice for homework every day or even twice a day. As with between-trial habituation, this goal is always best achieved through careful selection of a practice schedule beforehand, because it is better to avoid such problems strategically than to try to correct them after they happen. The ability to select the right exercises and assign them on the proper practice schedule is obviously a therapist talent that can take time to develop.

SIX

Nobody Likes Exposure

Think back to a time when you were most afraid in your life. Maybe it was a fire in your home, a car accident, a terrible storm, or a family member undergoing risky surgery. When you were overwhelmed with fear, you probably had difficulty performing effectively. If you have not had such experiences, consider the following scenarios and try to imagine the feelings in your body and the thoughts in your mind:

- You open your eyes in the morning and notice your own bed sheets heavily soaked with blood. Your hand moves to draw back the covers.
- Upon hearing a terrible and unfamiliar sound in the night, you search your house to find that all of your family members are missing.
- You turn the key in the door to your house as you come home. As the door swings open, there are strangers in your home, and the furniture is overturned.

Stop and imagine the feeling for a moment. It is sudden, overwhelming, and painful. It can involve feelings of confusion, weakness, and even unreality. This is anxiety, and whether the source is these terrible events or simply that you cannot ride the school bus, the phenomenology of the experience is the same. As outlined in Chapter 1, false alarms and true alarms do not differ in their emotional intensity, only in the rational basis for their onset.

This awful feeling is not unlike what you ask a child to experience each time you practice exposure—and, oddly, you expect them to come back for more! Plain and simple, active participation in CBT for anxiety may be one of the hardest things an anxious child will ever have to do. This chapter provides some strategies to assist with making the protocol more successful in that regard.

BUILDING RAPPORT

Rapport-building exercises are an implicit part of any good CBT approach. Even in some of the earliest studies on the treatment of phobias, it was a common assumption that a therapist should create a positive context within with to conduct any therapeutic activities. For example, in a study by Bandura et al. (1967), children's participation in exposure was preceded by a party involving cookies, party hats, prizes, balloons, and stories. In another study by Kanfer et al. (1975), the experimenters visited students and played games with them for up to 2 hours over a 1-week period prior to starting exposure.

Given that rapport building is such an integral part of setting the stage for success, one might wonder why this protocol does not include a module for building rapport. The reason is that designing such a protocol would be nearly impossible—and comparatively weaker than what most skilled therapists could improvise. As any good therapist knows, no one game, activity, conversation, or exercise fits or appeals to all children. These are the skills that often come most naturally to those who have chosen human service positions, and it seems imprudent for me to prescribe a limited and potentially less imaginative set of steps.

Here the CBT therapist is encouraged to be creative and spontaneous in drawing on his or her best skills in connecting with a child. At the beginning of the protocol and throughout its course, the therapist should always monitor the degree of engagement and whether sessions are sufficiently fun and interesting to compel the child to challenge him- or herself. In our program, rapport-building activities include games, pictures, walks, conversations about hobbies, and trips to get ice cream—but the full list of possibilities is theoretically infinite.

That being said, it should be remembered that although rapport sets the stage for success, it is not the primary goal of therapy, nor is it the primary therapeutic activity. As with every technique that is part of this protocol, the goal is to *decrease anxiety through exposure*, and all exercises are ultimately aimed at making exposure happen correctly. It can be challenging for some therapists who are particularly skilled at connecting with and engaging children and families to keep in mind that the goal is to get to exposure as quickly and efficiently as possible. The art is in keeping the child motivated and excited while always moving ahead to the next step. In other words, engagement for engagement's sake is unlikely to help.

On that note, a potential risk is worth mentioning. If too much of the initial work with the client and family is simply engagement based, without a clear eventual goal of active participation in exposure, problems may arise. For example, if a child and family experience 8 weeks of supportive listening and rapport building, they will come to see those attributes as the character and function of the therapeutic relationship. When the therapist later decides to shift gears, resentment may result. For that reason, it is advisable to make the purpose of therapy clear from the very beginning and to connect activities back to that central theme of decreasing anxiety through exposure.

PSYCHOEDUCATION

One of the best ways to keep that goal in focus is through psychoeducation. In the "Learning about Anxiety" module, the therapist works on a variety of exercises designed, directly or indirectly, to increase engagement. This module outlines the purpose of the therapy, provides a rationale for exposure practice and self-monitoring, and clearly defines the collaborative and active nature of the therapeutic relationship from the outset.

Another important aim of psychoeducation is to normalize the problem. Quite often there is a great reduction in the overall anxiety level of the child and family simply by reassuring them that anxiety is a normal and natural emotion. A family might have been worrying that the experience meant that the child was "crazy" or likely to have a life-long disability. In our program, I have encountered parents who were concerned that developmentally inappropriate fears were a precursor to childhood schizophrenia, for example, which is highly unlikely (i.e., approximate odds: 1 in 40,000). Thus, simple and straightforward information about childhood anxiety disorders, their course, developmental influences, and risks can sometimes provide a welcome relief to a family.

It is also important to instill a sense of hope. Providing knowledge about the emotion of anxiety demystifies it, in essence making the emotion more manageable for children and families. Psychoeducation can give parents and children a language with which to talk about the different parts of the problem, thereby creating a common and observable entry point for a solution.

Another way to instill hope can be to talk about the strong base of research support for CBT. Early in therapy it is useful to mention that all anxiety disorders, from separation anxiety to obsessive–compulsive disorder to posttraumatic stress disorder, are treatable, and all have documented evidence of being helped by cognitive-behavioral procedures (Chorpita & Southam-Gerow, 2006). When having this discussion, however, one must be cautious not to instill a false sense of hope, which can ultimately lead to problems or mistrust. It is important to be clear that there are no guarantees about what will and will not work for a particular child and family, but one can state, in a genuine manner, that (1) CBT has tremendous scientific support for its efficacy, (2) CBT is the first-line choice for treating anxiety disorders, and (3) CBT, on average, leads to substantial improvements in children with anxiety.

Finally, it is important to mention to families that the biggest predictor of failure for CBT is failing to participate actively or dropping out altogether. Children and parents should be told that their odds of improvement are much higher if they can make the intervention a priority for the short term and really dedicate themselves to participating in all of the skills and exercises.

INOCULATION

In addition to offering information about anxiety and its treatment, it is also helpful to predict difficulty for a child and family. CBT for anxiety is challenging and even somewhat aversive at times. It is better to let the child and family know up front that you expect such a challenge, rather than let it be a surprise. The reason for this admonition draws from what we already know about anxiety and cognition. By the time you get started, the child with whom you are working obviously has problems with anxiety. In addition, there are above-average odds that the parents with whom you are working have elevated anxiety as well. Thus, as we know from Chapter 2, their collective interpretation of difficult periods and setbacks is more likely than average to be overly negative and catastrophic in nature (e.g., "This means I can't do it," "It's not going to work for my child"). The best way to prevent that extreme conclusion is to predict difficulty and normalize it. In other words, you interpret the difficulty for them before it happens, in a much more neutral manner.

Taking that strategy one step further, it is sometimes helpful to let families know that CBT would not work as well if it were easy. Recall from Chapter 5 the premise of emotional processing theory, which suggests that a high level of anxious arousal is important for the child to learn to see a feared stimulus in a new way. So, for example, with younger children I have sometimes found it helpful to tell parents that crying can be a sign that the technique is working and that it is being done correctly. In truth, it is far more challenging to work with a child who does not get anxious in a therapy session. If we cannot make the child anxious, we are not doing exposure properly. Having laid the groundwork of psychoeducation with a family, it can then be important to help them reinterpret what would naturally be signals of failure to them (e.g., crying and distress) as signs of success. So crying and distress mean we have "activated the fear structure," and (as long as we observe the proper patterns of habituations) everything is proceeding according to the plan.

In an interesting experimental analysis of parent involvement, Knox, Albano, and Barlow (1996) evaluated the effectiveness of CBT with and without parent involvement for pediatric obsessive–compulsive disorder. The research design called for some children to be treated without parent involvement, and others to be treated conjointly. Thus, in the first condition, exposures were conducted without the parents receiving any rationale or understanding of what the treatment was or how it worked. As cases were being evaluated and piloted for this study design, it was observed that this approach created tremendous stress for parents in the "not involved" condition. For example, in one case the therapist would go over to the home and perform a very anxiety-provoking exposure exercise with the child while the parents sat in another room. According to that protocol design, children also received imaginal exposure, which involved the therapist reading a frightening script, custom-written to involve the child's unique fears. The script was then tape-recorded and left with the child to listen to each night, alone, for homework. Needless to say, it did not take much for some parents in this situation to raise complaints or withdraw from the program, given that all they saw from their perspective was someone making their child cry each time they met, and then leaving a scary tape behind that made the child upset every night.

This research finding is intended to drive home the point that uninformed families will not know what to make of CBT. Particularly given the popular stereotype that talk therapy is uniformly warm and supportive, parents are likely to feel that they have made the wrong choice. Again, build on the strong foundation you have laid with the Learning about Anxiety module, and let them know that what you are about to do together will be difficult, but it will also be worth it.

A CLEAR SUCCESS

Experienced therapists in our training program are familiar with the "turning point" that usually comes in the first weeks of CBT for anxiety. This turning point most often occurs after the first or second exposure exercise, when there is a true success, sometimes accompanied by some surprise or disbelief. Up until that point, most everything has involved discussion and explanation, with little or no real demonstrations of the potential power of exposure. After the first successful exposure exercise, in which the child can see that his or her own fear ratings have decreased, there are often spontaneous and excited statements by the child (e.g., "I really did it," "Wow, I'm not scared of that anymore"). Although not universal, this turning-point phenomenon appears to be more likely when therapists select and design the earliest exposure practices with great care. Picking something that is sufficiently difficult to instill a sense of accomplishment but easy enough to ensure a high probability of success takes some careful thinking and judgment.

Particularly helpful in this regard are those exposure exercises that are related to higher degrees of functional impairment or family problems. For example, the first time a child rides the bus to school, goes to sleep without crying out for reassurance, or orders food at a fast food restaurant can be a real cause for celebration for the child and family. In other words, this is an opportunity to solve a tangible problem that has been plaguing the family, and success usually goes a long way toward building the trust and commitment that will carry a child and family through the rest of the protocol. And if the parents are not terribly expressive or enthusiastic, it is always possible to recruit someone else who is. For example, on one occasion, I asked a girl who was phobic of bugs to call her grandmother at the end of a session to say that she had just caught an insect with her hand. The grandmother could not have reacted more positively than if I had I written a script for her. Just remember, it helps tremendously to give a family an early success and to encourage self-praise, celebration, and excitement.

STAY SENSITIVE AND CONCERNED

Any good therapist already knows that sensitivity, warmth, and concern will go a long way toward making the protocol more successful. However, as outlined in the beginning of the chapter, one area that can be particularly challenging with the treatment of anxiety in children is to remain sensitive to the magnitude of the emotion, which can seem trivial to others. Exposure exercises can become quite boring for some therapists, and there is a natural tendency to become impatient. Thirty minutes is a long time to sit quietly while a child pets a dog, sits in a darkened room, or reads aloud from a book. At such moments, it is helpful to remember that rushing a child can ruin the exercise, and if this sometimes very slow pace and extraordinary patience felt natural, the parents probably would have solved this problem already. As always, the art is in finding a proper balance—the pace that keeps a child on a clear and observable trajectory for success without being overwhelming. Maintaining this balance, as with many aspects of CBT, is something that improves with experience.

Sometimes personal experience can be the best way to teach this kind of patience. As a graduate student, I once walked across a suspension bridge that spanned a very high gorge in Western New York State (Letchworth State Park). The bridge was meant for trains, with a narrow walkway for daring pedestrians, so it was essentially just railroad ties laid across a steel beam structure. This meant that there were the customary gaps between railroad ties, through which I could view an 8-inch slice of the Chasm of Death (not its real name), which became deeper with each step closer to the center of the bridge (600 feet at the lowest point of the canyon). Despite all my training in anxiety and false alarms, I just waited for my body to be sucked through the gaps to an inevitable and unimaginably violent ending below. My wife, who is not afraid of heights, stood behind me telling me to keep going, occasionally putting her hand on my back and nudging me a bit. My fear level went from extremely high to nuclear. If someone discovered a "Stage 3" alarm—something beyond panic—I felt sure I was in it. When I get impatient with exposure now, I remember that bridge.

CULTURAL CONSIDERATIONS

Because knowledge regarding cultural factors is believed to be an important part of successful treatment, this particular protocol was developed and tested successfully in a highly multicultural environment. Unfortunately, the research on cultural factors related to childhood anxiety is limited, with the available data mainly suggesting uniformity across groups. For example, some research suggests that the nature and amount of fears among European American and African American children are relatively similar (Ginsburg & Silverman, 1996; Treadwell, Flannery-Schroeder, & Kendall, 1995). On the other hand, some cross-cultural studies of fears have revealed that although fears related to survival (e.g., fear of animals, fear of separation) appear in children of all cultures at approximately the same time, others fears can vary from culture to culture. For example, Eastern cultures that stress conformity over independence have been shown to increase certain fears, such as those related to social evaluation (Ollendick, Yang, King, Dong, & Akande, 1996).

Regarding treatment engagement, an important difference across cultures appears to be the tendency for families of children from minority groups not to seek help from mental health professionals (Neal & Turner, 1991). Members of many cultures, particularly those that are collectively or family oriented, are more likely to involve clergy, a medical doctor, or a family member for help with anxiety (e.g., Hatch, Friedman, & Paradis, 1996). Such considerations are particularly important with CBT, given evidence that some children from minority groups are more likely to terminate this type of treatment prematurely (Kendall & Flannery-Schroeder, 1998). This observation highlights the issues raised above regarding establishing success early. The flexible, modular nature of this protocol should allow the therapist to get to apply expeditiously those strategies that will create a success experience. For example, if the child is disruptive, a time-out program might be offered early to help get conditions under control for the family. Or if social skills are a significant and noticeable problem, they can be addressed in early sessions. Asking a family that may already be engaged in a culturally unfamiliar process (i.e., therapy) to delay or rush working on particular issues could create a breaking point.

Thus, more generally, a major consideration of any therapist should be sensitivity to the cultural background of the child and family. Efforts should be made to engage family members and to build a partnership of trust, which can be facilitated by the therapist's display of openness and respect for a diversity of beliefs and values. Understand what clients' goals are and do not assume that they will be the same goals as yours (e.g., the reduction of anxiety). Without this foundation of understanding, the likelihood of treatment success may be limited.

SEVEN

Skillful Design of Exposure

It cannot be said often enough: Exposure sounds easy, but it is not. There are hundreds of different ways to implement exposure properly, and it is not possible to provide examples for all circumstances or contexts. Nevertheless, the goal of this chapter is to outline the scope of possibilities and to reiterate the notion that creative and skillful design of exposure is where most of the "game" is won or lost.

DIAGNOSTIC CONSIDERATIONS

As outlined in Chapter 2, anxiety disorders are conceptualized here as having a core underlying process amenable to treatment with exposure. However, the anxiety disorders themselves are rather heterogeneous, and the exposure exercises can require considerable individualization. Some examples of typical approaches for the different disorders are outlined here.

Separation Anxiety Disorder

Recall that separation anxiety disorder is characterized by age-inappropriate anxiety about being separated from a caregiver. One particularly interfering consequence of separation anxiety can be the refusal to attend school or stay in school once there. This problem can involve tantrums on the way to school, frequent phone calls home, trips to the nurse's office or the principal's office, or outright refusal to go to school at all. Some common items children with separation anxiety write on their fear ladders include:

- Going to school (for part or all of the day)
- Sleeping over at a relative's house
- Staying home with a babysitter
- Going to bed at night without someone in the room
- (for adolescents) Staying at home alone while Mom or Dad runs an errand in the neighborhood

Generalized Anxiety disorder

What can be challenging about generalized anxiety is that it is often difficult to identify the feared stimulus itself. For example, if a child worries about taking a test, it is unclear whether the true fear is of being scolded by parents, thought poorly of by teacher, or laughed at by peers. With exposure exercises for generalized anxiety, it is helpful to take the time to "extend out" the stated worries in order to identify the ultimate feared consequences. It is those consequences—not the anticipatory worries—that make the best material for exposure exercises.

In many instances, the exposure practices for generalized anxiety might have to be contrived in some way. For example, through careful collaboration with a teacher, it could be possible for the child to be given a series of tests that are impossible to pass, as part of an exposure to failing. In this instance, the tests would not count toward anything, but the child would experience that when getting many items wrong, the teacher does not frown and parents do not yell. Learning to feel that less is at stake will help the child perform more optimally on real tests taken later. Alternatively, if the child fears criticism from peers about failing a test, exposure to teasing might be help reduce the worries about tests.

In our program imaginal exposure is used more often with generalized anxiety than with some other anxiety disorders because some of the exposure items are too difficult to implement *in vivo*. For example, it is difficult to conduct real exposures for such things as worrying about becoming sick, a parent passing away, or an accident happening to someone. In such instances, one could either attempt to administer exposure to eliciting cues (e.g., if child worries about an accident happening to a family member who drives a car, that family member could go out for a drive where the traffic is particularly bad), or to administer imaginal exposure to the feared event (e.g., in this case, an imaginary scene in which the accident happens, the family goes to the hospital, the person is injured and may die).

Some sample items for exposure practices with generalized anxiety include:

- Having someone in the family get sick
- Saying the wrong thing
- Making a mistake on a project
- Not being on time for school
- Taking a test

Social Phobia

Typically, exposure exercises for social phobia progress from practices with the therapist (e.g., role play) to practices involving peers in naturalistic settings. One particular challenge with social phobia occurs when the child is too phobic to speak with the therapist. In such cases, the problem is treated like any other exposure item, and patient and steady encouragement are important facilitators of progress.

Another possible concern with social phobia can involve the increased opportunity for failure experiences. For example, because the child will eventually be asked to practice items involving peers, care should be taken—especially early on—to ensure that the peers selected for exercises are those likely to have a neutral or positive response to the child's attempts to start a conversation, ask questions, or otherwise interact with them. Because sending a child off to interview the school bully on the first exposure practice can be a recipe for disaster, it might help to talk with teachers or parents to "prescreen" some of the intended participants for exposure.

Some social anxiety can be related to legitimate problems with social skills deficits. The relation between poor social skills and anxiety can be reciprocal in nature, with poor social skills leading to situational awkwardness that increases anxiety, and anxiety, in turn, decreasing the child's social skills further. In any case, it is important to keep in mind that some children do not have the basic steps in their social repertoire, and these should be provided first before initiating an exposure. For example, before starting a conversation with someone at school, a child should know, at a minimum, (1) how to say hello, (2) how to ask questions, (3) how to take turns in a conversation, and (4) how to say goodbye. In addition, competent use of nonverbal skills (e.g., smiling, eye contact) can be important as well. These may need to be rehearsed with the therapist prior to exposure exercises. For problems with social skills, two modules are included in this protocol to target conversational and nonverbal deficits.

Some sample exposure items from children's fear ladders for social phobia include:

- Writing on the board at school
- Calling someone on the phone to ask about homework
- Asking a store clerk a question
- Talking in front of the class
- Starting a conversation with someone I don't know very well

Specific Phobia

Specific phobia is characterized by excessive and disabling fear of an object or situation and can be organized into a number of basic areas: animal (e.g., dogs), natural/environmental (e.g., swimming), situational (e.g., crowds), blood–injury–injection (e.g., getting a shot), and other (e.g., fear of choking on food). Treatment of blood–injury–injection phobia, when accompanied by fainting, requires an additional procedure not described in this protocol, called "applied tension," which involves practicing tensing of the extremities to maintain cerebral blood pressure and avoid fainting. Otherwise, exposure exercises for specific phobias are usually the most straightforward to implement. A fear ladder for specific phobia is usually based on many variations of experiencing a single feared situation or object, for example (from easiest to hardest):

- Looking at cartoon pictures of dogs
- Watching a TV program about dogs
- Seeing a dog at a pet store or pound
- Seeing a dog across the room
- Petting a dog
- Feeding a dog from my hand

Obsessive–Compulsive Disorder

The treatment of obsessive–compulsive disorder may require more frequent contact initially, with exposure sessions occurring as often as two or three times per week. Exposure practice also involves a strategy called "response prevention," which consists of explicit instructions from the therapist that the child does not perform any rituals during exposure. An important goal of treatment for obsessive–compulsive disorder is to teach the child that the passage of time has the same effect as performing the ritual: the anxiety will go away. Teaching children to wait until their anxiety subsides on its own thereby reduces their need to perform the compulsions. In addition, unlike the performance of rituals, the strategy of "waiting it out" means that the anxiety is less likely to return later. Imaginal exposure is sometimes used, particularly with obsessions that are not associated with compulsions.

Elements of a fear ladder for obsessive–compulsive disorder can be quite diverse, as in the following example:

- Eating something that someone else touched
- Touching my sister's bed
- Walking through a doorway just once
- Throwing out some papers
- Having someone move my shoes from their "proper" place

Panic Disorder

Panic disorder involves a cycle in which a sensation of anxiety (e.g., fast heartbeat) leads the child to feel like an attack might begin, which is followed by an escalation of anxiety, which intensifies the sensations, further escalating the anxiety, and so forth, until the emotion spirals out of control. To break this cycle, the treatment of panic disorder primarily involves exposure sessions aimed at reducing the fear of "triggering" sensations associated with anxiety. In that sense, the treatment of panic disorder can be conceptualized a bit like the treatment of a specific phobia of physical sensations.

In building the fear ladder for panic disorder, it is important to identify as many feared sensations as possible. Because children and adolescents do not always have clear insight into the sensations that cue or trigger panic attacks, it may help to have them perform some interoceptive exposure exercises, such as breath holding, running in place, or spinning, to get a sense of whether any of the resulting sensations are important triggers. If so, these exercises should be part of exposure practice throughout treatment. These exposure exercises are first performed under controlled conditions with the therapist. As treatment progresses, the exposure exercises are eventually practiced in the natural environment (e.g., school, at the mall, in the car), particularly when agoraphobia is involved. Sample items for panic disorder are as follows:

- Running in place for 2 minutes (*creates breathlessness, rapid heartbeat*)
- Holding the breath (*creates breathlessness, dizziness*)
- Using a tongue depressor (*creates a gagging sensation*)

- Breathing through a coffee stirrer or narrow straw (*creates breathlessness*)
- Spinning in place (*creates dizziness*)
- Dressing in overly hot clothing in a hot room (*creates feeling of stuffiness, suffocation*)

Posttraumatic Stress Disorder

Depending on the nature of the trauma, the treatment of posttraumatic stress disorder might need to proceed more slowly, because it may take the child some time to build sufficient trust to disclose enough information to build a fear ladder. Exposure practice can involve writing down, reading aloud, or drawing aspects of the traumatic event. Imaginal exposure can also be helpful to reduce anxiety about some aspects related to the traumatic event or events (e.g., riding in a car, being at home alone). An important "subgoal" can also involve helping the child arrive at healthy conclusions about the experience, such as "it was not my fault" or "it is not likely to happen to me again." Imaginal exposure is sometimes used as well. Exposure for posttraumatic stress disorder can include such items from fear ladders as:

- Thinking about visiting my father
- Being in my room by myself
- Going to bed alone
- Being with a babysitter
- Mom going on a date with someone
- Riding in a car on a busy highway
- Swimming in the ocean

School Refusal

School refusal, sometimes called "school phobia," is not a true diagnostic syndrome. Some experts have suggested that the term "school phobia" is problematic in that most anxious children who refuse or resist going to school do not have a specific phobia (e.g., Kearney, 2001). Rather, anxious children who refuse school often have other diagnoses, such as social phobia or separation anxiety disorder. The treatment of these disorders when school refusal is involved often requires the inclusion of situations related to school attendance on the fear ladder. In addition, a primary goal of treatment should be to get the child to be at the school, even if not with other children or in class. For example, some children may only be capable of coming to school and working in the library for an hour with a therapist. This arrangement is far preferable, however, to therapy at home or at a clinic. If tutoring is needed because the child is at risk of falling behind academically, it is best to have the tutor work with the child somewhere at school rather than at home. Gradually, the time spent in the classroom can be increased through exposure practices, and the tutor can be faded out as the need subsides. School refusal requires great patience and flexibility on the part of the school personnel, and their thorough understanding of the treatment plan can be critical to its success. In addition, rewards can be helpful in getting the child to the school initially, until the exposure practices make attendance a more comfortable experience. An important rule to establish with school-refusing children is that each time a certain degree of progress is made (e.g., attending two classes a day), the child should not be allowed to backtrack. Finally, it is important to keep vacations and holidays in mind, as these can interfere with progress. Even long weekends can present stumbling points for school-refusing children. Goals for full attendance should target times that are not likely to be interrupted by a large vacation or holiday, and if treatment is beginning late in the school year, it may be advisable to consider enrolling the child in summer school or delaying treatment until a few weeks prior to the onset of following school year.

MAKING SMALL STEPS ON THE FEAR LADDER

One particularly important skill with exposure involves knowledge of how to take a feared stimulus or item and break it down into smaller parts. Without incremental steps, some items are simply too challenging to perform and thus cannot otherwise be addressed. Breaking down a stimulus requires one to consider the many features of a situation that could possibly vary to make things more or less anxiety provoking.

For example, a child might explain that he or she has a fear of giving a talk in front of peers. Although it is fine to have that item on the fear ladder for eventual practice, it is unlikely to happen as an initial step and would probably be an unwise choice if it did. The best place to start is to consider features of the situation that can be varied. In this example that would include length of speech, preparation time (e.g., surprise topic or prepared topic), audience size, audience composition, audience reaction, location, availability of supports (e.g., note cards), and position of speaker. With all of these factors in mind, the therapist can get to know which ones matter to the child and which do not. Those that appear to make a difference in the expected fear level can then be altered. As a result, a highly anxious child might begin with a 1-minute talk, sitting, using note cards in front of his or her mother, who responds with encouraging smiles. From there, it is simply a matter of how large a step to take next, until the final situation can be performed.

Throughout the protocol, the therapist should work to get to know these various situational features associated with any of the feared stimuli, noting which ones are most and least challenging for the child. In that way, the therapist can most easily design the proper emotional "entry point" that is neither too high nor too low.

BEING CREATIVE

Often what separates an average exposure exercise from a good one is the creativity and thoughtfulness that goes into its design. The same approach used in breaking down exercises into steps can be used to find the most efficient and therapeutic ways to conduct exposure. By manipulating some of the many features of feared events, objects, or situations, some truly effective exercises can be developed for what might otherwise be challenging items. Again, the goal is to create anxiety at a level that is high enough to afford progress without being overwhelming, all the while ensuring that within- and between-trial habituation occur. Within those parameters, there is a lot of room for creativity. Some examples follow.

Kristi

Recall that 14-year-old Kristi was afraid of both separation from her mother and social evaluation, particularly eating in front of others. While she was working on gradually increasing her time at school, one particularly helpful exposure exercise unrelated to school involved having her go to a food court at the mall with her mother, who would leave her for 30 minutes to order food, sit by herself in a central location, and eat the food she had ordered. Occurring about 6 weeks into treatment, this exercise was particularly useful because it involved simultaneous exposure to at least three of her fears: separation from mother, eating in front of others (eating alone was especially anxiety provoking), and talking to an adult to order the food. She was free to pick whatever food she wanted, which helped to motivate her to try this exercise. After three exposures in 1 week, she no longer found the exercise challenging—an accomplishment that offered much to talk about with respect to countering her apprehension about school.

Doug

Ten-year-old Doug frequently experienced panic attacks while riding in his parents' car. One of the exposure exercises used with Doug involved having him hyperventilate while riding in the car, which caused him to feel tingly and uncomfortable in a way that he associated with the onset of his panic attacks. While one parent drove, the other took fear ratings on a practice record. The driver was instructed to choose many one-way streets, which made Doug feel trapped, and to behave as if the family had gotten lost and did not know where to drive next. Doug was able to learn that even when he felt anxious and uncomfortable, the car never got trapped on a one-way street, and his parents were always able to find their way home. These exercises became easy for him after two weekends of practice.

Mary

Seven-year-old Mary was intensely afraid of the dark, and although her exposure exercises were relatively straightforward, some interesting possibilities emerged. Mary progressed from sitting in a dim room in a clinic setting, to a darkened room, to a darkened room with the door closed, ultimately working on going to sleep without a night light at home. During the course of treatment, it became clear that Mary was especially afraid that something scary was going to come out of her closet and "get" her. Final exposures at home thus involved her lying in her darkened bedroom at night, with the closet door partially open, just enough so that she could not see clearly what was in there. She then had to go and open the closet without turning on the lights, feel around to see that it was only her clothes and some toys, and then return to her bed. She was able to do this with a therapist and parent in the room at first, then quickly progressed to independent performance, with a parent issuing prompts from the hallway. This kind of "overexposure" can be really helpful in ensuring that the child's anxiety will be less likely to return.

Therapist Point of View: Diane

"A therapist's job is to be creative in applying the principles of the protocol to mold each module to make it fit for the client. One example that jumps to my mind when I had to be creative was when I was working with my client with severe social anxiety and selective mutism. This case involved an especially challenging preadolescent who had never spoken in school. My task was to adapt the exposure procedures to fit her level of readiness. At the beginning, Diane was unable to speak a word, let alone whisper. I had to be creative and devise a way for her to practice speaking without actually speaking.

"This plan was accomplished by breaking down speaking into small and manageable steps. We began by just opening and closing our mouths, sticking out our tongues, or smiling and frowning. Eventually, we worked our way up to mouthing letters. The breaking point came when I finally got her to whisper "n," then "o." We began pairing the two so quickly together that she said her first word, "No." After that, Diane was able to work her way up to speaking words and phrases, and then having conversations. Although this was a long road, Diane achieved goals that had been out of reach for years. It became clear to me that my job was to take the principles in the protocol and be creative to make them work for my client."

—KII KIMHAN, therapist,
University of Hawaii Center for Cognitive Behavior Therapy

Therapist Point of View: Donna

"A child I worked with had extreme social anxiety and could not call people by their names. Donna and I started out exposures by playing a card game—a version of Go Fish that I created for her with names of family members and famous people written on the cards. Every time one of us got a matching pair, we had to say the names that were written on the cards. Eventually, this game prompted her to start saying names in a way that got more comfortable over time.

"Donna and I also practiced having conversations together in sessions and eventually worked up to going outside to a nearby courtyard and "yelling" our conversation while standing over 30 feet away from each other. Donna also feared having people laugh at her, so we practiced conversations while she did something silly, such as stand on the table in the conference room with a stuffed animal on her head. She quickly got over feeling anxious about it and realized that ordinary conversation was easy compared with some of the things we had practiced."

—KIMBERLY BECKER, therapist,
University of Hawaii Center for Cognitive Behavior Therapy

Therapist Point of View: Kevin

"I was working with Kevin, a 15-year-old male with obsessive–compulsive disorder, separation anxiety, and two specific phobias. The obsessive–compulsive disorder involved hoarding food, clothing, and garbage items in bags to ward off anxiety about being separated from his home and mother. By the time he entered treatment Kevin was carrying around a large duffle bag, a backpack, and various other bags (e.g., plastic shopping bags and travel bags) full of garbage, clothes, and rotting food. The main problem with Kevin was that he was unwilling to do any exposure (e.g., throwing away items from his bags) outside of session.

"To address this area, I told him that I did not have any magic tricks. I told him that the majority of his gains would be made *outside* of the therapy room, outside of seeing me. He seemed quite puzzled but eventually grasped my point after I broke it down into percentages for him: We drew it on paper, and I showed him that I see him only 2 hours per week, which is at most 1% of his week, 1% of his life. On the other hand, unlike me, he is with himself 24 hours per day; 100% of the time. I always told him that I would do my best to guide him, but that he would need to work hard and make practice a part of his lifestyle. I would not be there when he gets dressed to go to school in the morning; I would not be there when he cleaned out his bag, etc. He needed to be strong on his own.

"Kevin was a talented and avid skateboarder. At one point, I told him that I did not want to talk about exposure for a little while and only wanted to talk about skateboarding. I had him generate a list of five skateboarding tricks (from hardest to easiest) on a folded piece of paper. As he explained to me all about skateboarding, he included the fact that if he did not practice constantly, he could not maintain his ability to do the hardest trick. I then unfolded the paper and drew to the right of the skateboard list five new items, from hardest to easiest: '0 bags, 1 bag, 2 bags, 3 bags, 4 bags.' That's when he really got it—and he began to practice on his own."

—Brad Nakamura, therapist,
University of Hawaii Center for Cognitive Behavior Therapy

Other Examples

A partial listing of additional examples is provided in Table 7.1 to illustrate further the range of options. As mentioned, there is no limit to the possibilities for success, as long as the basic principles of exposure are kept in mind: The exercises should provoke anxiety and should allow for within- and between-trial habituation. In all of the examples in Table 7.1, the participants were able to perform the exposures without difficulty by the third or fourth day of practice—many sooner.

SUMMARY

As outlined throughout Part II, the main principle to keep in mind is that exposure is the central component of the intervention. The therapist should work to obtain both within-

TABLE 7.1. **Example Exposure Practice Items for Selected Children's Fears**

Clinical scenario	Sample exposure used
"Worry that my appendix will burst"	The final exercise used an imaginal exposure script, involving an upset stomach that progresses to sharp pains, parents calling the ambulance, a confusing ambulance ride, and blacking out in the emergency room.
"Fear that looking at things related to cancer will cause me to develop cancer"	A final exercise involved making cookies, writing the word "cancer" on them with icing, and eating them.
"Fear of catching germs from doorknobs or other objects in public"	One exercise involved the therapist's disinfecting a doorknob prior to the session, then, without providing any information to the child, asking her to place her hand on the doorknob and then to lick her hand. The therapist does not answer questions about who touched the doorknob or whether it is clean.
"Fear of vomiting in car on the way to school"	One final exercise involved using a tongue depressor to create a gagging sensation, while riding in the back seat.
"Fear of thunder and lightning"	Exercises included watching videos about lightning storms and listening to a tape of thunder through headphones while in bed at night.
"Fear that eating food might lead me to choke"	Exercise included eating a variety of foods whose textures were challenging; the final exercise involved swallowing very small candies without chewing (about the size of vitamins).
"Fear of separation"	One exercise included the mother going out somewhere without saying where she would be or when she would return.
"Fear of talking to adults or looking foolish"	Exercises included buying a shirt at a store and returning it after 2 minutes to the same salesperson, and asking a store clerk standing next to a large clock what time it is.
"Fear of swimming"	The final exercise included swimming across a pool with eyes closed.

and between-trial habituation, taking the steps necessary to keep the child engaged in the exercises. Creativity is a must and should begin with a review of all possible features of the feared objects or contexts that can vary (e.g., size, proximity, audience). The therapist, child, and family should then work together to cover as much ground as possible while maintaining interest and enthusiasm and documenting and reviewing progress along the way. If these core principles are upheld, the chances of success will be maximized.

PART III

WHEN THE GOING GETS TOUGH

EIGHT

Basic Concepts of Modular Treatment

Sometimes things do not go as planned. Despite a committed approach to the basic treatment strategies, there is no progress. This lack of progress probably means that following the core plan is no longer a viable option; this is where things can get more complicated. When we begin to entertain the idea of flexibility in treatment, a whole host of possibilities come into play, some of which may be good, and some not. It is a tricky business to establish a set of guidelines for how to adapt or individualize a protocol without opening up options that are difficult to evaluate against one another. This chapter is intended to introduce the basic concept of modularity and its role in flexible treatment planning. This chapter is then followed by a more detailed chapter on the "nuts and bolts" of how to implement a treatment flexibly. For an overview, it is best to start with some examples of how this issue of strategic treatment flexibility has been addressed in other contexts.

STRATEGIES FOR INDIVIDUALIZING

Some contrasting approaches, developed with principles of adaptation and flexibility in mind, have emerged over the past decade or more. The majority of these fall under the heading of "prescriptive" approaches. One good example from the adult depression literature is the work of Beutler and colleagues on "prescriptive psychotherapy" (e.g., Beutler & Harwood, 2000; cf. Norcross, 2002). This approach is designed to work across theoretical orientations and to allow the therapist to match particular strategies or styles to client characteristics. Beutler and Harwood (2000) outlined an overarching set of guiding principles and identified different approaches in how to apply to these principles to different types of individuals.

Similarly, Persons and colleagues (Persons & Tompkins, 1997; Persons 1989) outlined a method for systematically developing an intervention based on a cognitive-behavioral case formulation. Building on strategies from the behavioral assessment literature, this approach requires the therapist to develop a working model of the client's problem and its modifiable internal and external influences. These factors are then addressed systematically in an effort to address the target problem.

Other structured approaches using a strategy of matching specific interventions to client characteristics draw from the work of Durand (1990) in targeting severe behavioral problems in children with autism. The essence of this approach is to determine, through a structured assessment, the function of the challenging behavior, which allows a therapist to train an appropriate functional substitute in the context of autism, using assistive technology for communication. Such work has been extended to a prescriptive model for treating anxious school refusal in children (Burke & Silverman, 1987; Kearney & Silverman, 1990), which prescribes specific cognitive or behavioral interventions that are based on a functional profile of the school-refusing behavior. Eisen and Silverman (1998) extended this work still further, showing that a particular cognitive or behavioral strategy (e.g., relaxation or cognitive restructuring) was successful when matched to different profiles of children with generalized anxiety disorder.

The collective ideas behind many of these approaches appear to make sense and reflect a long tradition of individualizing interventions to fit client problems. Although some of the literature is positive regarding these strategies, there is not uniform support for the idea that flexibility of this nature enhances treatment effects, and debates have continued on both sides of the flexibility controversy (e.g., Jacobson et al., 1989; Persons, 1991; Schulte, Kuenzel, Pepping, & Schulte-Bahrenberg, 1992; Wilson, 1996; Wolpe, 1989). It is this controversy, by the way, that leads us back to the emphasis on the core treatment plan—in other words, we should always try the most well-tested strategies first, as outlined in earlier chapters.

HOW THE MODULES REALLY JUST SUPPORT THE CORE TREATMENT PLAN

In fact, the flexibility in the protocol is less for individualization per se than it is for actually supporting the core strategies. In other words, therapists using this protocol are encouraged to be flexible *for the explicit purpose of getting back to the core strategies*. Along those lines, Schoenwald and Henggeler (2003) have argued that the time or effort to maintain the integrity of core strategies is related to positive outcomes, whether an intervention is flexible or not. Thus, with the current protocol, flexibility in implementation is thought of as the road *back* to exposure, taken only when threats to the core treatment plan arise.

Figure 8.1 builds on the core plan introduced earlier by demonstrating how sources of interference might arise that could challenge the therapist's ability to administer exposure successfully. If we imagine that the core four procedures must be delivered, some set of procedures must therefore become available for dealing with these "interference" circumstances. Calling on a new set of therapeutic strategies conditionally is part of the answer. For example, one might say that when exposure does not work, try some behavior management techniques or social skills training. The new challenge is how to introduce this flexibility while ensuring that the therapeutic procedures themselves are all being performed with proper integrity—remember the *fundamentals*. In other words,

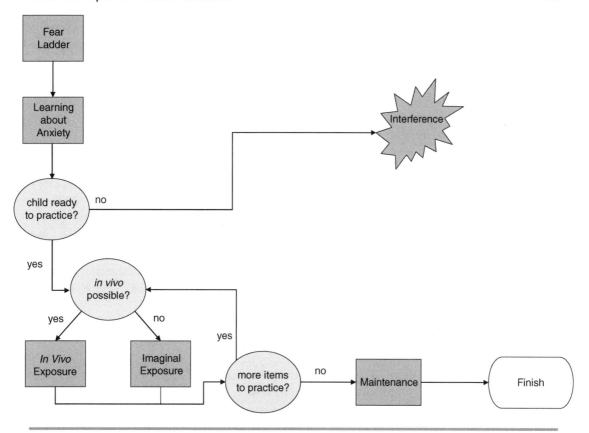

FIGURE 8.1. Flowchart for a modular CBT protocol.

we need to make sure that when the protocol is not working as planned, we do not suddenly turn to "clinical improvisation." Supports must be at hand for both reformulation of the case and descriptions of any new procedures to be implemented.

MODULARITY

As noted earlier, this delicate balance of structure and flexibility is achieved in this protocol through the use of modules—that is, self-contained descriptions of the specific therapeutic techniques to be used. The concept of modular treatment is not entirely new (e.g., Jacobson et al., 1989; Lazarus, 1974; Liberman, Mueser, & Glynn, 1988), and modular applications exist for a variety of psychological conditions (e.g., Annon, 1975; Falloon, 1988). Recently, however, the principles of modular psychotherapy design have been formalized to propose a set of core properties and to outline its potential advantages (Chorpita, Daleiden, & Weisz, 2005b). Central among these advantages, in terms of application, is this notion of structured flexibility. Because they can be selected and arranged in a variety of sequences, modules afford much more potential flexibility than a narrative set of protocol instructions; they can be delivered as needed, based on the characteristics of the child, family, and context. On the other hand, in contrast to many highly flexible treatment approaches, the use of modules assures that the therapy content for each procedure is highly specified, so that explicit procedures, when chosen, can be implemented with a high degree of integrity. This emphasis on *fundamentals* draws from the evidence that structured application of specific approaches is associated with greater treatment effects (Weisz, Donenberg, Han, & Kauneckis, 1995; Weisz, Donenberg, Han, & Weiss, 1995).

In this protocol, then, modules are arranged according to an overall guiding flowchart, which represents not only the core treatment plan but also the conditional use of other procedures, as needed. As noted, the design of this protocol was born out of a response to the challenges encountered when applying more structured CBT approaches in a public mental health context. As we began bending the rules of the protocols in our training program, the new set of decision rules was mapped over time, and the clinical procedures were codified in self-contained modular "handouts." In 1998 these handouts were integrated into a formal set of treatment modules, the first successful test of which was eventually documented 6 years later (Chorpita, Taylor, Francis, Moffitt, & Austin, 2004).

How Is Modularity Different?

The unique design features of a modular protocol are perhaps best illustrated in contrast to a more structured manualized approach, in which a set number of treatment procedures are typically delivered in a fixed sequence. The treatment plan for such an approach would look something like Figure 8.2. According to this design, a child would participate in a full set of therapeutic strategies in a given order.

In a sense, the treatment plan for such a static approach is based on the notion that many of these techniques have some evidence of being helpful for anxiety, and that interference is likely to be handled by delivering all of the techniques available in order. For example, challenges to successful exposure arising from poor social skills would be handled "in advance" by administering every child social skills training in the fourth session. Advantages of such an approach are its simplicity and the lack of generalization required when moving from research tests to clinical practice (i.e., the form of the protocol is completely preserved). Disadvantages, however, involve possible inefficiency and a lack of flexibility when critical interference arises.

Modular Treatment Planning

The treatment planning flowchart offered by this protocol is outlined in Figure 8.3 (and is reproduced in Chapter 9 and Part IV for convenient reference). Note that the formulation in the lower left is preserved as the core set of strategies (*in vivo* and imaginal exposure). When such strategies encounter obstacles or interference, however, a new set of strategies becomes available. Each strategy is contained in a module, whose conditions of use are well specified. For example, a therapist working with a child who shows poor motivation to participate in exposure should consider the rewards module, which

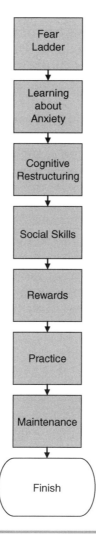

FIGURE 8.2. Flowchart for a standard manualized CBT protocol.

details how to set up a reward program to encourage new behaviors (in this case, most likely participation in exposure practices).

This idea can be illustrated best with Doug's case example. Recall that although Doug's principal concerns involved panic and agoraphobia, he also had a history of depression. Not surprisingly, Doug frequently showed very low motivation to go to school—perhaps some of which was due to fear of panic attacks, and some of which was due to the anhedonia commonly associated with depression. In addition, rather than tell his parents that he was afraid of school, Doug would typically complain of stomachaches, dizziness, or feeling out of breath. The typically resulting pattern was that his mother would end up driving him to school while engaging in a drawn-out discussion about how sick he felt, which then led his mother to encourage him to go to the school nurse or to give him permission to come home early. To her credit, Doug's mother used her best negotiating skills, daily, to get him to endure the car ride to school and to step out of the car when they arrived in the morning.

Doug's full case history through the 12th week of therapy is graphed on the clinical dashboard shown in Figure 8.4. Note that the first few sessions involved the core sequence prescribed in Figure 8.3: building a fear ladder, followed by education about anxiety for the mother and child ("Learning re Anxiety–C," "Learning re Anxiety–P," here combined in a single session), followed in turn by exposure ("Practicing," at about day 15). Both mother and child had difficulty with the first exposure, which for Doug involved going for a car ride with his parents. His mother and father could not get him to cooperate in these planned exercises without first enduring a great deal of complaining and resistance.

The guiding flowchart in Figure 8.3 suggested two possibilities. First, it seemed that Doug's overall low motivation—not uncommon with depression—might be addressed through the use of rewards. Second, Doug's frequent complaining and arguing might benefit from his parents' getting training in a strategy of ignoring, which is intended to extinguish mild, unwanted behaviors, such as whining, in children. Given Doug's previ-

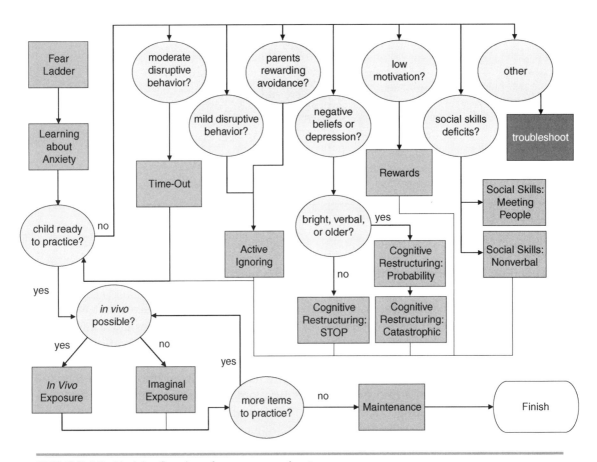

FIGURE 8.3. Modular flowchart for treatment planning.

MCBT Individual Case Supervision Form   **Client: Doug**

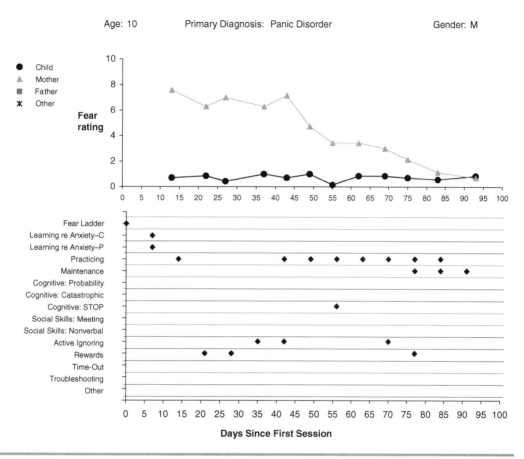

Age: 10   Primary Diagnosis: Panic Disorder   Gender: M

FIGURE 8.4. A clinical "dashboard" for Doug.

ous history with depression, and given that ignoring procedures can frequently be frustrating for parents and children at first, it was decided that starting a rewards program for Doug would make the most sense. Thus a program was established that allowed Doug to earn points that he could exchange for such things as time with his hand-held video game, a later bedtime (15 minutes), or renting a favorite movie on the weekend. As shown in Figure 8.4, this rewards program was developed over the course of two sessions and allowed Doug initially to be rewarded for simply repeating the exposure exercise first outlined in the third session (car rides).

Once the rewards program was in place and working adequately, the next two sessions were spent training his parents in how to handle the complaining and arguing that accompanied exposure practices during the week. These procedures were covered with the mother for one session and then with both parents and Doug in a second session. That second session also introduced some new exposure exercises for Doug to try (as indicated in Figure 8.4). Toward the middle of therapy, Doug experienced some difficulties when a new and particularly challenging kind of exposure greatly increased his resistance to participate further. At that time, Doug was given a single session involving cognitive procedures, which helped him reframe the exposure exercises and give them a try.

Thus three additional modules were selected and implemented to deal with specific circumstances that were interfering with successful exposure experiences. These were introduced over the course of about 3 weeks, at which point the focus returned as quickly as possible to the core strategies. In this case, the choices were successful: Doug was able to engage in exposure with far less difficulty after about 6 weeks, and then his progress was relatively straightforward.

Data in the progress pane support the success of the treatment plan as well. Doug's fear ratings, as reported by his mother, only began to make substantive progress when exposure was going well by week 6. Interestingly, because Doug chose to characterize his panic attacks as transient feelings of sickness, his fear ratings were never elevated. Fortunately, in this case, his mother's ratings were available to us as an index of progress. The main ideas illustrated here are (1) how the formulation of the case can be revised to handle therapeutic barriers, and (2) how these barriers can be overcome using the supplemental modules designed to address them. More detail is provided in the next chapter on when and how these supplemental techniques are chosen.

Beyond Flexible Treatment Planning

The current protocol is meant to allow flexibility not only with respect to treatment planning but also to a variety of other treatment characteristics. Again, these are best illustrated in contrast to the idea of a traditional manualized treatment approach. Some examples of these points of difference are summarized in Table 8.1.

SUMMARY

So far, the case has been made that anxiety disorders share common features, characterized by negative affect, misinterpretation of threat (i.e., "false alarms"), and related behavioral avoidance. This protocol aims to target these core features, regardless of the specific anxiety disorder in question or the presence of comorbidity. The approach outlined here is designed to capitalize on the strong empirical basis supporting a core treatment plan in which exposure is used as the core element of the treatment. Further, because the treatment strategies are packaged in self-contained modules, an individualized delivery of techniques is possible, allowing for new options to address specific therapeutic challenges. Knowing what those options are, it now makes sense to think through the details of which option to choose at what moment.

TABLE 8.1. Major Points of Difference between Modular and Standard Manualized Treatments

Standard manualized protocol	Modular protocol
Frequency of sessions may be fixed at once or twice per week.	Frequency of sessions is child centered.
Parent involvement can be absent, limited to specific sessions, or mandatory in all sessions, as determined by the manual chosen, not by the family's needs or the child's problem.	Parent involvement is fully variable; it can be intensive, if needed, or even omitted when parents are unavailable or not significantly involved in the formulation of the problem.
Duration of sessions is typically 45–50 minutes.	Duration of sessions is determined by attention span of child and the complexity of the exercise to be practiced; for example, a session can involve 15 minutes of review or 4 hours of guided *in vivo* exposure.
Pace may be fixed by protocol (typically one skill covered in one session).	Pace is determined by child; a child covers a new skill until it is adequately acquired or until there is compelling evidence that mastery is unlikely.
Setting is typically in a clinic office, although presumably could be elsewhere.	Setting can be anywhere (e.g., clinic, school playground, home); therapists are encouraged to choose the setting that best fits the exercise to be covered and that is consistent with family engagement strategies.
Children receive every component of manual.	Children receive only those techniques that fit their needs, nothing more; this allows a complete focus of attention on only those skills and strategies determined to be necessary.
To address disruptive behavior in children with anxiety, typically another manual is required, or "non-manualized" sessions are introduced, as designed ad hoc by the therapist.	Children can be selectively administered manualized strategies for disruptive behavior.
Intervention ends after a fixed length of time determined by manual content.	Intervention ends when goals are achieved or determined, jointly by child and therapist, to be unreachable using this approach.

NINE

What Are the Other Modules For?

The emphasis up to this point has been on coordinating the therapeutic activities to support repeated exposure to reduce fear and anxiety. Under ideal conditions, a child might need only the core four procedures of psychoeducation, self-monitoring, exposure, and maintenance. However, as noted earlier, in many circumstances challenges or issues will arise that disrupt one's ability to move smoothly through the four core modules. Although the concept of selectively applying supplemental modules may be clear, little has been said so far about how and when to select these other strategies. This chapter therefore outlines the specific steps for determining when therapeutic interference arises, and how to select the best module to address that interference.

PATTERNS OF USE

A small pilot study involving observations on patterns of manual use was drawn from children and adolescents completing an open trial during the early development phase of this manual. The inclusion criterion was a principal diagnosis of an anxiety disorder, as determined by a structured clinical interview. Children referred to the University of Hawaii Center for Cognitive Behavior Therapy are drawn from the existing state pool of children requiring mental health services through their public schools and thus represent challenging clinical cases that are typical of many community clinical settings.

Out of 26 children attending a full course of treatment for anxiety, the percentages of cases involving the use of particular modules were as follows: Fear Ladder (100%), Learning about Anxiety (100%), Exposure (imaginal or *in vivo*, 100%), Maintenance (100%), Troubleshooting (77%), Rewards (54%), Active Ignoring (46%), STOP (15%), Cognitive Restructuring (probability and catastrophic, 15%), Social Skills (meeting people or nonverbal communication, 15%), Time-Out (8%). These data are consistent with the design feature of this protocol, in that all children participated in the "core four" modules (Fear Ladder, Learning about Anxiety, Exposure, and Maintenance), and many were selectively administered some of the other procedures. This pattern reflects the notion that the intervention is primarily exposure based, with other techniques coming into play as needed. The data also showed considerable variability in which modules were administered to different children, with the majority receiving no formal cognitive procedures. More than half of the children required a reward program, almost half of the children's parents required formal training in differential reinforcement, and two cases required a formal time-out program. Two cases (15%) were successful using only the core treatment plan, in which the core four procedures were followed. Although the sample size is too small to provide reliable estimates of the relative probability of administering any one module, the data suggest that some kind of threat (i.e., interference) to the core plan could be the rule, not the exception. Thus it is important to understand how this interference is identified and handled.

TYPES OF THERAPEUTIC INTERFERENCE

Figure 9.1 shows the full flowchart, which includes various modules for addressing those situations in which exposure might not be the ideal choice. Note that the primary question is whether or not the child is ready to practice. Therapists using this approach

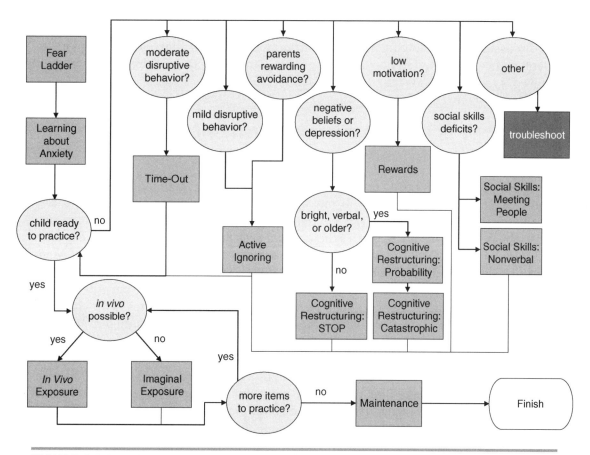

FIGURE 9.1. Modular flowchart for treatment planning.

are cautioned not to jump past this question to evaluating the criteria contained in the circles at the top of the figure (e.g., "mild disruptive behavior"). In other words, although many children might show mild disruptive behavior, or might have negative beliefs, it is only when those issues *interfere* with the successful application of exposure that they need to be addressed in this context.

The therapist should also keep in mind that one of the best ways to deal with a child who appears not to be ready to participate in exposure is to redesign the exposure (see Part II), rather than to shift to adjunctive techniques immediately. For example, a child who is less motivated to perform exposure might become more motivated if the exposure were merely simplified or modeled by the therapist. Such a solution would likely be more efficient in that it would require less time away from those activities likely to be of greatest benefit in reducing anxiety.

In making the determination that a child is not "ready to practice," a therapist should nearly always have attempted to design an exposure exercise and usually will have attempted to implement it. When clear evidence of interference is observed, then a choice can be made of how to address that interference. In our applications of this protocol, these sources of interference most commonly manifest, and are addressed, after several sessions of exposure have been performed, rather than in the early sessions of therapy. There it is preferable to wait for clear evidence to support the notion that exposure is either made impossible or severely undermined by complicating factors. Those factors are discussed in the following material, starting with modules that address the most frequent sources of interference and progressing to those that address less frequent sources.

SUPPLEMENTAL STRATEGIES

Rewards

The Rewards module is used under two conditions, which together are relatively common. The first condition, which in our applications is the more routine of the two, involves a child's very reluctant or halfhearted participation in exposure. As we now know, the best circumstances occur when a child sees the results produced by exposure and participates eagerly in anticipation of observing more progress or success. Many times, however, a child might feel pushed into each and every one of the exposures and is barely motivated to continue. This can be particularly true when the benefits of exposure are less obvious at first or do not generalize to situations important to the child. For example, when Mary was first told that she would need to practice sitting in the dark, she tried to participate, but it was clear that she was only yielding to pressure from adults. She showed little true interest in the practice sessions and did not seem to think that the goal—sleeping in the dark—was worth much effort. To address her low motivation, her therapist arranged for her to have extra time before bed to play with her pet mouse, and when she reached her goal, she could pick out a new toy for her mouse's cage. These strategies were introduced at about the third week of therapy, over the course of two sessions (see Figure 9.2). This use of the Rewards module was sufficient to get her to practice with greater effort and quickly led to important therapeutic gains.

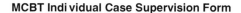

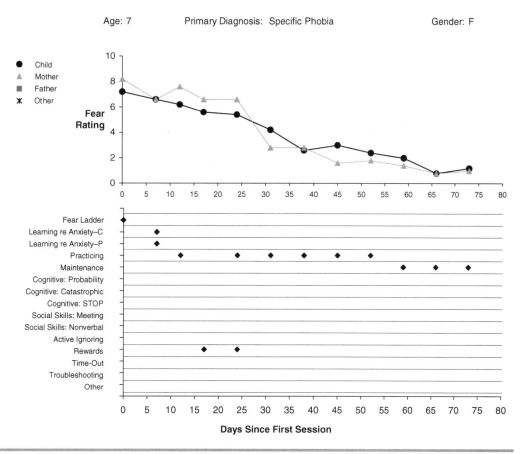

FIGURE 9.2. Clinical dashboard for Mary.

Motivation can also be a problem when exposure is intrinsically paired with other consequences that might be unrewarding. For example, exposure exercises for anxious children who are refusing to attend school at some point involve time in the classroom. Although it might be rewarding to the child to see his or her anxiety reduce over time, the short-term, immediate rewards of being in the classroom might be comparatively small or not obvious. In such instances, introducing a reward program that serves to increase motivation and approach can be quite helpful. To reinforce the successful sustainability of the rewards program, care should be taken over time to develop the child's awareness of natural reinforcers as well. For example, seeing friends at school or participating in favorite classes or activities should eventually contribute to the child's motivation to continue attending.

The second condition under which low motivation arises is actually just an extreme of the first condition: that is, a complete refusal to participate in exposure. When it occurs, this pattern is often evident at the beginning of therapy but could also emerge later, as the child becomes frustrated or exhausted during the course of the protocol. This circumstance is not difficult to notice because the child usually makes it clear that he or she is unwilling to practice something. In the previous example, had Mary completely refused to participate in practice exercises, her therapist would have had to introduce a set of rewards. It might be tempting to think that children who outright refuse to practice might need larger rewards than children who practice halfheartedly; however, one should always start with small and frequent rewards in determining the ideal schedule and rules for a rewards program (as outlined in the Rewards module in Part IV). More information about how to fine-tune a rewards program is discussed in Chapter 10.

Cognitive Procedures

As outlined in Chapter 2, the patterns of thinking that are characteristic of anxiety often involve misperceptions about threat that are overly negative in nature. When such patterns are extreme, they can interfere with successful exposure in multiple ways. For instance, children who feel overly hopeless and pessimistic (as is common with comorbid depression) will often predict that "practice will not work," so they might not see the value in it. The child's negative self-talk becomes an obstacle to participation in exposure and a barrier to corrective learning about feared objects or situations. Remember that at the end of the Learning about Anxiety module, the child should feel prepared and understand the reasons for practice. If the level of doubt and threat perception is too high, then cognitive procedures should be considered.

With Doug, negative thoughts were a source of interference early in the treatment. He felt that there was little room for improvement, and that the symptoms he was experiencing would be with him for the rest of his life. Given such beliefs, it did not seem worth it to "make himself feel even worse" by placing himself in feared situations. Using the STOP module, Doug learned how his thoughts could be inaccurate at times and that he might be able to come up with different ways of thinking about something. Most importantly, Doug learned that when he is unsure of the validity of his beliefs, the best way to find out is to test them out and see what happens. Doug was able to make an agreement with his therapist to try some exposure to see if it would improve his bad feelings. Using the STOP procedures, he identified thoughts about the exposure exercises (e.g., "Nothing will help me"), came up with alternative thoughts (e.g., "I've never tried this before, so maybe it could work"), and engaged in the appropriate behaviors to discover which thoughts were true.

One of Doug's exposure practices toward the middle of therapy was interoceptive in nature—that is, involving exposure to his own sensations. He was asked to breathe in and out repeatedly in order to recreate the feeling of dizziness that came when he experienced panic attacks. After repeated practice in a session, his anxiety ratings came down, and he was then asked by his therapist which of his thoughts or predictions was truer. He could easily see that his alternative thought ("maybe it could work") had more support, and he learned the even greater lesson that he needn't trust his first thought about something that is anxiety provoking—there might be a different way to see things.

One other way in which negative thoughts can interfere with exposure involves disqualifying or discounting the benefits and success. Our 14-year-old separation-anxious Kristi, who had comorbid social anxiety, was often "beating up on herself" cognitively following her exposure exercises. For example, although she performed quite well at exposures related to going to school, she was concerned that she "felt too anxious" or "didn't do a good enough job" at them. These thoughts appeared to stem from her social anxiety and were limiting the rate at which she could consolidate gains from her successful practicing. Until her therapist was able to address her manner of evaluating her own performance, Kristi was only willing to take small steps forward on her practices. Following one session of the STOP module, she was able to adapt her thinking and catch herself before being too critical of her gains. Realizing this pattern, Kristi soon began to move forward more quickly, rehearsing such thoughts as "It doesn't matter how well I do, it just matters that I practice things on my list." Kristi's clinical dashboard appears in Figure 9.3.

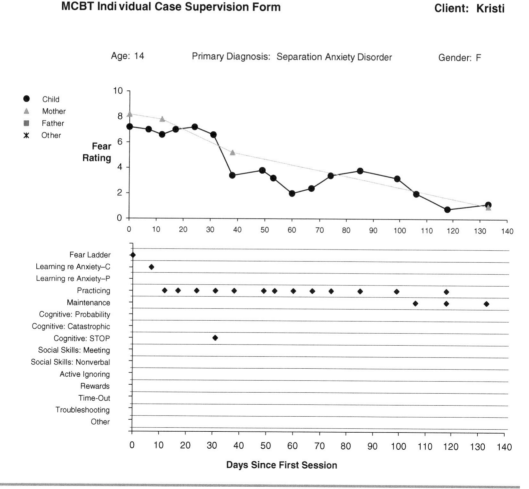

FIGURE 9.3. Clinical dashboard for Kristi.

Active Ignoring

Sometimes anxiety is accompanied by behaviors that are rather effective in eliciting reassurance, assistance, or even opportunities for escape from a demanding situation. With anxious children, these behaviors take the form of whining, crying, or repetitive questioning. Just as a good therapist would not terminate an otherwise routine exposure in the middle because a child is complaining, so parents, too, must learn to give the child the opportunity to experience the feared object or situation in order to learn that it is not a true threat.

The Active Ignoring module, then, is used in those situations for which it is likely that the child will elicit attention, assistance, reassurance, or escape using maladaptive coping behaviors (e.g., whining, tantruming, reassurance seeking). Such behaviors will make it unlikely or impossible for exposure practices to be performed outside of sessions in a way that would allow therapeutic gains. Children and parents who persist in maintaining the pattern of (1) anxiety (2) leading to complaining (3) leading to escape will only strengthen that chain of behaviors. The Active Ignoring module teaches parents to shift the manner in which they attend and communicate such that exposures can run their proper course, and interference is minimized or extinguished. Although none of the children in our three examples required this procedure, our use of the Active Ignoring module is rather common, particularly with younger children and children refusing to attend school.

Social Skills

In some circumstances a child might be ready to perform practices from an emotional standpoint but is not ready in terms of his or her set of actual skills. For example, asking a child to practice having a conversation with friends at school when his or her social skills are truly lacking may simply create an opportunity to fail and could thereby increase the anxiety over time. No child is expected to have perfect social skills, but there should be a minimal level of competence observed before a child is asked to perform social exposure exercises with peers.

The Social Skills modules are rarely used outside of the context of treating social anxiety, and even with social anxiety, their use can be limited. Because the initial exposure exercises for social anxiety typically involve role playing between therapist and child, it will become clear to the therapist whether these modules will be needed or not prior to the involvement of peers. Remember that exposures are always designed to maximize success, so if there are serious doubts about a child's social performance, it might not hurt to review these skills.

Time-Out

Although the Time-Out module is not used often in the context of treating anxiety (only about 10% of anxiety cases in our university clinic), when it is needed, this procedure can be a lifesaver. Time-Out is best used when a child's avoidance strategies involve aggression or severe tantrums that are difficult to ignore. For example, one child with obsessive–compulsive disorder who received services from our university program would hit her mother or pull her hair when her mother discouraged her from performing her compulsive rituals (i.e., ritualized sniffing of her own fingers). Because the treatment plan involved a combination of exposure and response prevention (i.e., the preclusion of rituals), her therapist could not see how exposure could be done successfully without some strategy to manage the aggression. The parents were therefore first trained in the use of time-out, and the mother was instructed to administer a time-out for any aggressive behaviors. After 2 weeks, this procedure was working quite well, and the family reported giving almost no time-outs due to the girl's rapid decrease in aggression. Once this context was established, the therapist then initiated the course of exposure and response prevention. Although occasional aggressive behaviors were noted, these were handled skillfully by the parents, who by then were experienced with managing such behavior.

Troubleshooting Therapy

Any good clinician knows that no matter how well laid out a plan, there is always a chance that the unanticipated or unfathomable will occur. The "troubleshooting" box in Figure 9.1 is designed to be a candid reflection of the fact that there will often be circumstances in which the formulation does not initially provide a clear answer. In our experience, almost every case involves at least one session devoted to troubleshooting. This "macro-level" troubleshooting is to be distinguished from troubleshooting specific modules or procedures (e.g., how to fine-tune a reward or time-out program). Rather, it involves larger and often idiosyncratic issues that seem to challenge the child's ability to move forward with the therapy altogether.

Because there is no clear way to codify this exercise yet, no specific module for troubleshooting exists in this manual. In our clinical program, these sessions have involved such varied situations and events as the following:

- Grief related to the loss of a pet or family member
- Child abuse
- Depression or substance use of other family members
- Specialized planning involving family vacations
- Managing academics (e.g., failing a course due to nonattendance)
- Divorce of parents
- Specialized comorbid conditions (e.g., enuresis that interferes with peer sleepovers)
- Suicidal ideation
- Hospitalization
- Lack of family engagement

Despite the wide variety of clinical scenarios that can elicit troubleshooting sessions, the one constant in our clinical program is that such sessions are preceded and followed by an increase in the usual amount of clinical supervision. Thus practicing therapists are encouraged to discuss with supervisors or peers (1) whether a significant issue has arisen that warrants direct attention and time away from the core modules, and (2) how that issue should be addressed in the context of the case formulation, such that the child and family can eventually get back on track with the core procedures. Remember, except under exceedingly rare circumstances (e.g., the emergence of a medical disorder; psychosis; the precedence of serious legal issues), the goal is to resolve the issue or incorporate it into the therapy program such that the child can continue to engage in successful exposure to reduce anxiety.

TEN

Back to Fundamentals

Even more common than troubleshooting the treatment plan or case formulation is the exercise of troubleshooting the fundamentals. The decision making framework of Figure 1.1 is reproduced, in part, in Figure 10.1 and shows that when there is a lack of therapeutic progress, one needs to ask whether the therapy procedures are being performed properly. Such attention must always be given to overseeing the integrity of the therapeutic procedures, and this need becomes even more pronounced when a procedure is newer to the therapist or when the child has a unique circumstance or style that complicates its use. Just as a portion of Part II was devoted to the proper executing and troubleshooting of exposure, this chapter is designed to address troubleshooting of the other therapy modules.

As the figure shows, it is important to note that a therapist who encounters obstacles has to determine whether there is a problem with fundamentals or with the treatment plan. A problem with fundamentals implies that a procedure (e.g., the Time-Out module) is not going properly and needs to be adjusted, whereas a problem with the treatment plan (the subsequent decision "poor plan?" in the overall framework) would imply that the module used was applied based on a faulty case formulation. As noted repeatedly above, it is good to be conservative about changing the treatment plan. That is, always consider first whether the module execution is correct. In fact, it is so commonly the case that a therapeutic procedure or module does not go perfectly the first time that skipping this review could lead to continual case reformulation in the face of poor progress. Do not skip this decision. Assume that there are likely to be problems with the execution of any strategy. To aid in this regard, this chapter outlines the common problems encountered with the fundamentals, along with their corresponding recommended solutions. For simple reference, these troubleshooting tips also appear again—in whole or in part—in the relevant modules.

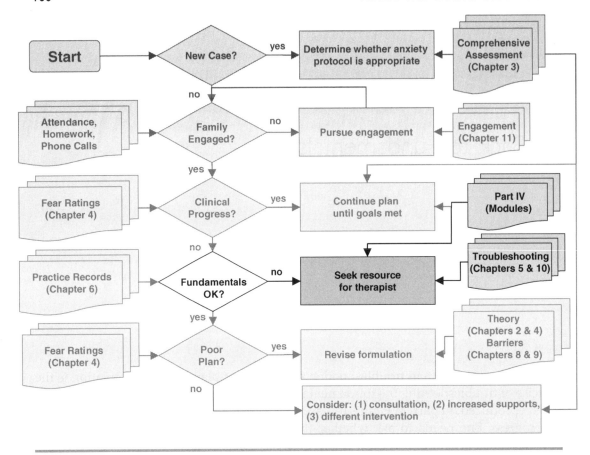

FIGURE 10.1. Working on the fundamentals.

FEAR LADDER

Problem 1: Ratings Are Not Working

The Fear Ladder module yields a list of fears whose average ratings are subsequently used as a key indicator of therapeutic progress. The fear ladder average is the main periodic outcome measure used to determine whether there is progress in the reduction of anxiety over time. In a reasonable number of cases, children simply cannot or will not use these ratings in a way that offers any clinical utility. For example, the ratings might be consistently low and not reflective of the anxiety level observable to others, as was the case with Doug, who frequently gave fear ratings of 0 for items that he was clearly afraid to practice. Other times the ratings are simply inconsistent, with a child guessing at numbers somewhat haphazardly. In either case, the ratings cannot be used to inform the kinds of clinical decision making outlined in Chapter 1.

Solution: Get Other Informants

One of the best ways to manage this problem is to recruit others who can provide better ratings. In Doug's case, we had his mother provide weekly fear ratings on a separate copy of the fear ladder. These worked well to indicate his overall level of fear from session to session.

Solution: Get Other Information

Sometimes additional informants are difficult to come by. Alternatively, they sometimes can be identified but can provide ratings or data that are of no better quality than that of the child. For example, a father giving ratings about his son's worrying might find it difficult to gauge the worrying with any accuracy, particularly if the child is fairly private and does not discuss these worries with the father. In such circumstances, it can be advisable to come up with a new index of progress. For example, in one case involving a child who would not eat solid food due to a fear of choking, we counted the number of seconds it took for the child to finish eating a standardized portion of food (e.g., two cookies). This rating was taken each week as a guide to overall progress, and individual ratings of fear ladder items were no longer taken.

PSYCHOEDUCATION

Problem 1: Feels Like School

The Psychoeducation module is designed to contain the greatest level of detail possible, with the rationale that it is easier to simplify than to add more detail during the session. Accordingly, much of the time there is the challenge of *not* overwhelming the child with facts and details about how anxiety works, how emotions, thoughts, and behaviors relate, etc. Because psychoeducation is one of the earliest modules covered, any lecturing could potentially interfere with the building of rapport or motivation.

Solution: Keep It Simple, Fun, and Slow

One option is to leave out much of the extra detail. The therapist should attempt to gauge the level of the child's aptitude and curiosity and should simply cover material in a way that is appropriate. This may mean leaving out entire pieces of the module or greatly simplifying their explanation. The therapist should also make sure the child is having fun. If the therapist is doing too much of the talking, that is probably a sign that the material should be simplified and that the therapist should be more interactive or use Socratic questioning to keep the child interested. Remember that lots of praise, high-fives, and other reinforcers will keep the child focused on learning. Finally, recall that modules can be covered in multiple sessions, so if a child is getting the material and enjoying it, but time is still running short, then it is best to cover this module over more than one session.

Problem 2: Missing the Rationale

Because there is much to cover in the Psychoeducation module, and because a therapist is usually focused also on managing the therapeutic relationship and establishing rapport, it can be easy to lose focus on the main principles of the module. By the end, a child may have limited understanding of how any of the material relates to what will happen in later therapy.

Solution: Keep the Focus

The function of the Psychoeducation module is to set the stage for exposure. If that is accomplished, then the module is a success. Achieving this success usually occurs in two broad steps. The first involves normalizing anxiety, which appears to have multiple benefits: It makes a child feel less different or abnormal, which, in itself, decreases anxiety and increases hope; it also shifts the child's goal of "eliminating" anxiety to managing it, which seems a lot more possible. By making the emotion more acceptable, normalizing also makes it more likely that a child will tolerate the temporary increases in anxiety that will come as a part of exposure. Thus there is increased hope and optimism and an increased range of opportunities for emotion management—both of which help to set the stage for exposure.

The second broad step in psychoeducation involves describing the program and its rationale. Even if a child does not understand the alarm metaphors, he or she is likely to understand that practice "makes things easier." With that knowledge in mind, it makes sense that the child and therapist will practice together until things get easier. One should not proceed to the Practicing module until the child has some basic understanding of its benefits.

REWARDS

Problem 1: The Rich Baseline

Probably the most common problem encountered in our clinical training program with respect to the Rewards module arises when the therapist attempts to design a rewards program with a family in which the child has free access to a wide variety of powerful reinforcers. For example, the child who plays video games all afternoon will hardly be motivated to perform new behaviors, such as exposure or homework, only to earn a token or small reward. For the "spoiled" child, the Rewards module faces impossible odds.

Solution: Focus on Earning

In this scenario, it is important to discuss with the family the basic notion that although love for children is unconditional, most good things in life are not. Good things usually must be earned. Thus much of what goes on the reward menu involves the behaviors in which the child already engages frequently (e.g., skateboarding, watching TV). If done hastily or improperly, however, this shift can come across as punishment or what is sometimes referred to as "response cost." For example, telling a child "Do your homework or I will take away your video games for the night" does not reflect the proper application of a rewards program.

Shifting the contingencies must be done within the framework of an open discussion about values related to effort and earning, with the idea that children do best in the long run if they learn how to get what they want through their own efforts. It is often helpful to have the child participate in some of this discussion as well. The child should know that he or she can have as many rewarding things as usual and that the overall level of rewards is under his or her control. It can be a subtle shift, but when done well ("Please finish your homework so you can still play your video game tonight"), it can increase the expected behaviors without creating resentment or withdrawal.

Problem 2: "I Don't Want Anything"

Because high negative emotionality is a common contributor to anxiety, many anxious children demonstrate a degree of anhedonia and withdrawal. When asked what they would want to earn on a rewards program, they sometimes say that they cannot think of anything. When asked, parents give a similar response, stating that they are not sure what their child likes.

Solution: Pick High-Frequency Behaviors

Look for behaviors that the child does often. Ask the parent or child what he or she does with free time. Usually, the answer will provide some clue as to what is rewarding. For example, a child who "just hangs out in her room" has probably found something there that is reinforcing, such as books, toys, a puzzle, or just a resting place. Further discussion and a little detective work will usually turn up some ideas.

Problem 3: The Distant Future

Parents and children sometimes suggest rewards that are far off in the future, such as getting a bicycle or going on a family vacation. Although of large value, such rewards often carry little motivational "juice" for children because they are too far off in the future. Further, this problem can overlap with Problem 1, in that most times these suggestions arise from a plan that was already in place for a family. For example, there was already discussion of purchasing a bicycle, or the family has already planned a vacation for next summer. Thus the reward is not only far off, but it might not seem novel, either.

Solution: Think Fast

Ironically, the best rewards are often those that cost little or no money and that can be delivered quickly. Examples include items such as trading cards (parents can buy a whole stack and give them out one at a time), stickers, or other little grab-bag objects from a "dollar store" or can include privileges such as picking what cereal to eat in the morning, getting to sit in the front seat of the car, or staying up an extra 15 minutes at bedtime. The therapist should make sure that most things on the rewards list can be delivered quickly and without great cost to the parents. If it is too difficult for children to wait or too difficult for parents to afford, the rewards program may break down.

Problem 4: Tangible Dependency

Some children appear only to be interested in working for rewards. That is, they seem to be dependent on the rewards, and when a request is made of them, they often ask

"What's my reward?" Related to this problem, such children can also develop the habit of begging. Often there is legitimate concern that the behaviors expected will not become sustainable or independent.

Solution: From Rewards to Praise from Others to Self-Praise

First, regarding begging, parents should be reminded that providing a reward in response to a child's request only rewards the request. Thus, in such cases, there should be ground rules that rewards are only delivered when the expected behavior (e.g., homework) is performed, and that the reward will be lost if a request is made. This means explaining to the child that to earn the reward, he or she must perform the appropriate behavior from the reward program *and* not ask for the reward.

The best way to address the larger issue of dependency is to encourage the introduction of social reinforcers initially. There should be more praise, pats on the back, high-fives, victory dances, smiles, hugs, and thumbs-up whenever there is good behavior—even if the child also gets a tangible reward. This pairing ultimately makes it possible to fade out some of the tangible objects and treats while maintaining the social rewards. Eventually, children can maintain their behaviors on a leaner tangible rewards schedule, while still working for praise.

Over time, the parents should encourage the praise to become internalized by the child. That is, they should progress from saying "You did a great job!" to asking "Didn't you do great?" to asking "How do you think you did?" Over time, the child should develop the capacity for self-praise, which can be applied even when there are no external rewards available. Finally, parents should take time to highlight the natural rewarding consequences of the child's good behavior (e.g., "Did you have fun with your friends at school today?"; "What did the teacher say when you got such a good grade?"). Ability to self-praise and to observe the natural rewards of one's behavior are the best insurance that those behaviors will become sustainable for the long run.

Problem 5: Bribery

Related to the above problem of dependency is some parents' concern that children should not need rewards to "do what is right." Sometimes this explanation comes with a description of when the parents themselves were children and were expected to do things without getting a reward. Ultimately, these parents may feel reasonable concern that they are simply bribing their children.

Solution: Give Rewards, Not Bribes

It can be helpful in this instance to point out to parents a major difference between bribery and rewards. Rewards are given after a behavior occurs, whereas bribes are given before. We never expect parents to give a reward first and then ask the child to perform a particular behavior as part of the deal.

Another matter to highlight is that all people work for rewards, including adults. It might be less obvious, in that adults are capable of waiting a long time for a reward (e.g., a paycheck, a vacation), but everyone is motivated by rewards. It might be helpful to have this discussion with parents in the context of their own lives and behaviors first. Whether it be a cup of coffee, a few minutes of TV, a scented shampoo or soap in the shower, a glass of wine with dinner, or a favorite pair of jeans on the weekend, rewards are common for everyone. The major difference is that these rewards are often self-administered, not externally delivered. But they are rewards, in that they follow some event or achievement and are anticipated with pleasure. Most adults don't start their day with the glass of wine or TV—these are rewards for a day of hard work. Coffee is a reward for getting out of bed, special soap for getting ready for the day, and comfy jeans a reward for working hard all week. Successful adults have multiple rewards throughout their day, and whether they know it or not, they have typically mastered the arrangement of their own routines (work, reward, work, reward) to maximize their performance and satisfaction.

It is not easy to develop such routines, and most children simply cannot teach themselves. Just like teaching them how to tie shoes and brush teeth, parents also need to teach their children how to self-reward so that they can be successful in the long run. The catch here is that for some children this training happens naturally, and for others the self-reward training starts with rewards delivered by parents. Children who need extra help start out by learning the connection between their behavior and consequences—good behavior leads to good consequences. Over time, these children can be taught to self-administer rewards in the above manner. Parents can be reassured that their children will not become spoiled or unappreciative as a result of using a rewards program (unless, of course, spoiled or unappreciative behavior itself is unintentionally rewarded—see previous Problem 4).

COGNITIVE PROCEDURES

Problem 1: No Thoughts

When asked what they are thinking when encountering a feared object, many children simply reply, "I don't know" or "Nothing." Such an answer gives the therapist precious little raw material to incorporate into cognitive restructuring exercises.

Solution: Turn Up the Volume

A child's stated anxious thoughts are really just verbal expressions of his or her expectations of the future state of the world. All people with an intact septal area, hippocampus, and Papez circuit (hence, all people who are capable of experiencing anxiety) are processing these expectations at any given moment—about 5–10 times per second, actually (Gray, 1987). So the problem is likely not that there are no "thoughts," but rather that a child has not been trained to notice them, or even more simply, to know what constitutes a thought. These children need to be given the opportunity to hear their own thoughts more clearly, and a variety of techniques may come in handy in this regard.

First, it can be useful to give examples of the kinds of thoughts people have when anxious. Being careful not to lead the child in a particular direction, one can give examples of the kinds of thoughts other children have when anxious, and then inquire whether these seem familiar. By normalizing these thoughts, such examples help to eliminate possible embarrassment about stating them, and they also give the child an idea of what a therapist means when asking about *thoughts*. Careful work using the thought bubbles included on the STOP Worksheet or using a similar game of thought guessing can be very helpful in teaching children what thoughts are and how to identify them. To make this training gradual, the STOP Worksheet progresses from identifying neutral thoughts, to other children's anxious thoughts, and finally to the child's own anxious thoughts. These exercises can be extended by asking children to "think aloud" by providing a running commentary during an exposure exercise. The therapist can then transcribe the material and review it with the child as evidence of the content of his or her anxious thoughts.

Problem 2: Thoughts Are Emotions

Some children cannot easily distinguish thoughts from emotions. When asked about an anxious thought, they might offer the example "I'm afraid." Again, this confusion creates some problems when training the child in cognitive restructuring, because the initial step involves identifying unrealistically negative predictions about the outcome(s) of the feared situation. A thought such as "I'm afraid" is simply an accurate verbal description of the child's emotional state at the time and therefore is not appropriate material for restructuring.

Solution: Go for Predictions

In general, this problem represents the child's inability to state anxious thoughts as negative predictions (related to the emotion of fear). The therapist's job is to use the statement given, "I'm afraid," as a starting point to help the child articulate the feared outcome. In the best scenario, the therapist might ask "What bad thing do you think will happen in that situation that would make you feel afraid like that?" In response, the child would offer a specific prediction, such as "I think other children will laugh at me."

When such specific predictions are hard to elicit, the therapist might simply have to work with thoughts about the feeling of anxiety itself. For example, the child might be prompted and encouraged to restate the thought as something like "If I'm afraid in this situation, that would be bad." The therapist could then ask why, and ultimately the child might arrive at a prediction such as "If I feel afraid, I'll be a weak person and others will notice." Because it is testable in exposure exercises, such a thought is ideal for cognitive restructuring.

ACTIVE IGNORING

Problem 1: Intermittent Attention

The essence of differential reinforcement strategies is to selectively attend to, or reinforce, desirable behaviors while fully ignoring undesirable behaviors. Such strategies are implicitly challenging because, in many circumstances, the child's undesirable behavior (e.g., crying) is a powerful stimulus that easily elicits attention from others. Often the behavior has been shaped over time to become maximally efficient in eliciting parental attention, such that unsuccessful attention-seeking behaviors have lessened in intensity over time, and the more successful ones have increased over time. This pattern makes it highly likely that parents or others will intermittently attend to a target behavior selected for ignoring. This is a particularly challenging problem, in that intermittent reinforcement schedules tend to produce more stable, robust behaviors than those schedules that reward a given behavior every single time (Ollendick et al., 2001). For example, when parents attend to (i.e., reinforce) swearing every other time it occurs, a child learns, in essence, that he or she must swear twice as much to get attention.

Solution: Use Full Strength

It is important to help prepare parents, teachers, or caretakers who intend to use active ignoring strategies of these risks. Those wishing to implement the technique should be told in advance that this is not a technique that can be used in a diluted fashion. A helpful analogy with parents or teachers is that of antibiotics. Patients are instructed to finish their entire dose of an antibiotic because failure to do so could cause not only a return of the problem, but a more resistant version of the problem. The same is true with active ignoring: Partial application can lead to more treatment-resistant behaviors than were present initially. In addition, it can be helpful (as outlined in the Active Ignoring module) to prepare parents for the possibility of an immediate worsening of the problem (i.e., an "extinction burst"), which is common upon removal of a reinforcer. Parents should be prepared to watch for this phenomenon and to remain committed to the strategy despite the temporary challenges. If all else fails, it can help to have parents or others use a diary to record the instances in which they respond to inappropriate behaviors selected for ignoring. These logs can be reviewed by the therapist, who can help strategize about how to improve the selective removal of attention.

Problem 2: Too Much Explanation

Another common problem with the active ignoring approach is parents' tendency to continue explaining the procedure to the child after it is put into place. For example, when a child is whining on the way to school, a parent might say, "Son, I am not going to pay any attention to this any more. We agreed, you know." Although overtly such a statement expresses the intention not to attend, the statement itself is, in fact, *attention*. This behavior (i.e., explaining) obviously neutralizes the chances of success of this intervention strategy.

Solution: Limit Explaining

It helps to warn parents of this tendency beforehand, giving amusing examples to highlight how common and yet unhelpful it is (e.g., "Some parents pull over their cars, turn off the motor, and talk at length with their fussing child about how they are no longer going to pay any attention to this kind of behavior—how helpful do you think that is?").

Families should then be encouraged to perform only a single review of the rules of active ignoring before they are implemented. If the rules need to be reviewed again, it must occur during a time when the family is calm and the child has not produced the unwanted behavior for some time.

Problem 3: Ignoring the Child

Some parents can take this procedure to the extreme and see it as license to ignore all behaviors produced by the child—in other words, to ignore the child. This approach will likely cause frustration and powerful extinction bursts on the part of the child, as he or she struggles to get any attention. The consequences can be worse than if no intervention were performed, particularly when the behaviors escalate to the point of eliciting parental anger. Ultimately parents can end up providing attention to the most extreme misbehavior, which then becomes a more common part of the child's behavior pattern.

Solution: Ignore Behaviors, Not Children

This problem is best prevented rather than handled after the fact. It must be stated clearly to parents that they are never to try to ignore their children. In fact, with active ignoring, the overall amount of attention and praise to the child might actually increase rather than decrease. The strategy is all about timing and focus of attention, not amount. If parents have difficulty with this concept, it must be reviewed regularly, and parents should role-play attending to positive behaviors.

SOCIAL SKILLS

Problem 1: Expecting No Anxiety

When engaging in social skills training, a child often forms the expectation that by increasing his or her skills, the anxiety associated with performance should go away. For example, teaching a child how to start a conversation might be assumed to eliminate that child's anxiety upon starting a conversation. However, in many instances, establishing or improving a set of performance skills and reducing performance anxiety are separate endeavors. Thus a child who is taught the basic steps of how to greet a peer and initiate a conversation may become frustrated when considerable anxiety arises during the performance of those new skills. As a result, such children frequently discredit their exposure exercises, concluding that their practice was a failure because they felt anxious.

Solution: "You Are Supposed to Feel Anxiety"

These children should be reminded that it would be unusual not to experience anxiety when practicing these new behaviors. On the contrary, the goal is to perform the skills or steps *while feeling anxious*. If a child can perform the appropriate skills or steps under these conditions, then the skills are considered well established and are likely to persist in new situations, despite some anxiety. Children should be reminded that—just like everything else they have learned—the anxiety will only come down over time with repeated practice.

TIME-OUT

Problem 1: Slow Starts

Because parents sometimes consider the use of time-out as a last resort, issuing a time-out can often be preceded by a considerable amount of discussion, negotiation, or even arguing. For example, an anxious child who throws something while having a tantrum about going to school might be told, "If you do that again, you will have to go to time-out." She then might kick something instead, eliciting yet another threat. With each interaction, the parent and child become increasingly upset and aggressive (Reid, Patterson, & Snyder, 2002). If a time-out is issued, it is usually done angrily and possibly inconsistently. Worse yet, parents may resort to hitting or yelling, dispensing with time-out altogether.

Solution: "Swift Justice"

Similar to the way that active ignoring must be used fully rather than in a diluted fashion, time-out also requires a certain level of commitment. Experts have suggested that the swiftness with which time-out is issued may be one of the best predictors of its effectiveness, and Russell Barkley has used the term "swift justice" to emphasize that aspect of the technique (e.g., Pfiffner, Barkley, & DuPaul, 2006). Parents should therefore be prepared to identify and review the time-out behaviors with the child in advance, and then enforce an immediate time-out upon their occurrence.

Problem 2: Time-Out Is Time In

Often parents will choose to send children to their room because it may be more convenient than establishing a dedicated time-out area elsewhere in the home. This scenario carries the high risk that the child will be surrounded by reinforcers during the time-out. For example, there are usually books, games, a computer, a bed on which to relax, and sometimes even a TV. Under such circumstances it is highly unlikely that the time-out procedure could be effective.

Solution: Time-Out from Reinforcement

Remind parents that the purpose of time-out is to remove all rewarding stimulation from the child for a brief period of time. Although it is possible to use a child's room for time-out, it can take a considerable amount of work to remove all reinforcers from that environment. It is usually easier to pick a place for the child to sit in some other part of the house, such as the kitchen or even a bathroom.

Problem 3: Fouling up the Follow-Up

Some parents end time-out by scolding the child or initiating an antagonistic discussion about the initial misbehavior. In many cases, this can reescalate the child and lead right to another time-out. Another common problem with finishing time-out is that parents may remove a demand that was previously in place before the time-out. For example, say that the child was instructed to get her backpack prepared for school, but she swore or was hostile to the parent, so a time-out would be issued. In some cases, parents will put the books and lunch into the backpack during the time-out to avoid another round of confrontation. This type of behavior also can diminish the effectiveness of time-out, in that it sends the message to the child, "Although you will have to do a time-out, you will not have to listen to my request."

Solution: Ending Short and Sweet

Parents should keep their interaction following time-out brief. For example, a parent might ask, "Do you know why you got this time-out?" but once the reason was clear, would not pursue further discussion. If a demand was in place previously, now is the time to repeat it. And the follow-through should not only be short but also sweet. That is, the tone should not be angry or aggressive but calm and matter-of-fact.

MAINTENANCE

Problem 1: Not Taking Credit

Even children who successfully complete the program may conclude at the end that the reason they improved was due to luck, or a special therapist, or something else other than him- or herself. This view can be a problem because the child will likely experience elevated anxiety after therapy is over, and if he or she has not come to understand his or her own role in managing that anxiety successfully, then there is an increased possibility that the child will feel helpless and distressed at the first sign of trouble.

Solution: It's the Child and the Skills

A therapist needs to emphasize throughout the program, and especially in the later stages, that the gains are attributable to the application of new skills and to the child's honest effort. This is best done using the Socratic approach; for example, "You know why this has gotten so easy for you?" At the end of the program the child should certainly be in the position to state that if something within the realm of reasonable problems comes up, dealing with it will not require reestablishing a relationship with the therapist or some other major intervention. Although a good therapist is necessary to teach the skills well, once established, the child then has his or her own internal coping skills that can always be marshaled. If not, the therapist may have more work to do.

Problem 2: Resuming Routines after CBT Ends

Some children and families expect that once the program is over, they can resume their old routines. Doing so can be a problem in that such a routine may facilitate avoidance of feared objects or situations and could thus allow unwanted anxiety to return and escalate.

Solution: The "Exposure Lifestyle"

A term popularized by one of the former expert therapists in our program, Brad Nakamura, the "exposure lifestyle" refers to a new way of identifying and handling challenges that one encounters throughout life. An exercise metaphor is appropriate in this case: it typically involves an intensive phase to "get in shape," but it also requires a maintenance program (i.e., a lifestyle of activity) to stay in shape. Similarly, life after CBT is not as intensive as when learning and applying the new skills, but children and families should be advised to monitor problematic anxiety and develop a plan to apply known skills as soon as is warranted. And in the best of circumstances, the child should consider all opportunities to approach unrealistically feared situations as a chance to improve his or her skill set.

Problem 3: Expecting Perfection

Many children and families feel some anxiety about termination and will raise examples of traces of anxiety that remain to be addressed by the therapist. It is possible that just as some of these last few items are addressed, new ones will surface. Ultimately, expecting that there will be no problematic anxiety left at the time of termination is probably unrealistic, and the notion that therapy must continue until all problems are fully resolved carries the false implication that problems can only be addressed under the therapist's careful watch. If the child is ever to manage his or her anxiety independently, then he or she must realize that some problems can be addressed without the help of others.

Solution: The "80/20" Approach

It can be helpful to raise the idea that it is an acceptable time to terminate when only 80% of the problems are successfully resolved. By design, it can be best to allow the remaining 20% of anxiety items to be worked on independently, so that there is a better chance of mastery and thus of maintaining future gains. Obviously, these are not magic numbers, but the idea makes sense that the child should terminate with at least one addressable challenge still in front of him or her. In general, improvements associated with CBT are likely to be larger 6 months after the program is over than right at termination, because the child has continued to apply CBT skills independently over time (Chorpita & Southam-Gerow, 2006).

ELEVEN

Supporting Families with Low Engagement

Being a parent is one of the greatest challenges many people ever face. Children are not easy; even "easy" children are not easy. Parents sacrifice a great deal physically, emotionally, and financially when deciding to raise children. They are usually far more tired and busy than before they had children. On top of that, parents of anxious children find themselves with the additional burden of worrying about their child's problem, and the odds are reasonable that at least one parent will disproportionately worry because of his or her own temperamentally elevated NA. Therapists must remain sensitive to the fact that, first and foremost, families need support. Because many families face multiple obstacles to engaging properly in the therapy program, an important goal of the therapy can be to understand and address engagement issues.

Engagement can be defined as the child and family's active and collaborative participation in the intervention. Engagement is a prerequisite for success, particularly in a therapy such as CBT, which holds active client participation and behavioral rehearsal as major strategies for change. Thus issues related to engagement and participation take precedence over more routine clinical issues. Stated more plainly, one should not attempt to follow the modules without first having sufficiently engaged the child and family. This prioritization appears quite clearly in the case formulation framework outlined in Figure 1.1.

Problems with engagement commonly manifest in one of two ways: impaired collaboration (often referred to in the literature as "noncompliance," the term "impaired collaboration" is used here due to its less pejorative connotations for families) or attrition risk. Impaired collaboration typically involves participation in some aspects of the intervention program without proper performance of particularly critical aspects, such as homework assignments, role plays, etc. For example, exercises might be done incorrectly, haphazardly, or not at all. In the strictest sense, "attrition" refers to the premature termination of the intervention; thus "attrition risk" involves the related phenomena of frequent appointment cancellations and "no-shows" (i.e., appointments missed without notice).

In general, engagement is a common problem in child intervention; attrition rates of 45% have been reported at community clinics (Armbruster & Fallon, 1994). With specific reference to anxiety, the literature shows that approximately 20–30% of children participating in clinical trials of CBT for childhood anxiety drop out of treatment (Chorpita & Southam-Gerow, 2006). This is particularly concerning, given that families participating in these university-based clinical trials are demographically at lower risk for attrition than those encountered in community clinic settings or public mental health systems (e.g., Southam-Gerow, Weisz, & Kendall, 2003; Southam-Gerow, Chorpita, Miller, & Taylor, 2006). In some clinical settings, therefore, engagement problems more likely could be the norm than the exception.

SOURCES OF POOR ENGAGEMENT

Although there is a scarcity of well-designed research on engagement, some key studies point to a variety of factors specifically related to attrition. Kazdin et al. (1997) studied 242 children participating in an intervention for aggressive or oppositional behavior. The major findings showed that (1) particular demographics predicted attrition, (2) perceptions of barriers to treatment predicted attrition, and (3) demographics and perceived barriers were relatively independent (i.e., perception of barriers to treatment did not mediate demographics). The demographics identified as risks for premature therapy termination included low socioeconomic status, membership in a minority group, having a single-parent family, being on public assistance, and the use of adverse childrearing practices. Specific factors representing perceived barriers that were found to be significantly related to attrition included perceived family stressors and obstacles, perceived treatment relevance, and relationship with the therapist. It is interesting to note that among these perceived barriers, relevance of the treatment had the highest effect size, and relationship with therapist had the lowest. This finding highlights the idea that engagement might not simply be a matter of the therapist's relationship with the family, at least in terms of predicting attrition. These findings are consistent with earlier research on engagement (Armbruster & Kazdin, 1994).

Far less is known about engagement with anxious children and families, and it is difficult to generalize from the more substantial literature involving aggressive children, because many of those interventions are primarily parent based. Whereas the issues regarding attrition risk might involve some overlap, given that parents often are responsible for taking their children to therapy sessions, the issues related to collaboration may not apply, given the greater involvement of the child in CBT relative to treatments for aggression. With respect to attrition, some findings from research on CBT for childhood anxiety suggested that single-parent families and minority status represent increased risk for attrition (Kendall& Sugarman, 1997), but these results were not replicated in a similar investigation (Pina, Silverman, Fuentes, Kurtines, & Weems, 2003). No studies so far have investigated the role of perceived barriers to treatment among children participating in CBT for anxiety.

COST–BENEFIT RATIO

Because many aspects of engagement can be conceptualized in terms of a perceived cost–benefit ratio for the child and family, this framework offers a useful heuristic for addressing both impaired collaboration and attrition risk. When engagement is poor, one can imagine that the child or family somehow perceives the cost of participating in therapy as being too great relative to the perceived value (not necessarily the monetary cost, but the "cost" in terms of dealing with intermediate problems, time needed, stress, etc.). Consistent with the principles of cognitive and behavioral theory, the goal then is to nudge this ratio toward a more favorable balance to elicit a collaborative response. A useful guideline for therapists is to consider a list of possible challenges related to the perceived costs and benefits, and to assess which of these might be related to engagement (see Table 11.1). Those factors identified should be investigated and become part of the overall case formulation.

TABLE 11.1. Summary of Types of Costs and Benefits in Therapy

Costs	
Complexity	Research generally has shown that new practices are less likely to be adopted to the extent that they are complex (Rogers, 1995). Some aspects of CBT can be complicated and can introduce costs to the child and family that are prohibitive.
Difficulty	The work of CBT is often challenging. In some instances, it might be too aversive for children to participate on their own (e.g., with *in vivo* exposure), or the homework assigned by the therapist might be too much to complete.
Therapeutic relationship	A long history of research has shown that qualities of the messenger are important determinants of whether and how a message is received (e.g., Heesacker, 1986; Cacioppo, Petty, & Stoltenberg, 1985). If the therapist is seen as too different, unfriendly, or insensitive, credibility and ability to elicit collaboration could be lost. These inhibiting factors can include strains in the relationship due to cultural differences or cultural insensitivity.
Stressors and obstacles	As shown by the work of Kazdin and colleagues (e.g., Kazdin et al., 1997), the presence of family stressors and obstacles (e.g., illness in family, moving to a new home, car problems) can interfere with the ability to participate in therapy.
Competing demands	Families balancing multiple priorities, such as extracurricular commitments, multiple jobs, or other family concerns might have difficulty protecting time to participate in CBT.
Benefits	
Impact	The potential to help might not be obvious or credible to the child and family. This difficulty can be related to the expected degree of change (high or low), as well as to the expected timing of change (fast or slow). Interventions that do not provide a rapid, positive response will be seen as having less benefit.
Value	It is sometimes possible for goals not to be valued as positive. This can be true for the child (e.g., returning to school in the context of social anxiety) as well as for a parent (e.g., having a socially anxious child become more assertive).
Relevance	The treatment as described might not seem logically connected to solving the problems faced by the child and family.

COLLABORATIVE STRATEGIES

The act of increasing engagement through collaboration can be conceptualized, in its simplest terms, as a form of persuasion. Thus the social psychology literature offers some useful guidelines about factors likely to increase the active participation of children and families. In general, both the qualities of the communicator (i.e., therapist) and the style in which the message is delivered can be important. The collective social psychology literature on persuasion suggests that a message is more likely to be accepted when the communicator is perceived as likeable, trustworthy, attractive, and expert. Similarly, acceptance is heightened when a message is delivered early, involves multiple communication channels (e.g., talking and reading), is emotional in nature (e.g., either delivered when the recipient is in a positive mood or is concerned about feared consequences), and stimulates thinking on the part of the recipient (Crano & Prislin, 2006).

The CBT therapist should keep in mind that the goal of engagement is not to enhance the quality of the relationship, per se, but rather to engage the child and family in the practices of CBT. Improving the relationship will be an important sub-goal sometimes, if the formulation suggests that a problematic therapeutic relationship is one of the primary costs perceived by the family, but the relationship is never the end goal itself. In fact, an overreliance on the therapeutic relationship can potentially interfere with a child or family's ability to incorporate CBT strategies and perform them independently. Likewise, a child might be prone to attribute success of a therapy program to the therapist or relationship, rather than to the cognitive and behavioral strategies learned and performed. These possible side effects of the therapeutic relationship should be carefully managed, and the therapist must remain committed to the goal of engaging the family in the therapy program, first and foremost.

Thus strategies to increase collaboration should generally involve a focus on the cost–benefit ratio and should involve a constructive, shared exploration of how to make this ratio more favorable for the child and family. Recently, Nock and Kazdin (2005) tested a program involving this type of collaboration to increase motivation among families seeking services for their children's oppositional, aggressive, or antisocial behavior. During the first, fifth, and seventh sessions with parents, selected therapists in the study elicited self-motivational statements from parents, systematically identified barriers to those goals, and then collaboratively developed plans to address barriers, including contingencies or "backup" plans. Nock and Kazdin found that participating in just these brief additional exercises with parents significantly helped to increase collaboration and decrease attrition risk. As noted above, less is known about whether such procedures are equally effective in the context of child anxiety, but so far our experience has suggested that the issues are more similar than different. Some specific suggestions related to collaborative approaches follow.

Simplify

As noted in the previous chapter, sometimes procedures must be greatly simplified to fit into the context of busy lives filled with competing demands. The therapist should ensure that the basic principles of any procedure or course of therapy are not compromised as a result. For example, a case involving anxious school refusal might proceed immediately to the use of exposure and rewards, with only the briefest psychoeducation beforehand. Alternatively, with some cases it might be advisable to work on only one of multiple fears—at least initially. For example, if a child is afraid of test taking, social events, and talking on the phone, and the parents primary concern is that the child is failing tests, it might be necessary to craft a treatment plan that simply addresses the test taking—particularly if the family has many other challenges or competing demands.

Simplification can also involve reducing the demand of the paperwork or monitoring associated with CBT. The most important part of the program is the practice or rehearsal. Forms and worksheets are designed to facilitate that component, but if they get in the way, they should be omitted or abbreviated.

Problem Solve

Working through a cost–benefit analysis with the family or going through basic problem-solving steps can enhance motivation or offer a new solution to address engagement barriers. Families that are plagued by multiple challenges might benefit from involvement in these exercises in order to map their priorities and to identify the steps to achieve them. Families challenged by divorce, poverty, racism, crime, bad schools, substance use, or other factors are likely to be in a weakened position of reacting to their environment, unable to get a foothold. Such families are often perceived to be continually in "crisis mode." A skilled therapist can create an opportunity to introduce a plan—which may or may not prioritize the needs of the anxious child, but nevertheless will clarify which next steps the family must take. This plan can serve as a road map to achieving the family's goals and hopes.

Go for High Impact

For many families, therapists will need to focus on making the success of the child as obvious and dramatic as possible. Frequent praise and review will serve to highlight the advantages and benefits of staying with the program. Sometimes it can help to go after the high priority targets first—that is, those fears that will have the greatest effect on impressing the family or alleviating their own worries.

Use Informed Consent

All therapists use informed consent to brief children and families on the parameters of therapy, but it may be necessary to emphasize the particular aspects of CBT that families will likely find challenging. CBT requires practice, and it usually requires at least some minimal observation or documentation of feelings, thoughts, or behaviors. Families can be told that this is a short-term/long-term tradeoff: The work and stress might increase in the short term, but the advantage is that the problems in the long run should be minimized. In many instances, providing this knowledge up front inoculates the family by framing the challenges as predictable and time limited.

Accept Partial Engagement

Sometimes these strategies will be insufficient to engage a child and family to participate fully at all times. Under such circumstances, it is nevertheless possible to achieve a positive outcome. For example, in the investigation by Chorpita, Taylor, Moffitt, et al. (2004) one of the participants had no parent willing to see or talk with the therapist. Nevertheless, a positive outcome was achieved. Let such families know that there are costs to minimizing parent participation, and that the effect size for CBT without including parents tends to be lower.

INTENSITY STRATEGIES

In addition to the collaborative goal-setting and problem-solving approaches of the type used by Nock and Kazdin (2005), there is another general type of strategy that has been used to facilitate engagement. This strategy often involves scaling the intensity of the therapist involvement to match the needs of the family. In a sense, intensity approaches are a possible outcome of the type of solutions that could be generated using the collaborative strategies noted above (e.g., decrease the "cost" represented in driving to the therapist's office by having the therapist come to the home). Nevertheless, intensity strategies merit their own discussion, given that they are potentially so effective and not traditionally considered in typical clinical settings.

In one of the only controlled trials of its kind, Santisteban et al. (1996) evaluated an intensity-based strategy designed to enhance engagement among families whose children were determined to be at risk for drug abuse. The engagement protocol outlined six levels of therapist intensity: (0) "polite concern," (1) "minimal joining" (encouraging a single family member to involve others), (2) "more thorough joining" (establishing a leadership position with family, deeper inquiry about family values and problems), (3) "family restructuring" through a single family member (having a family member negotiate with other family members and assume accountability for the engagement of other members), (4) "lower level ecological engagement" (e.g., restructuring through multiple family members), and (5) "higher level ecological interventions" (e.g., home visits, involvement of significant others to help in restructuring).

The design of the study allowed the engagement condition to use levels 0–5, as needed, whereas in the control group, only levels 0 and 1 were permitted. Santisteban et al. (1996) found that 81% of families in the engagement condition attended the first treatment session as compared with an average of 60% among controls. Once engaged (i.e., defined as attending first session), this 81% of families was able to maintain attendance as well as those 60% in the control group, suggesting that the effects on the additional 21% were durable beyond the first session. Interestingly, Santisteban noted that all of the successes in the experimental group occurred with the use of levels 2–4, suggesting that there is much room for engaging families without having to conduct home visits.

On the other hand, Henggeler and colleagues have focused heavily on level of contact—especially home visits—as a strategy to engage families with delinquent adolescents (Henggeler, Schoenwald, Borduin, Rowland, & Cunningham, 1998). Their intervention, multisystemic therapy (MST), emphasizes principles of therapist action, accountability, and daily contact with families. Henggeler et al. (1986) provide anecdotal evidence of the need for this level of intensity with their target population, noting that the intervention was originally to be tested as an office-based model delivered by graduate students in the psychology building of Memphis State University. Due to attrition and no-shows, the intervention was adapted to become a home-based model, which Henggeler et al. (1998) described as being "born of necessity" (p. 238).

The ideas behind both of these examples suggest that the level of support should match the family needs and capitalize on strengths and relationships that are likely to enhance engagement. MST, in particular, emphasizes the need for therapists to adhere to a core set of principles, around which flexible multidomain assessment and problem solving occur on a regular basis to keep the program moving forward. Again, although little is documented about how such principles generalize to internalizing populations, our experience working with families of anxious children in the Hawaii public mental health system suggests the benefits of such approaches are rather universal (Chorpita et al., 2004). Given these theoretical and practical considerations, some of the common intensity strategies used to facilitate engagement with this protocol are described next.

Go to the Problem

Connecting with a child and family can go well beyond a therapist's sensitivity and warmth. Often it is necessary to get out of the therapy office. Go to where the problem is—at least initially—to observe the family ecology and the context that has created obstacles to success. These obstacles can become short-term targets for the intervention, sometimes before any of the procedures in this manual can even be implemented. In some instances the therapist must create a formulation of the initial problem: The family cannot participate successfully in a therapy program. As noted above, obstacles may include car trouble, multiple jobs, illnesses, or a host of other factors. These need to be addressed head on in order for the program to have the best chance for success.

Going to a family's neighborhood or home can also have the effect of decreasing the social distance of the therapist and thereby increasing his or her relevance and credibility with the family. As noted, similar techniques have been recommended as part of family therapy protocols and often fall under the rubric of "joining" (e.g., Minuchin & Fishman, 1981).

"Whatever It Takes"

Practitioners of MST (Henggeler et al., 1998) use the phrase "Whatever It Takes" to describe their approach to problem-solving challenging cases. This approach often involves using basic problem-solving skills to understand the broader context of engagement and motivation, and being willing to address the underlying factors in whatever way is necessary. This could mean enlisting other family members, helping a parent get a job or find a reliable means of transportation, going to school to work with teachers, or going to work in a family's home—in essence, whatever it takes.

Users of this manual are encouraged to take that sentiment to heart. This manual spells out the principles and basic procedures of CBT for childhood anxiety, but research documents that such procedures work best in the context of an engaged and motivated family. This again is an area where a therapist must draw upon his or her reservoir of experience and marshal the talent, creativity, and discipline to deliver the skills of CBT to the anxious child. For now, how that is done will likely differ from family to family, and from therapist to therapist. The understanding and documentation of those methods will clearly be the subject of the next generation of child anxiety treatment research (Chorpita & Southam-Gerow, 2006).

PART IV

TREATMENT MODULES

TWELVE

Use of the Modules

Following a thorough assessment and the solid understanding of what is needed to engage the child and family in the practice of CBT, therapists should begin using the modules according to the guiding algorithm. Along with the procedural choices to be made, the therapist should be prepared to individualize the intervention even further according to the dimensions of *"face, place, and pace."* The intervention "face" represents the "look and feel" of the intervention to the child and involves selection of metaphors, characters, examples, and style of language to implement the procedures. That is, therapists should consider embellishing the protocol with images that would be appealing to children, based on their culture, age, gender, and community. For example, in Hawaii—where the protocol was developed and piloted—it is common to use examples related to surfing or swimming in discussions involving bravery, true alarms, and false alarms. This is where the skill of an experienced clinician comes heavily into play, inasmuch as there is only so much of this kind of detail that can be formalized about how to individualize and to engage children. More likely than not, to dictate a particular style or presentation would constrain therapists' natural ability to engage and connect with a child. Therapists are encouraged to use their own experience with what fits a particular child in terms of the overall "look and feel." That said, it is always important to keep in mind that although the protocol can have different "faces," the body of the CBT program is the same, and the basic principles and procedures should not be altered.

Individualization with respect to "place" implies that the therapist should have worked with the family to gain an understanding of the most appropriate setting or settings for the intervention. For some families, this might be in their homes; for others, at school. Sometimes such considerations will be determined by the nature of the problem. For example, in cases involving compulsive bedtime rituals, it might be helpful to schedule a meeting at the home in the evening to observe the problem and rehearse cognitive or behavioral strategies *in vivo*, perhaps with parents observing and learning. Other times, the choice might be related to engagement issues, as noted previously. For example, for children who repeatedly miss meetings due to problems with parental consistency in findings transportation, scheduling meetings at the school might be a reasonable solution. As mentioned in Chapter 11, going to the home is sometimes another way to deal with engagement issues. Although such practice has sometimes been described as "rewarding no-shows," the experience of our research team has been that such is not typically the case. Preliminary data comparing completers versus noncompleters in our program showed statistically significant differences in rate of cancellations and no-shows (of 21 cases, mean cancellations = 13% for noncompleters, 4% for completers; mean no-shows = 13% for noncompleters, 4% for completers). Our experience as well as related research (e.g., Cunningham & Henggeler, 1999) has suggested that scheduling immediate additional sessions and "going out to find the child" (as opposed to waiting another week to see if he or she comes to the clinic or office) yield important differences in whether families with challenges ultimately complete the therapy program.

Finally, individualization regarding pace suggests that the modules should be covered at the speed necessary to allow acquisition of the core skills. Therefore, it is important to keep in mind that the contents of a module need not be equated with a therapy session, although the general outline supports that application. In other words, a module can be covered over multiple sessions. For example, in our experience the Psychoeducation module can take several sessions for some children. Other modules can be covered in a part of a session, such as brief coverage of the differential reinforcement (Active Ignoring) module with parents following some exposure with the child. Modules can be repeated as many times as necessary, as typically happens with the exposure module (i.e., Practice). Overall, the basic idea is to go at the fastest pace possible that allows acquisition of the skills needed by the child and family. Sometimes acquisition will require lots of repetition and rehearsal; other times, not. In line with the principles outlined in the previous chapter on engagement, modules can also be simplified, and there are guidelines in each module for what elements should not be skipped when simplifying or working under time pressure.

Use of this intervention in our program generally reflects a high degree of flexibility regarding "place" and "pace." Over the past hundred cases, over 70% involved more than four sessions outside a clinic office (e.g., at a home or school), and approximately 40% of cases involved meeting more than once per week for at least some part of the protocol. These parameters of use are consistent with the design principles of the manual and are also related to the issues involving engagement.

MAIN FEATURES OF THE PROTOCOL

A concise summary of the most important features of the program is outlined here:

Toolbox Approach

The idea behind using modular treatment is that therapists use a "toolbox" in working with the child and family. Each tool in the box is represented by one of the individual modules. Although each module is self-contained in its design, modules can be combined together in multiple ways. Not all children or families need all of the tools, and the manner in which modules are selected is outlined in the flowchart, as noted previously.

Exposure

As discussed extensively, exposure, or practicing feared situations, is conceptualized as the main ingredient of treatment. It is what is required for change to occur. In essence, the subgoal of the treatment program is about making exposure happen. All other modules in the toolbox are designed to support exposure. For example, "Learning about Anxiety" is designed to make exposure credible and acceptable to the child by providing a rationale. The module "Rewards" is used when the child's motivation for exposure is too low; "Active Ignoring" is used when whining and resistance behaviors interfere with exposure; "Cognitive Restructuring" is used when the child's expectations for exposure are too negative; and so forth. In essence, the therapist should always be trying to solve the problem of making exposure happen, and when it happens, to make sure it happens properly.

Forms

The use of forms is considered an important part of maintaining the integrity of the treatment. The forms are designed to ensure a consistent experience for the child in the delivery of each technique. Forms come in three different types: Worksheets, Records, and Handouts. *Worksheets* are designed as in-session or homework exercises for the child; they incorporate and integrate material learned in therapy and are intended to be fun as well as educational. *Records* are used to track progress or events that are important to therapy. The most important record is the Fear Ladder, used to track fear ratings throughout treatment. Finally, *Handouts* are educational sheets for parents and teachers, designed to reinforce information about a technique that has been reviewed in session. Handouts are intended to serve as a reference for parents and teachers participating in the child's therapy. Throughout the modules, the names of all forms are written in **bold type**. A summary of forms can be found in Table 12.1). Note that some forms are used across multiple modules (e.g., Parent and Teacher Observation Records, Parent and Teacher About Anxiety Handouts).

Session Length

Modules do not have a fixed length, such that some modules may not be finished within a single meeting. Other modules may take less than one meeting and can be combined with still other modules. There is no prescription for session length, other than what makes sense clinically. For example, to cover information in "Learning about Anxiety," it might be best to meet daily with a child for three sessions of half an hour each. Other techniques, such as exposure, are sometimes best done in one large session of several hours. The main point is that the session length should be dictated primarily by the manner in which skills are being learned and exposure practices are progressing with the child, and secondarily by what is practical for the child and family.

TABLE 12.1. **A Listing of Forms Corresponding to Each Module**

Module	Worksheet	Record	Parent handout	Teacher handout
Making a Fear Ladder	—	Fear Ladder (Parent and Child)	—	—
Learning about Anxiety	Feelings Record, Thoughts Record (Child or Teen)	—	About Anxiety; Principles of Success	About Anxiety
Practice: *In Vivo*	Anxiety and How It Works	—	Discrete Practice Record; Continuous Practice Record	Practice
Practice: Imaginal	—	Discrete Practice Record	Practice	Practice
Maintenance and Relapse Prevention	What I Took Back from Anxiety	—	Building on Bravery	Building on Bravery
Cognitive Restructuring: Probability Overestimation	—	Two-Column and Five-Column Thought Record	About Anxiety	About Anxiety
Cognitive Restructuring: Catastrophic Thinking	—	Seven-Column Thought Record	About Anxiety	About Anxiety
Cognitive Restructuring: STOP	STOP Worksheet	STOP Record	About Anxiety	About Anxiety
Social Skills: Meeting New People	Meeting and Greeting Worksheet	Meeting and Greeting Record	—	—
Social Skills: Nonverbal Communication	Nonverbal Skills Worksheet	Nonverbal Skills Record	—	—
Active Ignoring	—	Parent Observation Record; Teacher Observation Record	Active Ignoring	Active Ignoring
Rewards	—	Parent Observation Record; Teacher Observation Record	Rewards	Rewards
Time-Out	—	Parent Observation Record; Teacher Observation Record	Time-Out	Time-Out

Frequency

Session frequency is also determined by the nature of the child's response to treatment. For example, if within-session gains are often lost between sessions, increased contact may be necessary. The goal should be to provide enough support and contact to ensure clear progress, while not overwhelming the child or family or providing more contact than necessary. As skills are incorporated more fully by the child and family, the frequency of contacts can be decreased to allow for greater independence in maintaining skills and for fewer complications related to termination.

Setting

The setting of the session is flexible. It should be convenient for the child and family, so that motivation remains high. Often exposure exercises will dictate a particular setting (e.g., school, pet store, home) in order to best approximate feared situations. Conducting these exposure exercises in their natural setting is encouraged as much as possible.

System Focus

Although CBT frequently focuses on working with the child's thoughts and behaviors, there will almost always be a need to address factors in the child's broader environment (Bronfenbrenner, 1986). Parents, teachers, peers, and other influences can often maintain, intensify, or otherwise affect anxiety and therefore hinder treatment progress. Therapists are encouraged to keep such factors in mind and when they present obstacles to progress, these factors should become the immediate focus of treatment. As always, such a focus is not intended to become a long-term digression from CBT (e.g., providing marital therapy for parents who cannot cooperatively supervise the child's exposure practice). Rather, a system focus is intended to address the obstacles that limit exposure-based practice, which always remains the main strategy of therapy. As part of this system focus, many of the parent modules were designed to be used with teachers as well. To the extent that teachers, parents, and other important influences are working together consistently, the chances for success are maximized.

Adaptation

Modules can be adapted. They need not be followed in a lockstep fashion, although major steps should not be omitted altogether. Children will differ by age, gender, diagnosis, hobbies, peer status, families, academic skill level, birth order, and many other important variables. Examples or exercises will often need to be adapted to fit the interest and cognitive level of the child. This type of adaptation is strongly encouraged, as it is best to try to make the steps of each technique as relevant and appealing as possible to the child.

STRUCTURE OF MODULES

Each module is organized according to a template that has a roughly uniform structure across the set of modules (Chorpita et al., 2005b). In our experience, this design feature helps therapists and children enter into the procedures more quickly, having become familiar with a consistent structure from session to session. Each module is organized as if the contents were to be covered in a singe session, even though—as noted—such an approach is not necessary. When there is not a one-to-one correspondence between a session and a module, the session structure should correspond with the structures outlined in the modules. With a few logical exceptions, the uniform parameters in each module include the following:

- A statement of objectives for the therapist
- A list of the core points if there are time constraints (cf. Weisz, Weersing, Valeri, & McCarty, 1999)
- A list of the materials needed
- A prompt to obtain the weekly rating(s)
- A prompt to set an agenda
- A set of procedures specific to each module
- The assignment of practice exercises
- A prompt to reinforce the child for in-session behavior
- A review of session information with the parents

The set of specific procedures includes some combination of examples, exercises, *in vivo* practices, and role plays. This set of procedures represents the "guts" of the module, and the materials that surround it are the typical steps that therapists are encouraged to use to structure any session.

Module contents are organized clearly according to the above list and use specific type sets and icons to maximize the efficiency of using the manual. These appear in Table 12.2, which shows each module parameter as associated with a particular heading format, a representative icon, and a definition of the parameter contents. Each module ends with additional "optional parameters," which can include a list of items typically overlooked, special considerations, troubleshooting ideas, specific diagnostic issues, and a listing of any evidence supporting the procedural contents of the module. These sections at the end of each module need be accessed only as needed. More generally, the therapist does not need to read all the modules or all parts of a single module in order to implement the protocol. Rather, given a basic understanding of the core logic, the therapist should become familiar with each module as needed, and he or she will gain experience through repeated applications.

TABLE 12.2. **Icon and Heading Table Corresponding to the Module Features**

Item	Format	Icon	Definition
MODULE NAME	Title heading		Name of the module
Objectives	Main heading	★	A list of the major points of the module
If Pressed for Time	Main heading	(clock)	The points most important to cover if some things need to be skipped
Who Is Needed	Main heading	(envelope)	The individuals who should be asked to participate in the meeting
Materials	Main heading	(pencil)	What forms and materials will be needed for the session
Weekly Rating	Main heading	(thermometer)	Instructions for taking a weekly rating
Assignment Review	Main heading	(document)	Instructions for reviewing homework or practices
Set the Agenda	Main heading	(calendar 1)	Instructions for setting the session agenda
Procedures	Main heading	(speech bubbles)	A detailed list of the module contents
Example	Boxed	(pushpin)	An example of a concept or dialogue
Exercise	Boxed	(weightlifter)	An exercise to practice—usually involves a Worksheet or game
In Vivo	Boxed	(clapperboard)	Naturalistic practice of a skill
Role Play	Boxed	(theater masks)	Rehearsal of a dialogue or interaction
Practice Assignment	Boxed	(house)	Homework for child or parent
End on a Positive	Main heading	☺	A reminder to end with some fun, rewarding activity or conversation
Brief the Family	Main heading	(people)	A reminder to review session contents with parents
CHECKLIST	Underlined heading	✓	A therapist review tool that prompts consideration of how successful the module was
DON'T FORGET!	Underlined heading	(pointing hand)	Important things to remember that sometimes can be overlooked
THINGS TO CONSIDER	Underlined heading	(i)	Details about ideas to try or about implementation under special circumstances
DIAGNOSTIC ISSUES	Underlined heading	(clipboard)	A guide for how to tailor interventions to specific diagnoses
TROUBLESHOOTING	Underlined heading	?	A guide for what to do if things are not working
WHAT'S THE EVIDENCE?	Underlined heading	(grid)	A summary of the evidence supporting a particular module

MAKING A FEAR LADDER

★ Objectives

The objective for this module is to construct a list of feared items that will form the basis for exposure exercise to come. This module is one of the "core four" modules.

⏱ If Pressed for Time

The priorities for this module are (1) to establish a list of feared items and (2) to avoid raising too much anxiety or concern about the items. It is less important that these items are all copied onto a form or sorted in an organized manner, because this can be done later. Also, there is no need to go into detail about how these items will be used for later practice. In fact, it might be better just to describe the fear ladder as a way to measure one's anxiety or fear level. If the child is having difficulty with this exercise, the fear ladder can be developed slowly over multiple sessions or meetings.

✉ Who Is Needed

Child
Parent(s), if possible

✏ Materials

Fear Ladder (parent and child)
Fear Thermometer
Index cards
Assessment materials from recent assessment (if possible)

[1] Set the Agenda

Meet with the child alone and talk with him or her about the various ideas and exercises you plan to cover in your meeting. Make sure these items are spelled out in order, with approximate time limits given for how long each part might take. This information will add to the predictability of the meeting and minimize uncertainty for the child. Ask the child if he or she has any issues to cover, and put these on the agenda as well. It can be helpful to write these items on a dry erase board or easel pad to serve as a visual reminder. Finally, be sure to point out that there will be an opportunity for a rewarding or fun activity at the end of the meeting.

🗪 Procedures

1. Continue to meet with the child alone. Emphasize the importance of being as honest and as thorough as possible. Explain that making a **Fear Ladder** is one of the most important parts of working together, and the better you do on this task together, the better the child will do with his or her anxiety.

🕯 Example

The work we are going to do today is really important. The better we do on this today, the more successful we will be in making the fear go away.

---

2. Make sure that the child is familiar with the use of the **Fear Thermometer**. You may need to practice once or twice with sample anchors to make sure that the child is giving accurate ratings. It is particularly important that the child be able to use the full range of the scale, not just the ends.
3. Next, you will work together to establish a list of feared stimuli within the domain of the primary diagnosis or main problem area. For example, if social phobia is the primary concern, the list should contain only socially related items. If the primary problem is panic disorder, the list should contain only cues related to the panic disorder. (Other problem areas should be targeted subsequently using a new **Fear Ladder**).

🕯 Example

Let's try to think of as many parts of this problem that make you feel afraid, scared, or nervous. What are some of the things that you can tell me?

---

4. Staying within the selected domain, identify as many feared stimuli as possible (e.g., situations, cues, sensations, obsessions). If targeting a discrete phobia (e.g., specific phobia or discrete social phobia), try to attempt as many gradations of the particular stimulus as possible. Otherwise, just generate a diversity of items, but always stay within the general target domain (i.e., stick to things that will be the target of treatment).
5. As you agree on each item, write it down on an index card and put it aside. Continue the process until you feel you have exhausted the domain.
6. If you do not have at least 10 items, consider the following options: (a) go back through the assessment or intake materials together to identify other items the child may have forgotten (e.g., many structured interviews have checklists for symptoms and cues); and/or (b) try to come up with variations of items already identified. This latter approach can be done by changing small features of the stimulus/situation (e.g., more/fewer people around, stimulus more/less proximal, escape more/less difficult).

⚡ Examples

- How would it be different if there were lots of other boys or girls around?
- What if you were not allowed to call home from school, even when you felt scared?

7. Once you have at least 10 items (the more the better), read them one by one to the child, each time getting a rating using the **Fear Thermometer**. Write down the rating on the card.

8. Once the child has rated each card, sort the cards in order of the fear ratings. If you do not have one card rated at almost every scale level from 2 to 9, go back to steps 4–6 (especially 6b) to generate items that fit into the missing scale points. The idea is to have a range of items with differing intensity levels.

9. *Praise the child* for doing well on this important task. Explain that you will now meet alone with his or her parent(s) for a few moments and then you will all meet together.

10. Shuffle the cards so that they are no longer in the order of the child's ratings.

11. Meet with the parent(s) alone. Make sure the parent(s) is familiar with the **Fear Thermometer**. *Without letting the parent know the child's ratings*, read each item and get a parent rating. Write down parent ratings on the card for each item, making sure to distinguish these ratings from the child ratings (e.g., circle all the parent ratings). If both parents are present and they disagree with each other, have them work together to come up with a number on which they agree.

12. Ask the parent(s) if there are any other stimuli or situations that he or she feels you or the child omitted. Write those items down on cards, and get parent ratings for those as well.

13. Bring the child into the session (everyone should be together at this point). If the parent(s) has added any new items, get fear ratings from the child for those final items.

14. Now you will need to select the items that will go on the ladder and be used to guide subsequent exposure exercises. Choose 10–12 items that (a) translate relatively easily into exposure or role-play exercises, and (b) suggest a logical sequence or progression of these exercises. Seek input from parent(s) or child when you are unclear about specific properties of an item being considered (e.g., how readily it can be practiced, if it is too similar to another item already on the ladder). In some rare cases, you will be forced to choose fewer than 10 items, but first be sure you have been as thorough as possible at steps 4–6.

15. If there is a very large number of cards, it helps to sort them into piles by "themes" when creating the ladder. For example, with social anxiety, try to put all the cards related to assertiveness together, then all the cards related to speaking in public, then all the cards related to conversations, etc. The number within each pile can then be reduced by taking out things that are too similar in content or severity. For example, it is best to keep for later practice exercises items within a theme that are different in severity rating or different enough in content to be important.

16. *Praise the child* again and thank the parent(s).

☺ End on a Positive

End the session on a fun note with a game, activity, or other exercise that will leave the child feeling positive about the work you have done together today. With younger children, be sure to provide extra praise for cooperative behavior during the meeting.

☞ DON'T FORGET!

- After the session is over, you will need to copy the items selected in steps 14 and 15 (but not the ratings) onto a blank child **Fear Ladder**. Items should be listed from highest to lowest intensity, according to the child's ratings. Copy these same items, without changing the order, onto the parent Fear Ladder. Make about 10 photocopies of each of the forms. Select one child and one parent form, date the forms, and enter the respective child and parent ratings from the index cards. Save the additional copies for future assessment.
- Each week (more or less frequently, depending on the need for feedback about progress), distribute an unrated, dated copy of the **Fear Ladder** to parent(s) and child before beginning a session and ask them to provide current ratings. Parent(s) and child should work independently to complete the forms, just as they did when the ladder was constructed. (If the child is over 12, it may not be necessary to have parent(s) contribute ratings.) Take the completed forms with you into the session. These will provide useful information about habituation patterns and formulation of homework exercises. If meetings are infrequent, the Fear Ladder can be completed over the phone, taken to school, or faxed to school.

✔ CHECKLIST

If two or more of the following items cannot be checked off, consider what problems may have arisen. Portions of the module might need to be repeated, or troubleshooting might be indicated to determine how to overcome or compensate for any challenges encountered.

_____ A **Fear Ladder** was constructed.

_____ Ratings were taken on the items, and the ratings showed acceptable range (not all too low or too high).

_____ Child understood that the **Fear Ladder** is a tool used to measure changes in anxiety.

_____ Child understood that the **Fear Ladder** would be used regularly to evaluate progress in overcoming fears and anxiety.

_____ A fun activity or positive time together was shared at the end of the meeting.

THINGS TO CONSIDER

- This is often the first session with the child, so care must also be taken to build rapport with the child and family. Be sure to provide extra praise and encouragement, and if possible, allow for some time in the session to get to know the child better. Particularly for younger children, working together on a game or a picture about his or her interests (e.g., family or hobbies) can facilitate this process. Some children with particularly high anxiety might need an entire session just devoted to getting acquainted. Such activities are not, however, a substitute for completing the Fear Ladder, and this eventual goal should be kept in mind.

DIAGNOSTIC ISSUES

- **Panic disorder with or without agoraphobia:** The items on the **Fear Ladder** should represent sensations and situations that cue panic attacks. It is important to realize that most children will not be forthcoming with information about feared sensations, so it is necessary at this point to ask what feelings a child might fear (e.g., feeling out of breath, holding breath, feeling dizzy, gagging, feeling lightheaded). These feared sensations will be induced via interoceptive exposure exercises in the **Practice:** *In vivo* module. If it is too difficult to determine which sensations provoke anxiety in the child, consider an interoceptive assessment session prior to completing the **Fear Ladder**. This would involve the following exposure exercises modeled briefly and then performed by the child: spinning in a chair, holding breath for 30 seconds, running in place for 1 minute, using a tongue depressor, staring at a bright light for 15 seconds and then reading a passage of text. Other exercises that might induce feared sensations can be added at the therapist's discretion. After each exercise, separate ratings of the maximum intensity of the sensation and the maximum level of anxiety should be recorded.
- **Obsessive–compulsive disorder:** Obsessive–compulsive disorder (OCD) can produce some of the longest **Fear Ladders**. Because the practices for OCD are numerous and very frequent, it is advisable to allow the ladder to be somewhat longer than usual. For example, a ladder with 20–25 items would be acceptable.
- **Generalized anxiety disorder:** The items on the ladder for generalized anxiety disorder should focus as much as possible on feared consequences of the worry. For example, it is better to have an item such as "getting a bad grade" than "worrying about schoolwork" because the treatment program will be directly targeting the fears about the consequences through exposure and possible cognitive exercises.

? TROUBLESHOOTING

- **Ratings are not working (1):** One of the best ways to manage this problem is to recruit others who can provide better ratings (e.g., mother, teacher).
- **Ratings are not working (2):** Sometimes additional informants are difficult to identify.

Alternatively, they are available but provide ratings or data that are of no better quality than that of the child. For example, a father giving ratings about his son's worrying might find it difficult to gauge with any accuracy, particularly if these worries are fairly private and not discussed with the father. In such circumstances, it can be advisable to come up with a new index of progress. For example, in one case involving a child who would not eat solid food due to a fear of choking, we counted the number of seconds it took for the child to finish eating a standardized portion of food (e.g., two cookies). This rating was taken each week as a guide to overall progress, and individual ratings of Fear Ladder items were no longer taken.

WHAT'S THE EVIDENCE?

- In many controlled studies of successful treatments for anxiety, self-monitoring is used as a central part of the therapy program (e.g., Barrett, 1998; Barrett, Dadds, & Rapee, 1996; Cobham, Dadds, & Spence, 1998; Goenjian et al., 1997; Kendall, 1994; Kendall et al., 1997; King et al., 1998; Pediatric OCD Treatment Study Team, 2004; Silverman et al., 1999).

LEARNING ABOUT ANXIETY

★ Objectives

Objectives for this module are to educate the child about how anxiety works in order to build a rationale for exposure practice, to instill optimism about the child's situation, and to encourage participation in treatment. This module is one of the "core four" modules.

⊙ If Pressed for Time

The main focus of this module is to convey the ideas that anxiety is our body's two-stage alarm system, that it is therefore not always bad to experience anxiety, and that problematic anxiety is similar to a false alarm.

⊠ Who Is Needed

Child
Parent(s), if possible

✐ Materials

Feelings Worksheet (optional)
Anxiety and How It Works Worksheet (child or adolescent)

⌁ Weekly Rating

Obtain the **Fear Ladder** ratings from both the child and his or her parent(s). Inspect the Fear Ladder for unusually high or problematic items. These might need to be discussed during the meeting.

[1] Set The Agenda

Meet with the child alone and talk with him or her about the various ideas and exercises you plan to cover in your meeting. Make sure these are spelled out in order, with approximate time limits given for how long each part might take. This information will add to the predictability of the meeting and minimize confusion. Ask the child if he or she has any issues to cover, and put these on the agenda as well. It can be helpful to write these items on a dry erase board or easel pad to serve as a visual reminder. Finally, be sure to point out that there will be an opportunity for a rewarding or fun activity at the end of the meeting.

🗫 Procedures

1. Continue to meet with child alone. State that you will be talking about anxiety today and begin by asking the child for his or her definition of anxiety. Elicit other words that might mean the same thing as "anxiety." Praise the child's definitions and incorporate them into your own.

2. Explain to the child that anxiety has three parts to it. One part is what we feel when we are anxious (i.e., physiological sensations), such as rapid breathing, having our heart pound, having our muscles become all tense, or becoming shaky and sweaty. To assist with this idea, it may help some children to work with you on a picture. You can use the **Feelings Worksheet**, or you can have the child (or help the child) draw a human figure—simple is OK (the **Feelings Worksheet** has separate boy and girl drawings for this first exercise—only one needs to be filled out). Then, by asking lots of questions (and pointing to areas, if necessary), help the child label each area that feels different with anxiety.

↳ Example

Can you point to parts of the drawing where you get feelings of anxiety or being scared? Does this part ever get those feelings when you are scared? What other parts of your body let you know that you are scared? What feelings do you get here? [Etc.]

3. The second part to anxiety is what we think when we are anxious (i.e., cognitive symptoms), such as thinking that something horrible is about to happen. At this point, it is a good idea to do some exercises to make sure the child knows what a thought is. It may help to use the third page of the **Feelings Worksheet** or to draw some of your own cartoon characters with empty "thought clouds" over their heads, and ask the child what thoughts go in those clouds. Try to get examples of some anxious thoughts the child has had recently.

4. The third part to anxiety is what we do when we are anxious (i.e., behavioral symptoms), such as leaving or escaping from places that make us scared or nervous. Ask the child what kinds of things people do and what he or she does when scared. Go through several examples, if necessary. Provide plenty of praise. If you feel you have spent a lot of time on the information up until now, this can be a good place to stop for the day.

5. Point out that anxiety is an emotion that all people experience. One way that we can think about anxiety is as an alarm. Ask the child if he or she can think of any other kinds of alarms (e.g., fire alarms, burglar alarms). Ask him or her what these alarms do (i.e., warn us that something bad or dangerous might be about to happen). Praise the child's efforts to come up with examples of alarms and what they do.

> **⚓ Example**
>
> That's right! Alarms protect us. They prevent bad things from happening by letting us know about danger.

6. Explain that anxiety is the body's alarm system, a very special one. It is so well designed that it actually has two stages to it. The first is a warning that danger may be coming, and the second tells us that the danger is here.

> **⚓ Example**
>
> So anxiety acts as our own alarm system, and it has two stages. The first stage of the anxiety alarm is a warning that something bad might be about to happen. It can be just like a yellow light that says "watch out." Have you ever felt like you knew something bad was going to happen? Yes, that was your warning alarm.
>
> The second stage of our alarm system tells us that the danger is here right now. This stage would be like a red light, which tells us that there is real trouble.

7. Make sure that the child understands the difference between the "yellow light" warning stage and the "red light" danger stage of the alarm system by asking him or her to restate what you have just discussed. Give some examples, as follow:

> **⚓ Example**
>
> If I were really scared of dogs, and I thought I heard a dog barking, what kind of alarm would I feel? Would it be the warning or the real thing? What if a dog jumped on me?

8. Ask the child whether he or she thinks anxiety is good or bad. Elicit the reasons why the child thinks this way about anxiety. Praise the response and indicate that the child is right, but then ask whether anxiety could really be both good and bad.

> **⚓ Example**
>
> **Therapist:** So, do you think anxiety is a good thing or a bad thing?
>
> **Child:** Anxiety is bad.
>
> **Therapist:** Why is anxiety bad?
>
> **Child:** It makes us afraid.
>
> **Therapist:** You're right. Sometimes too much anxiety can make us afraid too often, and that can be a bad thing. But can anxiety sometimes be a good thing, too? What ways might anxiety be good for us?

9. If the child is uncertain about how anxiety might be good, use further questioning to arrive at the functional nature of anxiety. Ask the child what would happen if we did not have anxiety. Illustrate this point by asking the child what would happen if he or she tried to cross the street without looking (i.e., the child might get run over by a

car, but he or she would be very calm while this was happening!). Emphasize the point that anxiety can serve many functions, and that it is often a very good thing to have because it prevents us from getting into dangerous situations or getting hurt.

⚓ Example

Most often, anxiety acts as an alarm that alerts us to do things that will help protect us from danger. And what do alarms do? That's right: The purpose of an alarm is to keep you out of trouble.

---

10. Point out that, whereas anxiety can serve many positive functions, sometimes it is not so positive, such as when people experience false alarms. Ask the child if he or she knows what false alarms are. If the child is unable to answer this question, explain that false alarms are alarms that go off when there is actually nothing bad happening, such as when a fire alarm goes off, but there is really no fire. Make sure that the child understands the difference between a false and a true alarm. It may help to draw a picture of a house with a smoke alarm going off and no fire and another house with a fire, or a picture of a bank with a robber outside and another without. Ask which one has the real alarm and which one has the false alarm.

11. Explain that when people experience a false alarm, it feels as real as if the dangerous thing were actually there, because they have the same kinds of scary feelings that they would have if the danger were really present. Point out that a lot of times people have false alarms, and that they get scared and nervous when there is really no danger. It is when people begin to have a lot of false alarms that their anxiety has gotten out of control, and it is in these cases that anxiety becomes harmful.

12. Tell the child that one of the goals in working together will be to get rid of the extra, or harmful, anxiety but not the good anxiety. Because anxiety is a good thing in many ways, it is important not to get rid of the alarms altogether. We can learn to help control the false alarms. Explain that one good way to deal with anxiety is to learn to tell the difference between a true alarm and a false alarm. Ask the child how he or she would find out if his or her anxiety is a false alarm or not (answer: by testing the alarm to see if it is true or not).

⚓ Example

What would happen if the smoke alarm went off? What do the firemen do? Do they check for fire?

---

13. Using the child's own fear domain, inquire as to how one could conduct such a test of true and false alarms.

⚓ Example

What could you do when your anxiety alarm goes off to see if the danger is real? How could you find out if there is anything to hurt you?

14. If the child is uncertain, explain that the best test to see if an anxiety alarm is true or false is to:
    • "Put yourself in the scary situation—situations that you are avoiding now."
    • "See if scary thing that you think will happen actually does happen."
15. Use questioning with the child to make sure that he or she understands how putting him- or herself in the situation is a test of whether the anxiety alarm is true or not.
16. Continue with this line of discussion to arrive at the point that conducting these tests is why practice is so important (i.e., "It lets you know whether you are having a true or a false alarm"). Ask the child why he or she thinks that practice, in any area, might be important (answer: to get better at things).

✏ Example

Therapist: What if I tried to teach you how to play a piano, and I told you everything about the piano; what the names of all the keys were, what the black keys did and what the white keys did, and how many of each color there were on the keyboard. After I told you everything there is to know about the piano, would you be able to play the piano really well?

Child: No.

Therapist: Why not?

Child: Because I never played the piano before.

Therapist: That's right, you would have never actually played the piano yourself before. What else would you need to do so that you could play the piano really well?

Child: Practice.

Therapist: And why would that be important?

Child: Because the only way to get better at things is to keep practicing them over and over again.

Other examples can be incorporated into the above discussion that are more applicable to the child, such as playing basketball or swimming, preferably something the child is skilled at and about which the child is not anxious. Use the above style of questioning to arrive at the point that the same principles that apply to learning how to play the piano or to play basketball are true for learning how to overcome unnecessary anxiety. Explain that only by practicing situations that make the child nervous right now will he or she be able to learn to control excess anxiety (the false alarms).

17. Indicate to the child that learning to control anxiety takes a lot of practice, and that there is no substitute for practice. Explain that practice will mean actually trying some of the things that the child is afraid of now, but that by doing these scary things, you and the child can test out whether his or her alarms are true or false

ones. Use examples to get the child to verbalize how something scary can be practiced, and how it can be practiced in a series of gradual steps.

18. Use questioning to arrive at the idea that practice can be gradual, and that small steps will be required until bigger ones can be taken.

✦ Example

Therapist: So, let's say I'm really scared of your dog [or something of which the child is not scared]. How would you make me less scared of your dog?

Child: I would tell you not to be afraid of it. I would tell you that my dog isn't scary.

Therapist: But how would you convince me that there is nothing to be afraid of about your dog?

Child: I would show you the dog and let you pet it.

Therapist: What if I was too afraid to pet it? What else would you do?

Child: I could get you to sit next to it.

Therapist: What if I was too afraid to sit next to it?

Child: Then maybe you could start off by just looking at it from far away.

---

19. Finally, introduce the idea of monitoring: Monitoring is like gathering clues or evidence.

✦ Example

Now, figuring out a problem like this can be like solving a mystery. What do detectives look for when solving a mystery? That's right—clues! We are going to work together to gather important clues to help us learn more about your anxiety. Sometimes when you practice, I will need you to write down some things (or your parents can help). This will tell us important things to help solve the mystery.

** Practice Assignment**

Remind the child about the **Fear Ladder** and how it will be used to gather clues, and explain that other forms will be added to help gather more ideas later. Give the child the **Feelings Worksheet** to complete at home. Explain that you will go over it together next time you meet.

☺ End on a Positive

End the session on a fun note with a game, activity, or other exercise that will leave the child feeling positive about the work you have done together today. With younger children, be sure to provide extra praise for cooperative behavior during the meeting.

Brief the Family

At the end of the session, it is helpful to meet with the parent(s). However, you should first ask the child if there is anything that he or she told you today that he or she does *not* want you to tell the parent(s). Be sure to honor the child's privacy within the appropriate limits of safety.

Have the child explain to the parent what concepts he or she has learned in the meeting today. You can add information as necessary, but try to allow the child to do as much of the work as possible. Provide plenty of praise and encouragement; this period with the parent(s) and child together is an ideal time to model for the parent(s) how to encourage and praise the child's behaviors. The main goal of this portion of the module is to familiarize the parent(s) with the concepts (as well as providing a good review for the child), so that the parent(s) can assist the child at home with using the new concepts and tools introduced in the therapy sessions.

 DON'T FORGET!

- Make sure that the child takes home the **Feelings Worksheet**.
- If your next module is the Learning about Anxiety—Parent Module, there is a chance the parent(s) might meet with you without the child. It can be helpful to ask about this arrangement beforehand, and if the child will not attend, make sure an extra Fear Ladder sheet is given to the child to take home and complete for the next meeting. The parent can then bring it to you next time.

✔ **CHECKLIST**

If two or more of the following items cannot be checked off, consider what problems may have arisen. Portions of the module might need to be repeated, or troubleshooting might be indicated to determine how to overcome or compensate for any challenges encountered.

____ The child understood the three parts of anxiety.

____ The child understood that anxiety is the body's natural alarm system.

____ The child understood that the alarm system has two "stages."

____ The child understood that too much anxiety is like a "false alarm."

____ The child understood the value of practice.

____ The child understood the strategy of taking measurements of anxiety to gather clues.

____ A fun activity or positive time together was shared at the end of the meeting.

(i) THINGS TO CONSIDER

- Many of the ideas in this module will be too challenging for some children. This module is often delivered in two sessions or more. If the child has difficulty with some aspects, it may be necessary to simplify the lessons, proceed more slowly, or cover only the basic parts. The most important steps in this module are the three parts of anxiety (steps 2–4) and the importance of practice and monitoring (steps 14–17). On the other hand, for some (e.g., adolescents), it may be possible to go into more detail. For example, those with generalized anxiety disorder can learn about how their "yellow light" is often stuck on. Those with panic disorder or specific or social phobia can learn about how their "red light" goes off at the wrong times. The more children/adolescents can apply these lessons to their own experience, the more likely they will integrate and remember the information.
- For younger children, many concrete examples are helpful to convey these ideas. It may also be helpful to allow for breaks to maintain the child's attention, or again, to break the module into several sessions.
- If the avoidance associated with the anxiety is leading to severe impairment (e.g., missed school), it might be best to abbreviate some of the material in order to get to the Practice module as soon as possible. Some of these concepts can be addressed later, once the avoidance is alleviated somewhat.

? TROUBLESHOOTING

- **"This feels like school"**: If the child feels the material is too boring or complicated, one option is to leave out much of the extra detail. The therapist should attempt to gauge the level of the child's aptitude and curiosity and should simply cover material in a way that is appropriate. This can mean leaving out entire pieces of the module or greatly simplifying their explanation. The therapist should also make sure that the child is having fun. If the therapist is doing too much of the talking, that is probably a sign that the material should be simplified and that the therapist should be more interactive or use Socratic questioning to keep the child interested. Remember that lots of praise, high-fives, and other reinforcers will keep the child focused on learning. Finally, recall that modules can be covered in multiple sessions, so if a child is getting the material and enjoying it but time is still running short, then it is best to cover this module over more than one session.
- **Missing the rationale**: If the child is missing the point of the exercises, then the therapist should make an effort to sharpen the focus. The function of this module is to set the stage for exposure, which is usually accomplished through two broad steps. The first involves normalizing anxiety, and the second involves describing the program and its rationale. Even if a child does not understand the alarm metaphors, he or she should understand that practice "makes things easier." With that knowledge in mind, it makes sense that what the child and therapist will do together is to practice until things get easier. One should not proceed to practice unless the child has some basic understanding of its benefits.

WHAT'S THE EVIDENCE?

- In many controlled studies of successful treatments for anxiety, psychoeducation with the child is used to prior to, or as part of, the main therapy procedures (e.g., Barrett, 1998; Barrett et al., 1996; Cobham et al., 1998; Cohen et al., 2004; De Haan, Hoogduin, Buitelaar, & Keijsers, 1998; Kendall, 1994; Kendall et al., 1997; King et al., 1998; King et al., 2000; Muris, Merckelbach, Holdrinet, & Sijsenaar, 1998; Öst, Svensson, Hellström, & Lindwall, 2001; Pediatric OCD Treatment Study Team, 2004; Silverman et al., 1999).

LEARNING ABOUT ANXIETY— PARENT MODULE

★ Objectives

Concurrent with, or immediately following, the presentation of the Learning about Anxiety module for children, some principles of practice and exposure can also be reviewed with parents. The main objectives are to build alliance with the parent(s) in order to build confidence in the intervention and solicit involvement with practice assignments to come. This particular review can be lengthened or abbreviated, as appropriate. Some parents will benefit from lots of time and detail, whereas others may only need the **About Anxiety Parent Handout** given to them and explained.

⏱ If Pressed for Time

The main focus of this module is to ensure that the parent(s) has a good understanding of the rationale for the therapy approach, and that he or she understands the importance of his or her involvement in the work that lies ahead.

✉ Who Is Needed

Parent(s)
Teacher(s), if indicated

✏ Materials

About Anxiety Handout (parent, teacher, or both)
Principles of Success Handout

🌡 Weekly Rating

Obtain the **Fear Ladder** ratings from the parent(s) and the child, if available. Inspect the Fear Ladder for unusually high or problematic items. These might need to be discussed during the meeting.

1 Set the Agenda

Meet with the parent(s) and talk about the various ideas and exercises you plan to cover in your session. Make sure that these are spelled out in order, with approximate time limits given for how long each part might take. This information will add to the predictability of the meeting and minimize confusion. Ask the parent(s) if he or she has any issues to cover and put these on the agenda as well. It can be helpful to write these items on a dry erase board or easel pad to serve as a visual reminder.

Procedures

1. Meet with the parent(s) alone and provide plenty of praise and reassurance.

> **Example**
>
> First of all, I want to thank you for meeting with me today. It is really clear that you are concerned about your child, and that you are interested in doing everything you can to help make things better. We are going to talk about some things today that I think can help provide a few extra strategies for you as a parent that can help your child overcome his or her challenges with anxiety.

2. Next, engage in a brief discussion of what does *not* work for anxiety. Basically, explain that although anxiety is fairly common in children, there are very few strategies that have been proven to help with anxiety problems. For example, telling a child "just relax" or explaining that his or her anxiety is unnecessary or does not make sense will not help. Also, with the exception of insignificant worries, "talking it out" has never been shown to help with any anxiety problems. Another common approach, "getting to the origin of the fears," has not been show to help reduce anxiety, either. This information might be somewhat surprising, due to misleading portrayals of therapy on television and in movies. Explain to the parent(s) that what all this means is that you will *not* be "talking it out" with the child and you will *not* be "searching for the root of the fears." It is very important that parents understand that those types of approaches are not likely to help.

> **Example**
>
> Have you ever been really worried about something and had someone tell you "just relax"? Did it make you relax? Why not? That's right, it is not that simple! You see, one of the things we have learned is that just talking about worries or telling people to relax doesn't really show them how to get started. So what we would like to try will be a bit different than just "talking it out" or saying "just relax."

3. Follow with an explanation of what *does* work. One of the only things that has been shown to help anxiety problems in children is *practice*: that is, practicing having the

fear and discovering that nothing bad happens. Ask the parent to give an example of how someone who is scared of something could get used to it by practicing (e.g., "Have you ever known someone who was scared to fly in airplanes? How would he or she get over that fear?"). Be sure to point out that practice involves getting used to something and learning that it is safe. Praise the parent(s) for good examples.

4. Explain that your job, then, is not to be just a listener but also a coach. Use an example from sports or exercise to explain how the coach's job is to (a) make sure practice is goal directed (e.g., children are not asked to stand around with a basketball during practice, they are asked to dribble or shoot baskets); (b) ensure that practice is safe (e.g., coaches make sure that children are warmed up and don't do anything that is too strenuous or extreme); and (c) keep the athlete feeling interested in practice (e.g., coaches often give pep talks, especially when practice is hard or things are not going well for a few days). This is what you will do as a therapist: plan, organize, supervise, troubleshoot, and give feedback about practice. If things are getting in the way of practice, your job is to help make practice easier.

5. Explain that another important goal is for the parent(s) to become the coach as quickly as possible. To the extent possible, the parent(s) will be asked to learn how to do all the practice exercises with the child, and to learn how to fix problems that arise. As soon as the parent(s) can start to take over, the therapist backs away a bit, providing support only when needed. Eventually, the family will be able to do all the practice without help and won't need the therapist any more. Remind the parent(s) that this is an active approach to treatment, and that children always do better when their parent(s) participates actively.

✎ Example

So remember, your child and I won't just be talking about how he [or she] feels each week. I am going to teach him [or her] skills to learn and practice, skills that you can help with, too. We are doing it this way because we don't know of anything else that has been shown to help with anxiety.

6. Explain why anxiety works this way by reviewing its nature. As you did with the child, point out that anxiety is an emotion that all people experience. One way that we can think about anxiety is as an *alarm*. In most cases, that alarm is helpful and protects us from danger. Ask the parent(s) to imagine what people would do if they felt no anxiety (the parent(s) should be guided to provide an answer that suggests that those people would not be able to avoid danger and would experience trouble). Then point out that, in the child's situation, the alarm is a little too sensitive—it goes off sometimes when it should not. Explain that the goal of therapy is to make sure that the child is better able to tell which fears are real and which dangers are only *false alarms*. The goal is not to help the child get rid of *all* anxiety, but rather to have him or her experience anxiety only when it is appropriate. Mention to the parent(s) that you will provide a handout explaining more about how anxiety works. (It is better to give the handout at the end of the meeting, not at this point.)

7. Answer any questions at this point and incorporate answers into the model of anxiety reviewed so far.

8. Introduce information about what makes treatment successful. Point out that we also believe we know about what makes practice work better for some children than for others.

♭ Example

So, we know how anxiety works, and we know why practice is important. Is there anything else that we need to know? We should also want to know what is the *best way* to practice, right?

---

9. At this point, you can give the parent(s) the **Principles of Success Handout**. Review the following principles:
   - In-session work is less important than homework. What happens at home and school is more important than what happens with the therapist. Just like with music lessons, the therapist just reviews progress and assigns more things to practice. If the child does not practice in-between meetings with the therapist, little progress will be made.
   - The therapist and parents are coaches. Things work best if parents take over an increasingly larger part of the coaching role as treatment proceeds.
   - Treatment works best if it is a high priority to the child and parent; if all are not committed to the program, results will not be so good. For now, the program might have to come first before other things such as school plays, sports, weekend trips, etc. One good thing, though, is that this approach is short term, so it usually only has to be a priority for a few months.
   - A minimum level of commitment is required. When a child's enthusiasm is low, the parent's enthusiasm must be extra high; similarly, if a parent's enthusiasm is low, the enthusiasm of the child must be very high. Refer to the illustration on the handout.
   - It is important to be willing to allow things to be hard in the short term so that life can be easier in the long term. For example, although the parent(s) could drop off their child at a place to have fun, leaving the child in a good mood afterward, the long-term anxiety problems won't go away. On the other hand, with extra work now, anxiety problems can be better later. This means that therapy will *not* necessarily involve doing only what makes the child most comfortable.
   - Things go better if the parent(s) remembers that practicing is safe and does not "rescue" the child from doing so. For example, sometimes a child might cry or complain during some of the practices. This response is perfectly normal, and the parent(s) should try to help his or her child "stick it out" in the tough situation and get used to whatever is difficult now. It is all right to be supportive, but it is not a good idea to stop the practice just because it is hard.
   - Child and parent willingness to meet with and speak on the phone with the therapist is extremely important. Without that, there is little chance of success.
   - When the parent(s) is anxious, treatment can often be more difficult; this is why

the therapist is the coach in the beginning and decides which pace is best for the child.

- Finally, it is common for many of these exercises to be difficult, and it is OK for families to talk about what is getting in the way of therapy. Parents who talk about what is not working for them and their family do better than families who are having trouble but don't tell anyone about it. Remember, the therapist is there to help solve problems, even with issues such as poor attendance, lack of enthusiasm, and doubts about progress.

10. Answer any questions at this time and provide the parent(s) with the **About Anxiety Handout** to take home.

☞ DON'T FORGET!

- Make sure that the parent takes home the **About Anxiety Handout**.

✔ CHECKLIST

If one or more of the following items cannot be checked off, consider what problems may have arisen. Portions of the module might need to be repeated, or troubleshooting might be indicated to determine how to overcome or compensate for any challenges encountered.

- ____ The parent understood the value of practice.
- ____ The parent understood the role of therapist and parents as coaches.
- ____ The parent understood the importance of his or her involvement in the program.
- ____ The parent had a chance to ask questions and have his or her concerns addressed and understood.

ⓘ THINGS TO CONSIDER

- Therapists should be careful when discussing commitment and motivation with families, so as to avoid suggesting that family members are "not interested" in the child's progress. Many families are motivated to see their children improve, but they do not have the time or resources to help make that improvement happen. A better approach is to describe that treatment must be an important goal for both the parent and the child, using the words "high priority" instead. The parent(s) should be encouraged to inform the therapist if they (i.e., child and parent) are not finding enough time to practice outside of session, as well as to discuss any other difficulties they are having with treatment as such difficulties arise.
- Try to discuss parents' roles in the anxiety problems in a nonblaming manner. Parents are often involved in the problem but should be viewed as respected resources with the most power and access to address the problems at hand.
- This is also a good time to encourage as many questions as possible from the parent(s)

about treatment. It is important to be sure that the parent(s) understands how things are going to work.

? TROUBLESHOOTING

- **Too much detail**: If the material is too detailed, remember that it is OK to simplify.
- **"Exposure seems too unpleasant for my child"**: If the parent(s) is uncomfortable with the idea of exposure, reassure him or her that anxiety is not harmful, and that the exposure exercises are carefully designed to optimize success and corrective learning.

WHAT'S THE EVIDENCE?

- In many controlled studies of successful treatments for anxiety, psychoeducation with the caretaker(s) is used prior to, or as part of, the main therapy procedures (e.g., Barrett, 1998; Barrett et al., 1996; Cobham et al., 1998; Cohen et al., 2004; De Haan et al., 1998; Kendall, 1994; Kendall et al., 1997; King et al., 1998; King et al., 2000; Pediatric OCD Treatment Study Team, 2004; Spence, Donovan, & Brechman-Toussaint, 2000).

PRACTICE: *IN VIVO*

★ Objectives

Objectives for this module are to review any practice exercises, troubleshoot their results, and introduce and perform new practice exercises, as needed. Practices should be conducted so as to allow habituation to occur, as evidenced by a decrease in fear ratings. This module (along with Practice: Imaginal) is one of the "core four" modules, and it is typically repeated throughout treatment until all ratings for feared items are sufficiently reduced.

⏱ If Pressed for Time

Have the child pick a feared situation or stimulus and practice exposure to it. The exercise should be set up to allow habituation to occur, and there should be a review of success.

✉ Who Is Needed

Child
Parent(s), if possible

✎ Materials

Fear Thermometer
Fear Ladder
Practice Record (discrete or continuous)
Practice Handout (parent, teacher, or both), if not given out already

🌡 Weekly Rating

Obtain the **Fear Ladder** ratings from both the child and parent(s). Inspect the Fear Ladder for unusually high or problematic items; these might need to be discussed during the meeting.

Assignment Review

Review any practice assignments that were given in the previous session. Discuss what was learned and consider rehearsing pieces of the homework together to consolidate the information. If the assignment was not completed, troubleshoot reasons why and consider the various options for handling whatever the obstacle might be. In all but the rarest of circumstances, do not proceed to new material if the assignment is not complete. It is better to take the planned session to perform the assignment together or to problem-solve how to accomplish it at home.

1 Set The Agenda

Meet with the child alone and talk about the various ideas and exercises you plan to cover in your meeting. Make sure these are spelled out in order, with approximate time limits given for how long each part might take. This information will add to the predictability of the meeting and minimize confusion. Ask the child if he or she has any issues to cover and put these on the agenda as well. It can be helpful to write these items on a dry erase board or easel pad to serve as a visual reminder. Finally, be sure to point out that there will be an opportunity for a rewarding or fun activity at the end of the meeting.

Procedures

1. Continue to meet with the child alone. If this is the first time starting exposure practice, review the fact that this next phase of treatment involves practicing in order to build new skills for coping with anxiety.
2. Assist the child in choosing a situation from his or her **Fear Ladder**—easy ones at first, harder ones later.

 In Vivo

Ask the child to visualize the situation and define overt behavioral goals for it (e.g., initiating a conversation, being in the room with a dog). If necessary, discuss and modify the goal so that it is not so hard that the child will refuse. Remember that small steps are OK. Goals can always be made easier to get the process started.

To the extent possible, practice the exposure together. If the situation is too unusual or difficult, the practice may need to be role-played or acted out. These challenges can also be addressed by conducting sessions in the location of the feared stimuli (e.g., child's home, the mall, school). If the exposure will involve discrete trials of behaviors, such as holding the breath or asking someone a question, it is best to use the **Discrete Practice Record**. For extended or continuous behaviors, such as standing in a dark room, giving a speech, or touching a feared object, it is best to use the **Continuous Practice Record**. Date the **Practice Record**, and write the name of the practice item in the leftmost empty space. Before the beginning, get a rating on the **Fear Thermometer** and record it on the appropriate **Practice Record**. During discrete exposure practice, take fear ratings only before and after each trial. During continuous exposure practice, take additional fear ratings at about 1-minute intervals during the exercise (intervals can be longer if the exposure might run longer than 15–20 minutes).

Continue the exposure until the fear rating is a 3 or less for items starting at a 5 or above, 1 or less for items starting at 4 or below, or until 30 minutes has elapsed. When finished, draw lines to connect the values within each trial and to connect the "before" values across trials.

If fear levels decreased during the exposure, ask the child what happened to his or her anxiety. Ask if the feared consequences occurred or if anything bad happened. Use the **Practice Record** to demonstrate that the anxiety did indeed go down over time.

If the fear did not decrease, point out that the child endured the anxiety without quitting and that the feared consequences did not occur.

❧ Example

You did a great job! And did anything really terrible happen to you? Nice job being so brave!

3. If there is time (if exposure was only 5–10 minutes), repeat the practice exercise again after a short break. Ask the child if he or she noticed that the second time was easier in any way.
4. Offer plenty of praise for the success, even if it is very small.

🏠 Practice Assignment

Assign daily exposure homework by filling out a new **Practice Record** (discrete or continuous, depending on the item to be practiced). Write the appropriate instructions and item names at the top (child should stop when fear rating is 3 or less for items starting at 5 or above, 1 or less for items starting at 4 or below, or until about 30 minutes has elapsed), and instruct the child to practice once every day or every other day, at a minimum.

Explain the **Practice Record** and its use, remembering to tie it back in with the idea of a detective solving a mystery. If the form is too difficult for the child to use, have the parents assist. It may be necessary to give parents a demonstration of how to use the form by doing a "mini-practice" together.

☺ End on a Positive

End the session on a fun note with a game, activity, or other exercise that will leave the child feeling positive about the work you have done together today. With younger children, be sure to provide extra praise for cooperative behavior during the meeting.

Brief the Family

At the end of the session, it is helpful to meet with the parent(s). However, you should first ask the child if there is anything that he or she told you today that he or she does *not* want you to tell the parent(s). Be sure to honor the child's privacy within the appropriate limits of safety.

Have the child explain to the parent(s) what concepts he or she has learned in the meeting today. You can add information as necessary, but try to allow the child to do as much of the work as possible. Provide plenty of praise and encouragement; this time with the parent(s) and child together is an ideal time to model for the parent(s) how to encourage and praise the child's behaviors. The main goal of this portion of the module is to familiarize the parent(s) with the concepts (as well as providing a good review for the child), so that the parent(s) can assist the child at home with using the new concepts and tools introduced in the therapy sessions.

⚡ Example

Now, figuring out a problem like this can be like solving a mystery. What do detectives look for when solving a mystery? That's right—clues! Each time you practice, you will be gathering important clues to help us learn more about your anxiety. That's why it is so important that you write them down.

☝ DON'T FORGET!

- Make sure that the family takes home enough **Practice Records**.

✓ CHECKLIST

If two or more of the following items cannot be checked off, consider what problems may have arisen. Portions of the module might need to be repeated, or troubleshooting might be indicated to determine how to overcome or compensate for any challenges encountered.

_____ The child practiced exposure to a feared stimulus or situation.

_____ Habituation was observed *within* practice trials, as measured by the fear ratings on the **Discrete** or **Continuous Practice Record**.

_____ Habituation was observed *between* practice trials (i.e., initial ratings went down each time a new trial began), as measured by the fear ratings on the **Discrete** or **Continuous Practice Record**.

_____ The child appeared to recognize the experience as a success.

_____ A fun activity or positive time together was shared at the end of the meeting.

(i) THINGS TO CONSIDER

- Practice should progress from easy items to more challenging items across sessions.
- If there is no habituation within practice sessions, consider making practice sessions longer.
- If there is habituation within practice sessions but not between practice sessions, consider making sessions more frequent.
- It is OK to add new items to the **Fear Ladder** if new ones arise.
- If the exposure is being conducted with a child who has had sessions involving cognitive techniques (e.g., STOP), then it can be helpful to have the child precede the exposure exercise by stating his or her anxious thoughts and going through the practice of restructuring or coming up with alternative thoughts. Following the practice, review with the child which thoughts proved to be true: the nervous thoughts or the restructured thoughts.

DIAGNOSTIC ISSUES

- If the exposure is being conducted with a child with OCD, be sure to explain the importance of refraining from the compulsions during and after the exercises. This may require asking the child periodically about whether he or she has performed the ritual or has had urges to do so, particularly in the instance of covert or cognitive rituals. Following the exercise, provide lots of praise for response prevention. Be sure to explain that the same rules for response prevention apply when practicing at home as well.

? TROUBLESHOOTING

- **No within-trial habituation**: If the child's ratings do not decrease during a practice exercise, consider longer trials, or if that is not possible, start with easier items.
- **No between-trial habituation**: If the child's beginning ratings do not decrease across practice exercises, consider more trials that are not spaced as far apart in time.
- **Child will not initiate the exposure practice**: Pick an easier item to practice or consider using rewards if there are no easier items to practice.
- **Child cannot expand on the practice**: If the child cannot seem to generalize the gains and show new behaviors (e.g., engages in the exact same conversation each time there is a social anxiety exposure), try introducing a "novelty requirement" in which part of the exposure is to improvise or expand on an initial behavior.
- **Dependence on a model**: Sometimes, it helps to demonstrate or *model* the practice first. Most children will develop an ability to repeat the practice behavior performed by the model, but some will become dependent on that same person demonstrating it every time first. In such cases, having a different person model the behavior can help break the child's dependence on the original model, ultimately helping the child to perform the practices spontaneously.

- **Aversive consequences could occur in the natural setting**: If it is possible that something aversive other than feeling anxious could actually happen during a naturalistic exposure (e.g., getting teased by a peer), extend the in-session rehearsal to prepare for these consequences by making the consequences part of the exposure or using cognitive strategies to decatastrophize them. Also, clarify the goal—that is, make sure that the child knows the object of the exercise: to complete the behavior, not (1) to avoid being anxious or (2) to avoid being teased.

WHAT'S THE EVIDENCE?

- In dozens of controlled studies, exposure in its various forms has demonstrated superior treatment effects relative to active treatments or no-treatment control conditions (e.g., Chorpita, Vitali, & Barlow, 1996; Mann & Rosenthal, 1969; Menzies & Clarke, 1993; Öst et al., 2001; Ultee, Griffioen, & Schellekans, 1982).
- Exposure has been a component of more than 97% of evidence-based interventions (Chorpita & Southam-Gerow, 2006), and 100% of clinically tested CBT programs for anxious children.

PRACTICE: IMAGINAL

★ Objectives

Objectives for this module are to practice exposure to feared items and to allow habituation to occur. This module (along with **Practice: *In vivo***) is one of the "core four" modules and is often repeated throughout treatment until all ratings for feared items are sufficiently reduced.

⏰ If Pressed for Time

Have the child pick a feared situation or stimulus and practice exposure to it. The exercise should be set up to allow habituation to occur, and there should be a review of success.

✉ Who Is Needed

Child
Parent(s), if possible

✐ Materials

Imaginal exposure script
Blank audiotape
Tape recorder
Fear Ladder (ratings filled in)
Discrete Practice Record
Fear Thermometer
Practice Handout (parent, teacher, or both)

🌡 Weekly Rating

Obtain the **Fear Ladder** ratings from both the child and parent(s). Inspect the Fear Ladder for unusually high or problematic items; these might need to be discussed during the meeting.

Assignment Review

Review any practice assignments that were given in the previous session. Discuss what was learned and consider rehearsing pieces of the homework together to consolidate the information. If the assignment was not completed, troubleshoot reasons why and consider the various options for handling whatever the obstacle might be. In all but the rarest of circumstances, do not proceed to new material if the assignment is not complete. It is better to take the planned session to perform the assignment together or to problem-solve how to accomplish it at home.

[1] **Set the Agenda**

Meet with the child alone and talk about the various ideas and exercises you plan to cover in your meeting. Make sure these are spelled out in order, with approximate time limits given for how long each part might take. This information will add to the predictability of the meeting and minimize confusion. Ask the child if he or she has any issues to cover and put these on the agenda as well. It can be helpful to write these items on a dry erase board or easel pad to serve as a visual reminder. Finally, be sure to point out that there will be an opportunity for a rewarding or fun activity at the end of the meeting.

 Procedures

1. Meet with the child alone and go over the self-monitoring forms and the **Fear Ladder**; check that they have been filled out correctly. Discuss progress since the last contact. Check that the homework practice was performed. Discuss ways to resolve any problems that occurred and answer any questions.
2. Inform the child of the exposure item for this session and describe the course of the session. Answer any questions.

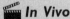 *In Vivo*

Begin the imaginal exposure by reading from the prepared script. The child should sit in a comfortable chair, with the **Fear Thermometer** before him or her. Instruct the child to allow him- or herself to feel as if the imaginal script were really occurring, as he or she would do when becoming involved in a good movie or book.

🕯 **Example**

Try to imagine the scene as clearly as you can. What color are the things around you? What kind of day is it? Try to picture as many of these things as you can, as if you were watching it on TV.

In Vivo (Continued)

Use a **Discrete Practice Record**, filling in the item and the date. Ask for a "before" fear rating. Start the tape and read the imaginal exposure script. At the conclusion of the script, pause the tape, obtain a fear rating, start the tape recording again, and reread the script.

If necessary, ask the child to delay any involved discussion until the end of the entire exercise.

If the child asks to abort the exposure, be sure to show empathy while stressing that sticking with it is the most effective way to decrease that anxiety. Sensitivity is needed in providing the child with information that will allow him or her to continue the exposure, without providing reassurance regarding the anxiety. Reassurance regarding the fears can potentially negate the effects of the exposure and will render imaginal exposure homework assignments more difficult for the child. (Very few children attempt to abort the exposure. Almost all children are able to complete the exposures without extensive reassurance.)

At the end of each reading of the scene, continue the exposure until the fear rating is 3 or less for items starting at 5 or above, 1 or less for items starting at 4 or below, or until 30 minutes has elapsed. When finished, draw lines to connect the values within each trial and to connect the "before" values across trials.

3. If fear levels decreased during the exposure, ask the child what happened to his or her anxiety. Ask if the feared consequences occurred or if anything bad happened. Use the **Discrete Practice Record** to demonstrate that the anxiety did indeed lessen over time.
4. If the fear did not decrease, point out that the child completed the exposure without quitting, despite high anxiety, and that the feared consequences did not occur.

Example

You did a great job, you were able to listen for all that time. And did anything really terrible happen to you? Nice job being so brave!

Practice Assignment

Discuss progress during the session, give the child the imaginal exposure tape, ask the child to return the tape at the next session, and assign daily exposure homework by filling out a new **Discrete Practice Record**. Write the appropriate instructions and item names at the top (child should stop when fear rating is 2 or less for items starting at 4 or above, 1 or less for items starting at 3 or below, or until about 30 minutes has elapsed), and instruct the child to practice once every day or every other day, at a minimum.

Explain the **Discrete Practice Record** and its use, remembering to tie it back in with the idea of a detective solving a mystery. If the form is too difficult for the child to use, have the parents assist. It may be necessary to give parents a demonstration of how to use the form by doing a "mini-practice" together.

> **↳ Example**
>
> Now, figuring out a problem like this can be like solving a mystery. What do detectives look for when solving a mystery? That's right—clues! Each time you practice, you will gather important clues to help us learn more about your anxiety. That's why it is so important that you write them down.

☺ End on a Positive

End the session on a fun note with a game, activity, or other exercise that will leave the child feeling positive about the work you have done together today. With younger children, be sure to provide extra praise for cooperative behavior during the meeting.

ᴪ Brief the Family

At the end of the session, it is helpful to meet with the parent(s). However, you should first ask the child if there is anything that he or she told you today that he or she does *not* want you to tell the parent(s). Be sure to honor the child's privacy within the appropriate limits of safety.

Have the child explain to the parent what concepts he or she has learned in the meeting today. You can add information as necessary, but try to allow the child to do as much of the work as possible. Provide plenty of praise and encouragement; this time with the parent(s) and the child is an ideal time to model for the parent(s) how to encourage and praise the child's behaviors. The main goal of this portion of the module is to familiarize the parent(s) with the concepts (as well as providing a good review for the child), so that the parent(s) can assist the child at home with using the new concepts and tools introduced in the therapy sessions.

☝ DON'T FORGET!

- Make sure that the family takes home enough **Discrete Practice Records**.

✔ CHECKLIST

If two or more of the following items cannot be checked off, consider what problems may have arisen. Portions of the module might need to be repeated, or troubleshooting might be indicated to determine how to overcome or compensate for any challenges encountered.

_____ The child practiced exposure to an imagined feared stimulus or situation.

_____ Habituation was observed within practice trials, as measured by the fear ratings on the **Discrete Practice Record**.

_____ Habituation was observed between practice trials (i.e., initial ratings went down each time a new trial began) as measured by the fear ratings on the **Discrete Practice Record**.

____ The child appeared to recognize the experience as a success.

____ A fun activity or positive time together was shared at the end of the meeting.

(i) THINGS TO CONSIDER

- Practice should progress from easy items to more challenging items across sessions.
- If there is no habituation within practice sessions, consider making practice sessions longer.
- If there is habituation within practice sessions but not between practice sessions, consider making sessions more frequent.
- It is OK to add new items to the **Fear Ladder** if new ones arise.
- If the exposure is being conducted with a child who has had sessions involving cognitive techniques (e.g., STOP), then it can be helpful to have the child precede the exposure exercise by stating his or her anxious thoughts and going through the practice of restructuring or coming up with alternative thoughts. Following the practice, review with the child which thoughts proved to be true: the nervous thoughts or the restructured thoughts.

DIAGNOSTIC ISSUES

- If the exposure is being conducted with a child with OCD, be sure to explain the importance of refraining from the compulsions during and after the exercises. This may require asking the child periodically about whether he or she has performed the ritual or has had urges to do so, particularly in the instance of covert or cognitive rituals. Following the exercise, provide lots of praise for response prevention. Be sure to explain that the same rules for response prevention apply when practicing at home as well.

? TROUBLESHOOTING

- **No within-trial habituation**: If the child's ratings do not decrease during a practice exercise, consider longer trials, or if that is not possible, start with easier items.
- **No between-trial habituation**: If the child's beginning ratings do not decrease across practice exercises, consider more trials that are not spaced as far apart in time.
- **Child will not initiate the exposure practice**: Pick an easier item to practice or consider using rewards if there are no easier items to practice.
- **Child cannot imagine**: If the child has difficulty participating in imaginal exercises (e.g., cannot relax, cannot picture scenes), it can be helpful to practice such exercises with pleasant imagery first. Being more relaxed initially can help the child to learn to

picture the images and focus on them. It can also help to ask questions about the imagery, such as "What color is the carpet?" "Are there other people nearby?" etc.

⊞ WHAT'S THE EVIDENCE?

- Imaginal exposure has proven superior to control groups in over 10 controlled clinical tests (Bandura et al., 1969; Barabasz, 1973; Bornstein & Knapp, 1981; Deffenbacher & Kemper, 1974; Johnson, Tyler, Thompson, & Jones, 1971; Kandel, Ayllon, & Rosenbaum, 1977; Laxer & Walker, 1970; Parish, Buntman, & Buntman, 1976; Saigh, 1986, 1987; Van Hasselt et al., 1979).

MAINTENANCE AND RELAPSE PREVENTION

★ Objectives

Objectives for this module are to demonstrate to the child that gains have been made, to review the skills that helped most, and to ensure that practice will continue after meetings with the therapist are over. It is possible that the child may have a few lingering fears at this point, but if he or she continues to practice after therapy has ended, additional improvements are expected. This module is one of the "core four" modules.

⏱ If Pressed for Time

The main objectives are to help the child take credit for success and to encourage continued practice.

✉ Who Is Needed

Child
Parent(s), if possible

✏ Materials

What I Took Back Worksheet
Building on Bravery Handout (parent, teacher, or both)

🌡 Weekly Rating

Obtain the **Fear Ladder** ratings from both the child and parent(s). Inspect the Fear Ladder for unusually high or problematic items; these might need to be discussed during the meeting.

📄 Assignment Review

Review any practice assignments that were given in the previous session. Discuss what was learned and consider rehearsing pieces of the homework together to consolidate the information. If the assignment was not completed, troubleshoot reasons why and consider the various options for handling whatever the obstacle might be. In all but the rarest of circumstances, do not proceed to new material if the assignment is not complete. It is better to take the planned session to perform the assignment together or to problem-solve how to accomplish it at home.

⎡1⎦ Set the Agenda

Meet with the child alone and talk about the various ideas and exercises you plan to cover in your meeting. Make sure these are spelled out in order, with approximate time limits given for how long each part might take. This information will add to the predictability of the meeting and minimize confusion. Ask the child if he or she has any issues to cover and put these on the agenda as well. It can be helpful to write these items on a dry erase board or easel pad to serve as a visual reminder. Finally, be sure to point out that there will be an opportunity for a rewarding or fun activity at the end of the meeting.

🗫 Procedures

1. Meet with the child alone and discuss and review some of the basic concepts from the Learning about Anxiety module and how this understanding fits his or her experience.
2. Make sure that the child is able to attribute gains to practice. Some children may benefit from working on a drawing to symbolize this progress; for example, a multipanel cartoon that involves the progression from anxiety to coping, with some scenes of the exposure in between.
3. Discuss the importance of continued exposure in everyday life. You can return to analogies of sports, exercise, or playing a musical instrument, etc., to make the point that without regular practice, people can get "rusty." Ask how the child thinks he or she will continue to challenge him- or herself day to day with "mini-practice" exercises.

🏋 Exercise

Complete the **What I Took Back Worksheet** by having the child first write all of the things that were difficult in the left column under the scary monster icon (for some adolescents, a simple two-column record would be appropriate). These can be items taken from the Fear Ladder and can refer to quality-of-life domains as well (e.g., family time, friends, hobbies). Then read each item to the child and ask, "Has this gotten better for you?" If the child answers "yes," have him or her cross it out and rewrite it in the second column. At the end of the exercise, most or all of the things should be under the right column. If any remain under the left column, ask the child how he or she plans to apply the same skills that worked for everything else to these areas. This is a great time for plenty of praise.

4. Bring parent(s) into session to discuss these same issues and have child explain the picture, if one has been completed. Review the **What I Took Back Worksheet** together.

5. Praise the child in front of the parent(s) and praise the parent(s) for his or her efforts as well. Make sure to point out that the progress was due primarily to the child and family's efforts, not to the therapist. It is important that the child take responsibility for the success that was experienced and attribute gains to his or her own effort.

6. Discuss the conceptions of a "lapse" and a "relapse." Explain that lapses are natural and involve minor steps backward. This discussion can involve the **What I Took Back Worksheet** by telling the child that some of the things in the right column might try to drift back to the left side. Remind the child that if that happens, these areas can simply be worked on with additional practice exercises. Lapses are more common during stressful times, and it is perfectly normal for some anxiety to return now and then or for some new stimulus to become the focus. This concept can be tied in with the Learning about Anxiety information regarding the idea that some anxiety is helpful. The goal is to avoid a "relapse": "Do not jump to the conclusion that you are back at square one and remember that all of the skills that you learned will always be a part of you. All you need to do is use them when some anxiety starts to bother you."

7. Talk with the family about how you will gradually decrease the number of sessions to a "checkup," progress review and question-and-answer every 2 weeks, and eventually down to once a month and then finishing. For some children, this progressive decrease in therapy may go quickly if they are successful at maintaining gains and implementing continued naturalistic exposure and if parent(s) have few questions about conducting and facilitating exposure. For others, the sessions may need to be tapered more gradually to allow time to facilitate generalization of gains.

8. Give the family the **Building on Bravery Handout**, if you have not already done so, and provide one for the teacher, if necessary.

9. On the session before the last, work with the child to plan a fun activity for the final session. This final session can involve snacks, playing a game, making a goodbye card, going for a walk (these interests and activities will differ widely by child and age). Use the last session to review concepts, answer questions, and say goodbye.

☞ DON'T FORGET!

- Make sure that the parent(s) and child take home any **Practice Records** or other materials they will need to work on their own.

✓ CHECKLIST

If two or more of the following items cannot be checked off, consider what problems may have arisen. Portions of the module might need to be repeated, or troubleshooting might be indicated to determine how to overcome or compensate for any challenges encountered.

____ The child was able to articulate basic concepts about anxiety.

____ The child attributes his or her gains to practice exercises.

____ The child sees the value of future practice exercises.

____ The child can articulate the domains of improved functioning by using the **What I Took Back Worksheet**.

____ The child and family understand the difference between "lapse" and "relapse."

____ The child and family intend to continue practice exercises after treatment ends.

____ A fun activity or positive time together was shared at the end of the meeting.

(i) THINGS TO CONSIDER

- It is a good idea to have the child make a tangible product to keep as a reminder of the work and to symbolize the gains made together. This can be a picture, a videotape or audiotape on which the child explains the value of the program, or some other creative work.

? TROUBLESHOOTING

- **Not taking credit**: If a child feels "lucky" that things are better or that the therapist should get the credit for his or her improvement, then the therapist should emphasize that the gains are attributable to the application of new skills and to the child's honest effort. This is best done Socratically—for example, "Do know why this has gotten so easy for you?"
- **Expecting CBT to end**: If the child seems convinced that things should return to life as usual, it may be important to point out that the skills obtained can be (should be) used now and in the future. The term "exposure lifestyle" is sometimes used to refer to a new way of identifying and handling the challenges that are encountered throughout life. An exercise metaphor is appropriate in this case: "Getting in shape" typically involves an intensive phase, but continuing a lifestyle of activity to stay in shape also requires consistent effort. Similarly, life after CBT is not as intensive as when learning and applying the new skills for the first time, but children and families should be able to monitor problematic anxiety and develop a plan to apply known skills as soon as is warranted.
- **Expecting perfection**: If children or parents feel that they are not doing well enough to end therapy, it can be helpful to raise the idea that it is an acceptable time to terminate when only 80% of the problems are successfully resolved. By design, it can be best to allow the remaining 20% of anxiety items to be worked on independently, so that there is a better chance of mastery and thus of maintaining future gains. Obvi-

ously, these are not magic numbers, but the idea makes sense that the child should terminate with at least one addressable challenge still in front of him or her.

⊞ WHAT'S THE EVIDENCE?

- In many controlled studies of successful treatments for anxiety, treatment typically concludes with a discussion of gains and how to maintain them (e.g., Barrett et al., 1998; Barrett, Dadds, & Rapee, 1996; Cobham et al., 1998; Cohen et al., 2004; De Haan et al., 1998; Kendall, 1994; Kendall et al., 1997; King et al., 1998; King et al., 2000; Pediatric OCD Treatment Study Team, 2004; Spence et al., 2000).
- Evidence generally favors the idea that getting individuals personally involved in an idea will increase the probability that they will adopt that idea (Petty & Cacioppo, 1984). Thus, getting children to discuss their gains and why treatment worked may help them maintain a positive attitude toward using their CBT skills after treatment has ended.

COGNITIVE RESTRUCTURING: PROBABILITY OVERESTIMATION

★ Objectives

Objectives for this module are to introduce the idea of thoughts and how they are related to anxiety, and to demonstrate a technique for correcting negative thinking. This module is typically used with older or more verbal children who frequently express overly negative or pessimistic ideas. This module is particularly important if the negative or pessimistic ideas appear to be interfering with a child's ability to engage in, or benefit from, exposure practice.

⏱ If Pressed for Time

Instill the notion that anxious thoughts are not always accurate and assign a basic strategy for how to test that accuracy.

✉ Who Is Needed

Child
Parent(s), if possible

✐ Materials

Two-Column and Five-Column Thought Records
Fear Ladder (for reference, as needed)

🌡 Weekly Rating

Obtain the **Fear Ladder** ratings from both the child and parent(s). Inspect the Fear Ladder for unusually high or problematic items; these might need to be discussed during the meeting.

📄 Assignment Review

Review any practice assignments that were given in the previous session. Discuss what was learned and consider rehearsing pieces of the homework together to consolidate the information. If the assignment was not completed, troubleshoot reasons why and consider the various options for handling whatever the obstacle might be. In all but the rarest of circumstances, do not proceed to new material if the assignment is not complete. It is better to take the planned session to perform the assignment together or to problem-solve how to accomplish it at home.

1 Set the Agenda

Meet with the child alone and talk about the various ideas and exercises you plan to cover in your meeting. Make sure these are spelled out in order, with approximate time limits given for how long each part might take. This information will add to the predictability of the meeting and minimize confusion. Ask the child if he or she has any issues to cover and put these on the agenda as well. It can be helpful to write these items on a dry erase board or easel pad to serve as a visual reminder. Finally, be sure to point out that there will be an opportunity for a rewarding or fun activity at the end of the meeting.

Procedures

1. Meet with the child alone and explain that you will be spending the next several sessions talking about different kinds of thoughts that make children feel upset, and that you will be teaching the child how to deal with these thoughts to make him- or herself feel better. Explain that these types of thoughts can be unpleasant and even scary, but that most children eventually feel better after learning the techniques you will be teaching.
2. Before beginning, make sure that the child has a clear understanding of what a thought is and how thoughts are distinguished from feelings. Introduce the idea that children's thoughts can cover a range of different topics, and that thoughts often include predictions about the future. Elicit some predictions of the future from the child to make sure that the child understands this concept, and praise him or her for these efforts.
3. Point out to the child that sometimes children predict that things will turn out well for them but at other times, they might predict that bad things will happen to them. Make sure that the child understands this distinction and elicit some examples of each. Let the child know that you want to focus on predictions that bad things will happen because many children predict that things will not turn out well when this is not always the case, and these are the kinds of thoughts that can make children feel upset.
4. Review the concept of probability. One way of explaining probability may be to provide different examples of events and ask the child which event is more or less likely to occur. For example, you might ask the child what the probability or chance is that he or she will get a cold in the next month, win the lottery, get a good grade on a test, or get a bad grade on a test. Have the child practice estimating the actual number. Using a continuum to mark probabilities from 0 to 100 can be helpful when teaching this skill. Point out that different events can be rated as being more or less likely to

occur, and that one of your goals is to help the child accurately estimate the probability of good and bad events. Elicit some examples of events and their probabilities, record these on the **Two-Column Thought Record**, and provide feedback if any probability estimates seem inappropriate.

5. Once the child understands the concept of probabilities, ask if he or she thinks that it is problematic for a person to *always* predict that things will go badly. If the child does not see that this situation is problematic, review how always expecting the worst possible outcome can make a person feel overly sad, upset, or anxious. To illustrate how such thoughts can be problematic, try to use the Socratic method with an example (preferably in the child's nonfeared domain). For example, if the child likes to swim at the beach, ask whether it would be good to spend all of his or her time *not* swimming because he or she was afraid a shark was going to bite him or her. Use Socratic questioning to lead the child to the point that he or she would likely feel sad, upset, or anxious with such thoughts, and that it is not in his or her best interest to become upset over something that is not likely to happen. Also consider pointing out that avoidance of fun activities may occur as a result of negative predictions, which is also not in the child's best interests. Emphasize that you are not trying to tell the child that he or she should have no anxiety at all; rather, your goal is to have the child evaluate the evidence for his or her predictions and minimize any anxiety that is excessive.

6. Ask if the child can think of any situations in which he or she predicted a negative outcome that did not occur. Find out how upset he or she became in this situation. Confirm that this kind of error is exactly what you are talking about.

♈ Exercise

Indicate to the child that you will be teaching a special set of questions to ask him- or herself (as indicated on the **Five-Column Thought Record**) when he or she starts to predict that something bad will happen. Refer to these questions on the **Five-Column Thought Record** as they arise. Tell the child that is it important to remember that thoughts about the future are not always true and should be treated as guesses or hypotheses about how things will work out.

   Column 1: Tell the child that the first question is "What is your thought/prediction?" and that indicate that this question asks him or her to write down the thought.

   Column 2: Tell the child that the next question asks him or her to indicate "How likely does it feel?" and that this is an estimate of the probability, as you explained earlier. Have the child estimate the probability of the thought with no help from you (i.e., do not coach the child yet to make an accurate prediction, because you are taking him or her through these steps for illustration) and write down the probability in column 2.

   Column 3: Tell the child that the third question asks "What are some alternative thoughts?" Explain that the goal here is to think of a prediction of how things might work out that is different from what the child has listed in column 1. Ideally, the goal is to have the child list as many alternative thoughts as possible to illustrate the point that people can have many different interpretations of the same event. If the child has some difficulty, use Socratic questioning to help him or her generate alternative thoughts.

Column 4: Tell the child that the fourth question, "What is the proof?", refers to the evidence supporting the alternative thought. Review the idea that it is best to think about the evidence when making a prediction, and have the child try to think of some evidence for (or against) this thought. Questions to help this process include:

"Has this ever happened to me before?"
"Is there any evidence that this won't happen?"
"Are there any facts that back this up?"

Explain again to the child that he or she is like a detective looking for clues and evidence, and that it is always better to consult the evidence before making any decisions/predictions. If the child presents "evidence" that is faulty, point out the problems with using the offered statements as evidence.

Column 5: Tell the child that the fifth question asks "How likely is it, really?" and explain that he or she needs to reestimate the probability of the thought in column 1, based on what he or she has learned from considering alternative thoughts and the evidence. Compare the probability ratings in columns 2 and 5. In the ideal scenario, the child will estimate a lower probability for column 5. If the probability estimates do not change or if the estimate in column 5 is higher, ask the child how he or she arrived at the probability in column 5 and use Socratic questioning, if needed, to lead the child to readjust the probability statement.

This is a great time for praise.

7. Throughout this process, the therapist should keep in mind that there are three reasons why probability overestimation errors continue to occur despite disconfirming experiences:
   • The child may feel that something bad did not happen this time, but that it will happen the next time, due to the law of averages.
   • The child may feel that he or she has things or people around to keep him or her safe (e.g., a significant other) and thereby discount the evidence for the alternative thought.
   • The child may make probability overestimation errors because of a current mood state (e.g., child is anxious).
8. Because each of these examples may not apply to every child, the therapist may benefit most from addressing these issues as they arise and using Socratic questioning to point out the faulty logic behind each of the presumptions.
9. Ask the child if he or she has any questions about what you just covered. Praise the child for his or her efforts.

🏠 Practice Assignment

If you have completed all the material in the module, explain and assign the **Five-Column Thought Record** for practice. If it was necessary to stop early, it is best to assign the **Two-Column Thought Record** for practice until the all the material in the module has been covered.

☺ End on a Positive

End the session on a fun note with a game, activity, or other exercise that will leave the child feeling positive about the work you have done together today. With younger children, be sure to provide extra praise for cooperative behavior during the meeting.

👪 Brief the Family

At the end of the session, it is helpful to meet with the parent(s). However, you should first ask the child if there is anything that he or she told you today that he or she does *not* want you to tell the parent(s). Be sure to honor the child's privacy within the appropriate limits of safety.

Have the child explain to the parent what concepts he or she has learned in the meeting today. You can add information as necessary, but try to allow the child to do as much of the work as possible. Provide plenty of praise and encouragement; this time with the parent(s) and child together is an ideal time to model for the parent(s) how to encourage and praise the child's behaviors. The main goal of this portion of the module is to familiarize the parent(s) with the concepts (as well as providing a good review for the child), so that the parent(s) can assist the child at home with using the new concepts and tools introduced in the therapy sessions.

☝ DON'T FORGET!

• Make sure that the child takes home the **Two-Column or Five-Column Thought Record** for homework.

✔ CHECKLIST

If one or more of the following items cannot be checked off, consider what problems may have arisen. Portions of the module might need to be repeated, or troubleshooting might be indicated to determine how to overcome or compensate for any challenges encountered.

____ The child understood what a thought is.

____ The child understood the concepts of probability and guessing about the future.

____ The child understood and collaboratively completed a **Thought Record**.

____ A fun activity or positive time together was shared at the end of the meeting.

(i) THINGS TO CONSIDER

- Once children have used this module, they should be encouraged to go through these cognitive procedures each time an exposure exercise is performed. Together you should review whether the negative thoughts came true and the implications of any corrective information.

? TROUBLESHOOTING

- **No thoughts**: If a child claims not to have any thoughts at all, it can be useful to give examples of the kinds of thoughts people have when anxious. Being careful not to lead the child in a particular direction, give examples of the kinds of thoughts other children have when anxious, and then inquire whether these seem familiar. By normalizing these thoughts, such examples help to eliminate possible embarrassment about stating them, and they also give the child an idea of what a therapist means when asking about thoughts.
- **Thoughts are emotions**: Sometimes a child is unable to state anxious thoughts as negative predictions. In the best scenario, the therapist might ask "What bad thing do you think will happen in that situation that would make you feel afraid like that?" and the child would offer a specific prediction, such as "I think other children will laugh at me." When such specific predictions are hard to elicit, the therapist might simply have to work with thoughts about the feeling of anxiety itself. For example, the child might be prompted and encouraged to restate the thought as something like "If I am afraid in this situation, that would be bad." The therapist could then ask why, and ultimately the child could arrive at a prediction, such as "If I feel afraid, I will be a weak person and others will notice." Because it is testable in exposure exercises, such a thought is ideal for cognitive restructuring.

⊞ WHAT'S THE EVIDENCE?

- In many controlled studies of successful treatments for anxiety, cognitive strategies are used prior to, or as part of, the main therapy procedures (e.g., Barrett, 1998; Barrett et al., 1996; Cobham et al., 1998; Cohen et al., 2004; De Haan et al., 1998; Goenjian et al., 1997; Graziano & Mooney, 1980; Kendall, 1994; Kendall et al., 1997; King et al., 1998; King et al., 2000; Muris et al., 1998; Pediatric OCD Treatment Study Team, 2004; Silverman, Kurtines, Ginsburg, Weems, Lumpkin, et al., 1999; Spence et al., 2000).
- In one very early study, children who merely used confident self-statements significantly reduced their fear of the dark relative to children who used other kinds of self-statements (Kanfer et al., 1975).

COGNITIVE RESTRUCTURING: CATASTROPHIC THINKING

★ Objectives

The objective for this module is to continue with cognitive restructuring as a technique for correcting negative thinking. This module almost always follows Probability Overestimation, and is used with older or more verbal children who frequently express overly negative or pessimistic ideas. This module is particularly important when a significant amount of the child's thoughts involve an exaggeration of the feared consequences, coupled with the feeling that the child cannot cope with a negative outcome.

⏱ If Pressed for Time

Instill the notion that even when bad things happen, they might not be as bad as they seem. Build this view into existing strategies for monitoring and testing the accuracy of ones' thoughts (e.g., using the **Thought Record**).

✉ Who Is Needed

Child
Parent(s), if possible

✏ Materials

Seven-Column Thought Record (Note: Last two columns pertain to catastrophic thinking.)

🌡 Weekly Rating

Obtain the **Fear Ladder** ratings from both the child and parent(s). Inspect the Fear Ladder for unusually high or problematic items; these might need to be discussed during the meeting.

Assignment Review

Review any practice assignments that were given in the previous session. Discuss what was learned, and consider rehearsing pieces of the homework together to consolidate the information. If the assignment was not completed, troubleshoot reasons why and consider the various options for handling whatever the obstacle might be. In all but the rarest of circumstances, do not proceed to new material if the assignment is not complete. It is better to take the planned session to perform the assignment together or to problem-solve how to accomplish it at home.

1 Set the Agenda

Meet with the child alone and talk with the child about the various ideas and exercises you plan to cover in your meeting. Make sure these are spelled out in order, with approximate time limits given for how long each part might take. This information will add to the predictability of the meeting and minimize confusion. Ask the child if he or she has any issues to cover and put these on the agenda as well. It can be helpful to write these items on a dry erase board or easel pad to serve as a visual reminder. Finally, be sure to point out that there will be an opportunity for a rewarding or fun activity at the end of the meeting.

Procedures

1. Meet with the child alone and explain that the session will be spent talking about certain types of thoughts that can make children feel upset, and that you will be going over ways to deal with these thoughts that may help him or her to feel better. Explain that such thoughts can be scary or difficult to talk about, but that it would be most helpful for you if he or she could be as honest as possible. You should already have covered Cognitive Restructuring: Probability Overestimation, so let the child know that these exercises will be somewhat similar to this material.
2. Before beginning, remember to discuss the idea that thoughts are like predictions or guesses about the future. Sometimes they are right, and sometimes they are wrong.
3. Introduce the idea that catastrophic thoughts are one type of thought, and that children often think catastrophically when they are feeling anxious or distressed.
4. Define a catastrophic thought as a thought in which the child fears that something terrible or dangerous will happen to him or her and that he or she will not be able to cope with it—in other words, believing the worst will come true. To illustrate, consider giving an example of a catastrophic thought that is salient to the child but is not in the feared domain. For example, if the child is not afraid of making a small mistake at a music recital, you might say:

↯ Example

One example of a catastrophic thought for some children would be "I am afraid to make a mistake at my music recital because if people heard my mistake, they would think I'm dumb."

5. Verify that the child knows why the example illustrates catastrophic thinking and ask him or her how catastrophic it would be to make a mistake at a recital that people noticed. Using the same example, go on to point out that catastrophic thoughts often predict a much worse outcome than would really happen. Also, point out that children sometimes fear that they will not be able to cope with a difficult situation when, in fact, they really could.
6. Inquire about the effects of having such a thought. Go on to mention that these bad effects are why we want to try to change these kinds of thoughts.

↯ Example

Do thoughts like this make things better or worse for you?

7. Help the child to identify a thought that is relevant to his or her **Fear Ladder** items by saying something like "I know you said that you feel worried about...," "What would be terrible for you about...?" Continue guiding this process with questions until you have a catastrophic thought with the negative outcome spelled out clearly. If the child only states one part of the thought, for example, "I'm worried that I'll do bad at my piano recital," you should question the child further for more detail about what would be so bad about making a mistake (e.g., "It would be terrible because people would hear my mistake," "It would be terrible because my face might turn red," and so forth). Praise the child for any efforts in this process.
8. When eliciting the child's sample catastrophic thought, keep in mind that certain thoughts may embody both (1) a probability overestimation error and (2) a catastrophic thinking error. In such a case, consider reviewing why the thought represents a probability overestimation error before addressing the catastrophic nature of the thought.

🏋 Exercise

Once you have identified the thought, praise the child and add that you want to write it down because what he or she said is important. Write down the catastrophic thought in column 1 of the **Thought Record**, using the child's exact words as much as possible and putting the words into a sentence form starting with the first person (e.g., "I'm afraid that I will make a mistake at my piano recital and that people will hear my mistake"). As you are writing the sentence down, repeat it back to the child to check see that you have understood him/her correctly.

Once the catastrophic thought has been recorded, teach the child the countering strategy by asking the question: "If the worst thing actually did happen, how terrible or catastrophic would it be?" or "So if [the worst thing] actually happened, what would be terrible about that for you?" You should write down the child's response (note that there is not a specific column on the **Seven-Column Thought Record** for this information). If the child lists a series of negative consequences, each can be explored, as illustrated in the example below.

Note that the child should also be asked about his or her ability to cope with the imagined aversive consequences. Questions to address this issue would be "If [the worst thing] actually happened, do you think you would be able to cope with it?" and "Can you think of any time when you have coped with something similar before?" and "Do we have any evidence that you could handle it? Have other people survived the same kind of thing?" Note that space on the **Thought Record** is provided to record the coping response in column 6, and to record evidence of being able to handle the problem in column 7. Once the child gives you an answer, write down his or her coping responses in these respective columns.

Provide plenty of praise.

♣ Example

Child: I would be afraid of making a mistake at my piano recital.

Therapist: And why would it be terrible for you to make a mistake at your recital?

Child: If I made a mistake, everyone would hear it.

Therapist: And if everyone heard the mistake, what would be terrible for you about that?

Child: I would feel embarrassed.

Therapist: So you're saying that you would feel embarrassed if people heard you make a mistake at your recital. I'm wondering, what would feel terrible for you about feeling embarrassed?

Child: It wouldn't feel very good.

Therapist: That's true, feeling embarrassed doesn't feel good. I'm wondering, though, how long that embarrassment would last and whether you think you could cope with those feelings for that length of time?

Child: I'd be embarrassed for a few minutes. I guess I could handle it.

Therapist: Yes, it sounds like you could handle it. I'm wondering now if you've ever been in a similar situation where you've been embarrassed and have coped with those feelings. Such a situation would give us more evidence that you'd be able to handle this situation.

9. Socratic questions are used in this manner to elicit all of the negative consequences imagined by the child and to guide the child to the conclusion that (a) the negative consequences might not be as aversive as imagined, or (b) that such consequences might be unpleasant and difficult, but effective coping was nonetheless possible. Make the point that you are not necessarily implying that all feared consequences are not as terrible as imagined. Rather, in situations where the outcome is unpleasant, the goal is to cope with it despite the presence of distress and anxiety.

10. During the restructuring process, there are several points to consider. First, in posing the questions to counter the catastrophic thought, it is important *not* to unduly force the child to endorse a particular conclusion. Rather, the strategy should be to guide the child to draw that conclusion on his or her own, because cognitive change is more likely to occur when the thoughts are self-generated.

11. Next, address whether the child imagines that the negative or unpleasant situation would last forever. If this idea is endorsed, it should be pointed out that the effects are time limited and manageable; you might consider asking, as a means of addressing this issue, about the amount of time the child would actually feel anxious, as was done in the above example. Make the point that that it would not be physically possible for the associated anxiety to escalate and continue indefinitely.

12. Remind the child that focusing on these types of feelings may produce more distress and anxiety initially because these thoughts are anxiety provoking. An increase in subjective anxiety is expected and normal. You can tell the child that some children react to this increase in negative thoughts by trying to distract themselves or avoid such thoughts, but that the thoughts first must be identified before they can be evaluated and challenged. The child can be reassured that anxious thoughts will eventually become less noticeable, less uncomfortable, and easier to challenge as he or she continues to practice cognitive restructuring. The process can be likened to learning how to ride a bike: Initially, it is hard to learn, but with practice, the skills can be applied more automatically. Tell the child that these questioning skills can be applied to different situations, and that it would be most helpful if he or she could apply these questions routinely, whenever catastrophic thoughts arise.

Practice Assignment

Assign the **Seven-Column Thought Record** for homework. It should be filled out each time the child has an anxious thought this week. Be sure the child can recite the homework back to you before finishing. Provide plenty of praise.

☺ End on a Positive

End the session on a fun note with a game, activity, or other exercise that will leave the child feeling positive about the work you have done together today. With younger children, be sure to provide extra praise for cooperative behavior during the meeting.

Brief the Family

At the end of the session, it is helpful to meet with the parent(s). However, you should first ask the child if there is anything that he or she told you today that he or she does *not* want you to tell the parent(s). Be sure to honor the child's privacy within the appropriate limits of safety.

Have the child explain to the parent what concepts he or she has learned in the meeting today. You can add information as necessary, but try to allow the child to do as

much of the work as possible. Provide plenty of praise and encouragement; this time with the parent(s) and child together is an ideal time to model for the parent(s) how to encourage and praise the child's behaviors. The main goal of this portion of the module is to familiarize the parent(s) with the concepts (as well as providing a good review for the child), so that the parent(s) can assist the child at home with using the new concepts and tools introduced in the therapy sessions.

☝ DON'T FORGET!

- Make sure that the child takes home the **Seven-Column Thought Record** for homework.

✔ CHECKLIST

If one or more of the following items cannot be checked off, consider what problems may have arisen. Portions of the module might need to be repeated, or troubleshooting might be indicated to determine how to overcome or compensate for any challenges encountered.

____ The child understood the concept of a catastrophic thought.

____ The child understood and collaboratively completed the **Seven-Column Thought Record**.

____ A fun activity or positive time together was shared at the end of the meeting.

ⓘ THINGS TO CONSIDER

- Once children have used this module, they should be encouraged to go through these cognitive procedures each time an exposure exercise is performed. Review whether the negative thoughts came true and the implications of any corrective information.

TROUBLESHOOTING

- **No thoughts**: If a child claims not to have any thoughts at all, it can be useful to give examples of the kinds of thoughts people have when anxious. Being careful not to lead the child in a particular direction, give examples of the kinds of thoughts other children have when anxious, and then inquire whether these seem familiar. By normalizing these thoughts, such examples help to eliminate possible embarrassment about stating them, and they also give the child an idea of what a therapist means when asking about thoughts.
- **Thoughts are emotions**: Sometimes a child is unable to state anxious thoughts as negative predictions. In the best scenario, the therapist might ask "What bad thing do you think will happen in that situation that would make you feel afraid like that?" and the child would offer a specific prediction, such as "I think other children will laugh at

me." When such specific predictions are hard to elicit, the therapist might simply have to work with thoughts about the feeling of anxiety itself. For example, the child might be prompted and encouraged to restate the thought as something like "If I am afraid in this situation, that would be bad." The therapist could then ask why, and ultimately the child could arrive at a prediction, such as "If I feel afraid, I will be a weak person and others will notice." Because it is testable in exposure exercises, such a thought is ideal for cognitive restructuring.

WHAT'S THE EVIDENCE?

- In many controlled studies of successful treatments for anxiety, cognitive strategies are used to prior to or as part of the main therapy procedures (e.g., Barrett, 1998; Barrett et al., 1996; Cobham et al., 1998; Cohen et al., 2004; De Haan et al., 1998; Goenjian et al., 1997; Graziano & Mooney, 1980; Kendall, 1994; Kendall et al., 1997; King et al., 1998; King et al., 2000; Muris et al., 1998; Pediatric OCD Treatment Study Team, 2004; Silverman, Kurtines, Ginsburg, Weems, Lumpkin, et al., 1999; Spence et al., 2000).
- In one very early study, children who merely used confident self-statements significantly reduced their fear of the dark relative to children who used other kinds of self-statements (Kanfer et al., 1975).

COGNITIVE RESTRUCTURING: STOP

★ Objectives

Objectives for this module are to introduce cognitive restructuring as a technique for correcting negative thinking. This module is typically used with younger children or less verbal or mature adolescents who appear to have overly negative or pessimistic ideas. This module is particularly important if the negative or pessimistic ideas appear to be interfering with a child's ability to engage in, or benefit from, exposure practice.

⏲ If Pressed for Time

Instill the notion that anxious thoughts are not always accurate, by covering as much of the worksheet as possible. Teach the steps that correspond to the acronym "STOP".

✉ Who Is Needed

Child
Parent(s), if possible

✎ Materials

Fear Ladder (for reference, as needed)
STOP Worksheet
STOP Record

🌡 Weekly Rating

Obtain the **Fear Ladder** ratings from both the child and parent(s). Inspect the Fear Ladder for unusually high or problematic items; these might need to be discussed during the meeting.

📄 Assignment Review

Review any practice assignments that were given in the previous session. Discuss what was learned, and consider rehearsing pieces of the homework together to consolidate the information. If the assignment was not completed, troubleshoot reasons why and consider the various options for handling whatever the obstacle might be. In all but the rarest of circumstances, do not proceed to new material if the assignment is not complete. It is better to take the planned session to perform the assignment together or to problem-solve how to accomplish it at home.

1 Set the Agenda

Meet with the child and talk with the child about the various ideas and exercises you plan to cover in your meeting. Make sure these are spelled out in order, with approximate time limits given for how long each part might take. This information will add to the predictability of the meeting and minimize confusion. Ask the child if he or she has any issues to cover and put these on the agenda as well. It can be helpful to write these items on a dry erase board or easel pad to serve as a visual reminder. Finally, be sure to point out that there will be an opportunity for a rewarding or fun activity at the end of the meeting.

🗩 Procedures

1. Meet with the child alone and explain that you will be spending the session talking about different kinds feelings that children have and how to identify those feelings in themselves and in other people. Tell the child that you will show him or her a way to stop those bad feelings. The technique is called "STOP," and it involves several steps that you will discuss together.

> ### ⵜ Exercise
> Show the child the **STOP Worksheet** and work though it with the child, according to the steps that follow.

2. Point out the stop sign in the upper left-hand corner, explaining that here it refers to the first step. Go through pages 1–4 of the **STOP Worksheet** to (a) elicit ideas about feelings from the child, (b) ask how he or she would be able to tell if someone were experiencing these feelings, and (c) find out when he or she has those feelings.
3. During these first four pages, discuss with the child the idea that feelings can be expressed. It might help to ask the child to practice expressing some feelings, using facial expressions and body movements, to see if you are able to guess his or her feelings.
4. When finishing page 3, discuss the idea that there are often many reasons that can explain nervous feelings in a person's body. This explanation should be tied to what was learned in the Learning about Anxiety module.

> ### ⚡ Example
> Remember, all these feelings are supposed to be part of the alarm system that is meant to help you when there is danger. Why do you think these feelings would happen?

5. Using as many questions as possible, point out that the alarm makes your heart beat faster, makes you breathe faster (so you might feel out of breath), and makes you sweat so you can cool off if you need to run away. You get butterflies or stomach-aches because your stomach stops working on food so your body can concentrate on the danger. Feeling shaky, dizzy, or blushing is often a result of all the increased energy that your body generates. Make sure the child sees that most of these feelings are things that people feel when they exercise hard, and suggest that feeling scared gets your body ready for some hard work in case you need to get out of trouble.

6. As you finish page 4, review with the child the feelings that he or she has when in situations that make the child feel nervous or scared. Remind the child that everyone has times when they are a little bit afraid. Ask the child to provide examples of times when friends or family members were scared or afraid. The goal here is to point out that it is OK to be scared sometimes (again, consistent with the idea that anxiety is natural and can often be helpful), and when you don't want to be scared, there are things you can do about it.

7. Review that the first step in overcoming scared or anxious feelings is to learn *how to identify when you are feeling that way*. Discuss with the child the first clue that he or she has when becoming frightened or scared. Tell the child that this first step is called Scared, and that's the first letter in "STOP." Refer back to the stop sign on page 4.

8. Indicate that the next step in working to overcome scared or anxious feelings is to talk about the kinds of thoughts that make children feel upset. Inform the child that you will be teaching him or her how to identify and deal with these thoughts to feel better. Explain that these types of thoughts can be unpleasant and even scary to think about, but that most children eventually feel better after learning the techniques you will be teaching.

9. Go on to page 5, making sure that the child has a clear understanding of what a thought is and how thoughts are distinguished from feelings. Introduce the idea that children's thoughts can cover a range of different topics, but that thoughts often include guesses about the future. Elicit some predictions of the future from the child to make sure that the child understands this concept, and praise him or her for such efforts. For some children, the idea of a fortune teller or crystal ball may be helpful.

> **꘎ Example**
>
> **Therapist**: Do you know what a fortune teller does?
>
> **Child**: They try to say what is going to happen.
>
> **Therapist**: Right! They make guesses about the future. That's just like the thoughts that you have. Your thoughts tell you what might happen in the future.

10. Go on to page 6, pointing out to the child that not everyone makes the same guesses or has the same thoughts in a situation. Some children guess that things will turn out well for them, and other children may guess that bad things will happen to them. Make sure that the child understands the idea that *thoughts can be wrong*. If you feel that the child can make the connection, then tie in the concept with the idea of a false

alarm. (Appropriate answers on this page should be future oriented, such as "The boy thinks that the dog will be fun to play with"; "The girl thinks the dog might bite her.")

11. Once the child has provided examples of good and bad predictions, discuss the ways in which different thoughts can lead to different feelings and actions. Use the example on page 6 to demonstrate how two different thoughts in the same situation can result in quite different feelings and actions.

⚲   Example

What would the girl do in this situation? What would the boy do? Why?

---

12. Explain to the child that some kinds of thoughts can help people cope with a situation, but that other thoughts can make the scared or nervous feelings even worse. Let the child know that you want to focus on thoughts that bad things will happen because many children predict that things will not turn out well when this is not always the case, and these are the kinds of thoughts that can make children feel upset. Inform the child that the second step in learning to overcome scared or anxious feelings is to learn how to identify the thoughts that might make him or her feel more anxious. Tell the child that this step is called *Thoughts*. Review with the child, using examples, the ways in which recognizing thoughts can help in anxious situations. Remind the child that the more he or she practices identifying his or her own thoughts, the better the child will be able to know what he or she is expecting to happen in a situation.

13. Tell the child that the next step in learning to overcome anxious or scared feelings is to think of things that he or she can do to feel less scared, more relaxed, and to begin having a good time. Note that this step is called *Other Thoughts*. Go over page 7 and be sure the child is able to come up with realistic assurances that the bad things will not come true (e.g., "My mom usually comes back on time"; "Those kids are probably laughing at a joke that someone told").

14. Complete page 8 and discuss the child's own ideas about what he or she can do in particular situations to help him- or herself better cope with the scared or worried feelings.

15. Discuss how each step covered so far can help the child feel less anxious by using examples.

⚲   Example

Therapist: Let's imagine that you are outside at recess and a child you recognize from class comes up to you on the playground. You would like to get to know this classmate better, but you feel nervous about talking to him. What would you do?

Child: I probably wouldn't be able to talk to him.

Therapist: Let's remember the first step. What is the *S* for? Are you feeling *S*cared? How can you tell that you're scared?

> **Child**: Well, my heart would be beating really fast, and I would feel like I had a bad stomachache.
>
> **Therapist**: OK. Are you having scared *Thoughts*? What are you worried about in this situation?
>
> **Child**: I'm worried that I might say something stupid.
>
> **Therapist**: OK. Now let's look at the third step. What are some *Other* thoughts that you might have that would make this situation less scary?

16. Praise the child for his or her efforts in this exercise. If time allows, ask the child to work through another situation in which he or she might feel anxious or scared, indicating how he or she would use each step on his or her own. Provide praise again.

17. Inform the child that now you will review the last step in helping to overcome scared and anxious thoughts. Tell the child that this step is called *Praise*, and discuss page 9 of the worksheet. Ask the child for some examples of children doing well at a task, and ask the child to suggest some things these children could tell themselves after doing so well (e.g., "It was hard but I did it—nice job!" or "I was really brave this time!"). It is OK to write some of these down on page 9 of the **STOP Worksheet**.

18. Indicate to the child that he or she has just learned a plan that can help him or her to cope with scared or anxious feelings. Point out that it is often difficult to remember all of the steps when feeling scared or nervous, and remind him or her that the first letter of each step spells out the word "STOP."

 Practice Assignment

Give the child the worksheet to take home if it has not been completed in session. Have the child take home the **STOP Record** to keep track of thoughts and responses.

☺ End on a Positive

End the session on a fun note with a game, activity, or other exercise that will leave the child feeling positive about the work you have done together today. With younger children, be sure to provide extra praise for cooperative behavior during the meeting.

👫 Brief the Family

At the end of the session, it is helpful to meet with the parent(s). However, you should first ask the child if there is anything that he or she told you today that he or she does *not* want you to tell the parent(s). Be sure to honor the child's privacy within the appropriate limits of safety.

Have the child explain to the parent(s) what concepts he or she has learned in the meeting today. You can add information as necessary, but try to allow the child to do as

much of the work as possible. Provide plenty of praise and encouragement; this time with the parent(s) and child together is an ideal time to model for the parent(s) how to encourage and praise the child's behaviors. The main goal of this portion of the module is to familiarize the parent(s) with the concepts (as well as providing a good review for the child), so that the parent(s) can assist the child at home with using the new concepts and tools introduced in the therapy sessions.

 DON'T FORGET!

- Make sure that the child takes home the **STOP Worksheet** and can explain it to the parent(s).

✔ **CHECKLIST**

If two or more of the following items cannot be checked off, consider what problems may have arisen. Portions of the module might need to be repeated, or troubleshooting might be indicated to determine how to overcome or compensate for any challenges encountered.

____ The child understood the concept of how thoughts affect feelings.

____ The child understood the concept of how thoughts can be inaccurate.

____ The child understood the concept of how other, new thoughts can generated.

____ The child understood and collaboratively completed the **STOP Worksheet**.

____ A fun activity or positive time together was shared at the end of the meeting.

ⓘ **THINGS TO CONSIDER**

- Once children have used STOP, they should be encouraged to go through the four steps each time an exposure exercise is performed. For example, before starting an exposure practice you can ask the child how he or she will know if he or she feels scared. Then ask what some of those scared thoughts might be, and write them down on the **STOP Record**. Next have the child generate other thoughts that might be more realistic and reassuring. At that point, suggest that the child recite some of those other thoughts to him- or herself during the practice. Complete the exposure exercise and then remember to praise and to encourage self-praise. These steps should be used for practice at home as well as those exercises done together.

? **TROUBLESHOOTING**

- **No thoughts**: If a child claims not to have any thoughts at all, it can be useful to give examples of the kinds of thoughts people have when anxious. Being careful not to lead the child in a particular direction, give examples of the kinds of thoughts other children have when anxious, and then inquire whether these seem familiar. By normalizing these thoughts, such examples help to eliminate possible embarrassment about stating them, and they also give the child an idea of what a therapist means when asking about thoughts.

- **Thoughts are emotions**: Sometimes a child is unable to state anxious thoughts as negative predictions. In the best scenario, the therapist might ask "What bad thing do you think will happen in that situation that would make you feel afraid like that?" and the child would offer a specific prediction, such as "I think other children will laugh at me." When such specific predictions are hard to elicit, the therapist might simply have to work with thoughts about the feeling of anxiety itself. For example, the child might be prompted and encouraged to restate the thought as something like "If I am afraid in this situation, that would be bad." The therapist could then ask why, and ultimately the child could arrive at a prediction, such as "If I feel afraid, I will be a weak person and others will notice." Because it is testable in exposure exercises, such a thought is ideal for cognitive restructuring.

⊞ WHAT'S THE EVIDENCE?

- In many controlled studies of successful treatments for anxiety, cognitive strategies are used to prior to, or as part of, the main therapy procedures (e.g., Barrett, 1998; Barrett et al., 1996; Cobham et al., 1998; Cohen et al., 2004; De Haan et al., 1998; Goenjian et al., 1997; Graziano & Mooney, 1980; Kendall, 1994; Kendall et al., 1997; King et al., 1998; King et al., 2000; Muris et al., 1998; Pediatric OCD Treatment Study Team, 2004; Silverman, Kurtines, Ginsburg, Weens, Lumpkin, et al., 1999; Spence et al., 2000).
- In one very early study, children who merely used confident self-statements significantly reduced their fear of the dark relative to children who used other kinds of self-statements (Kanfer et al., 1975).

SOCIAL SKILLS: MEETING NEW PEOPLE

★ Objectives

The objective for this module is to teach basic skills for meeting new people. This module is commonly used with children whose poor social skills interfere with their ability to develop successful peer relationships. For the child who has both social anxiety and poor social skills and is willing to engage in exposure practice, it is nevertheless important to address the social skills first, so that subsequent practice exercises reinforce the proper behaviors for social interaction. This module is often used in conjunction with Social Skills: Nonverbal Communication.

⊙ If Pressed for Time

At a minimum, teach the child how to say hi and ask questions and rehearse at least once.

✉ Who is Needed

Child
Parent(s), if possible

✏ Materials

Meeting and Greeting Worksheet
Meeting and Greeting Record

🌡 Weekly Rating

Obtain the **Fear Ladder** ratings from both the child and parent(s). Inspect the Fear Ladder for unusually high or problematic items; these might need to be discussed during the meeting.

Assignment Review

Review any practice assignments that were given in the previous session. Discuss what was learned, and consider rehearsing pieces of the homework together to consolidate the information. If the assignment was not completed, troubleshoot reasons why and consider the various options for handling whatever the obstacle might be. In all but the rarest of circumstances, do not proceed to new material if the assignment is not complete. It is better to take the planned session to perform the assignment together or to problem-solve how to accomplish it at home.

1 Set the Agenda

Meet with the child alone and talk about the various ideas and exercises you plan to cover in your meeting. Make sure these are spelled out in order, with approximate time limits given for how long each part might take. This information will add to the predictability of the meeting and minimize confusion. Ask the child if he or she has any issues to cover and put these on the agenda as well. It can be helpful to write these items on a dry erase board or easel pad to serve as a visual reminder. Finally, be sure to point out that there will be an opportunity for a rewarding or fun activity at the end of the meeting.

Procedures

1. Meet with the child alone and discuss the importance of having the skills to meet new people and engage in conversations.

> **Example**
>
> Do you think it is good to meet new people? What are some ways that you can meet new people? Having conversations with new people helps you to discover whether you like each other and want to become friends.

> **Exercise**
>
> Go over the first page of the **Meeting and Greeting Worksheet**. Explain that these are the steps for meeting someone new. Conduct a brief role play in which the child introduces him- or herself. If the child does well, try another in which you do not say your name unless asked to demonstrate that it is OK to ask the other person's name if that person does not say it. Practice this introduction until successful.
>
> Go over the remaining pages of the **Meeting and Greeting Worksheet**. Point out that the steps to having a conversation involve taking turns asking/telling/saying something and listening. These steps can be repeated until the child is no longer interested in talking, and then the child can make a closing remark.

Role Play

Role-play with the child a situation in which the child meets a new person. For example, you could role-play two children meeting each other in the school cafeteria. Introduce yourself first, allow the child to introduce him- or herself, and ask him or her about teachers and classes and his or her likes and dislikes. Find a topic in common to discuss and focus the rest of the conversation on this topic. Discuss the role play after it ends. What went well? What could be done better next time? Praise the child for doing well on this task.

2. If things are going well, introduce the idea of changing the subject in a conversation. Point out that most people don't ask and say things about the same topic over and over before they get tired of it. Discuss some ways to shift the topic in a conversation. Try a role play in which the child is asked to change the topic after a minute of conversation. Discuss the role play after it ends. What went well? What could be done better next time? Praise the child for doing well on this task.
3. If it can be arranged, have the child practice a role play for meeting a new child with a confederate or cooperative peer. Discuss the role play afterward with the child alone.

 Practice Assignment

For homework, give the child the **Meeting and Greeting Record** and ask him or her to have at least one conversation at home and one at school using the steps on the bottom of the worksheet. The conversation at school can be with someone the child already knows or with someone he or she doesn't know well. Tell the child that a good way to get hints about what to discuss with other children is to observe others' conversations at school. Note what things others talk about, their interests, and what they do in their spare time.

☺ End on a Positive

End the session on a fun note with a game, activity, or other exercise that will leave the child feeling positive about the work you have done together today. With younger children, be sure to provide extra praise for cooperative behavior during the meeting.

🏃 Brief the Family

At the end of the session, it is helpful to meet with the parent(s). However, you should first ask the child if there is anything that he or she told you today that he or she does *not* want you to tell the parent(s). Be sure to honor the child's privacy within the appropriate limits of safety.

Have the child explain to the parent(s) what concepts he or she has learned in the meeting today. You can add information as necessary, but try to allow the child to do as

much of the work as possible. Provide plenty of praise and encouragement; this time with the parent(s) and child together is an ideal time to model for the parent(s) how to encourage and praise the child's behaviors. The main goal of this portion of the module is to familiarize the parent(s) with the concepts (as well as providing a good review for the child), so that the parent(s) can assist the child at home with using the new concepts and tools introduced in the therapy sessions.

☝ DON'T FORGET!

- Make sure that the child takes home the **Meeting and Greeting Worksheet** and the **Meeting and Greeting Record**.

✔ CHECKLIST

If two or more of the following items cannot be checked off, consider what problems may have arisen. Portions of the module might need to be repeated, or troubleshooting might be indicated to determine how to overcome or compensate for any challenges encountered.

- ____ The child understood the importance of social skills.
- ____ The child was able to role-play a greeting successfully.
- ____ The child was able to role-play taking turns in a conversation successfully.
- ____ The child understood and collaboratively completed the **Meeting and Greeting Worksheet**.
- ____ A fun activity or positive time together was shared at the end of the meeting.

❓ TROUBLESHOOTING

- **Expecting no anxiety**: Sometimes children feel disappointed when they are anxious during a role play. These children should be reminded that anxiety is expected when practicing new behaviors. In fact, the goal is to perform the skills or steps *while feeling anxious*. If a child can perform the appropriate skills or steps under these conditions, then the skills are considered well established and are likely to persist in new situations, despite some anxiety. Children should be reminded that—just like everything else they have learned—the anxiety will decrease over time only with repeated practice.

▦ WHAT'S THE EVIDENCE?

- Social skills training has been shown to significantly reduce anxiety in children with social phobia (Beidel, Turner, & Morris, 2000; Miller, Barrett, Hampe, & Noble, 1972; Spence, Donovan, & Brechman-Toussaint, 2000).

SOCIAL SKILLS: NONVERBAL COMMUNICATION

★ Objectives

The objectives for this module are to increase awareness about nonverbal communication and teach basic skills for improving conversation. This module is commonly used with children whose poor social skills interfere with their ability to develop successful peer relationships. For the child who has both social anxiety and poor social skills and is willing to engage in exposure practice, it is nevertheless important to address the social skills first, so that subsequent practice exercises reinforce the proper behaviors for social interaction. This module is often used in conjunction with Social Skills: Meeting New People.

⏱ If Pressed for Time

Pick the most relevant skills from the **Nonverbal Skills Worksheet** and cover only those. Rehearse at least one that can be practiced before the next session.

✉ Who Is Needed

Child
Parent(s), if possible

✐ Materials

Nonverbal Skills Worksheet
Nonverbal Skills Record

🌡 Weekly Rating

Obtain the **Fear Ladder** ratings from both the child and parent(s). Inspect the Fear Ladder for unusually high or problematic items; these might need to be discussed during the meeting.

Assignment Review

Review any practice assignments that were given in the previous session. Discuss what was learned, and consider rehearsing pieces of the homework together to consolidate the information. If the assignment was not completed, troubleshoot reasons why and consider the various options for handling whatever the obstacle might be. In all but the rarest of circumstances, do not proceed to new material if the assignment is not complete. It is better to take the planned session to perform the assignment together or to problem-solve how to accomplish it at home.

1 Set the Agenda

Meet with the child alone and talk with the child about the various ideas and exercises you plan to cover in your meeting. Make sure these are spelled out in order, with approximate time limits given for how long each part might take. This information will add to the predictability of the meeting and minimize confusion. Ask the child if he or she has any issues to cover and put these on the agenda as well. It can be helpful to write these items on a dry erase board or easel pad to serve as a visual reminder. Finally, be sure to point out that there will be an opportunity for a rewarding or fun activity at the end of the meeting.

Procedures

1. Meet with the child alone and discuss the importance of nonverbal communication.

> **Example**
> Today we're going to talk about things that we need to do with our bodies when we are talking to other people. We may not even notice doing these things, but if we don't do them, other people can feel uncomfortable.

2. Discuss "talking distance." Describe that people generally stand a certain distance apart when talking—not too far, not too close.

> **Exercise**
> Go through the talking distance activities on the **Nonverbal Skills Worksheet**.

> **Example**
> One important thing to do when talking to someone is not to stand too close or too far away. Why do you think that is important? Let's go through some exercises together to learn more about this area.

3. Following the exercises, lead the child to see that the optimal distance to keep between people when having a conversation is neither too close nor too far. Also discuss that there are different needs for personal space in different situations (e.g., crowded vs. empty elevator) and with different people (e.g., brother or sister vs. someone you just met).
4. Discuss eye contact as an important way to show respect and interest. Depending on the social and cultural context, it is important to strike a balance between too much eye contact (i.e., staring) and too little.

Y Exercise
Go through the eye contact activities on the **Nonverbal Skills Worksheet**.

Example
Another important thing to do when talking to someone is to look him or her in the eye. One important reason for this is to let the person know that you are paying attention to him or her and not someone else. Let's go through some more exercises to learn about eye contact.

5. Following the exercises, lead the child to see that the optimal amount of eye contact for most situations is about half the time. Too little eye contact shows no interest, and too much can make things uncomfortable. Praise the child for doing well on this task.
6. Discuss speaking voice, helping the child understand that it is important not to talk too loudly or too quietly. Ask the child what each of those talking styles might mean to a listener (e.g., a loud style might be overwhelming and an overly quiet style might be annoying).

Y Exercise
Go through the speaking voice activities on the **Nonverbal Skills Worksheet**.

Example
It is also important to use the right voice when talking to others. What would happen if you were too quiet? What about if you sounded sad? Let's go through some exercises to learn about how to use your best speaking voice.

7. Following the exercises, help the child to see that it is important to speak loud enough to be heard and to show interest by sounding happy or excited. Praise the child for doing well on this task.

Role Play
Spend the remainder of available time together role playing a conversation, working on each of the skills, in turn, and then putting them together. It is helpful for the therapist to alternately model the skill, then observe it in the child. There should always be lots of praise, even when the performance was less than expected.

🖋 Example

"I like the way you made eye contact that time, and you were standing just the perfect distance. Nice going! Now we're going to try that one again, and this time I'd like you to try talking just a tiny bit louder. Think you can do that? All right!"

🏠 Practice Assignment

For homework, give the child the **Nonverbal Skills Record**. Assign at least two situations and explain how the sheet should be filled out. Make sure the child understands how to use the **Nonverbal Skills Record**.

☺ End on a Positive

End the session on a fun note with a game, activity, or other exercise that will leave the child feeling positive about the work you have done together today. With younger children, be sure to provide extra praise for cooperative behavior during the meeting.

👪 Brief the Family

At the end of the session, it is helpful to meet with the parent(s). However, you should first ask the child if there is anything that he or she told you today that he or she does *not* want you to tell the parent(s). Be sure to honor the child's privacy within the appropriate limits of safety.

Have the child explain to the parent(s) what concepts he or she has learned in the meeting today. You can add information as necessary, but try to allow the child to do as much of the work as possible. Provide plenty of praise and encouragement; this time with the parent(s) and child together is an ideal time to model for the parent(s) how to encourage and praise the child's behaviors. The main goal of this portion of the module is to familiarize the parent(s) with the concepts (as well as providing a good review for the child), so that the parent(s) can assist the child at home with using the new concepts and tools introduced in the therapy sessions.

 DON'T FORGET!

_____

- Make sure that the child takes home the **Nonverbal Skills Worksheet** and the **Nonverbal Skills Record**.

✓ **CHECKLIST**

_____

If two or more of the following items cannot be checked off, consider what problems may have arisen. Portions of the module might need to be repeated, or troubleshooting might be indicated to determine how to overcome or compensate for any challenges encountered.

_____ The child understood the importance of distance when talking.

_____ The child was able to role-play the appropriate distance when talking successfully.

_____ The child understood the importance of eye contact.

_____ The child was able to role-play eye contact successfully.

_____ The child understood the importance of voice level.

_____ The child was able to role-play voice level successfully.

_____ The child was able to integrate these skills in a role play.

_____ The child understood and collaboratively completed the **Nonverbal Skills Worksheet**.

_____ A fun activity or positive time together was shared at the end of the meeting.

(i) THINGS TO CONSIDER

• This module can be administered in a highly flexible manner. Not all children may need all three exercises, or at least not equal emphasis. The module can also broken up into three different parts and gone over more slowly for children whose skills are not highly developed in this area. In this manner, the **Nonverbal Skills Record** could be assigned with only one column at a time for homework, for example. The goal is to go at the pace that will best help the child incorporate these skills and start practicing them in different situations.

? TROUBLESHOOTING

• **Expecting no anxiety**: Sometimes children feel disappointed when they are anxious during a role play. These children should be reminded that anxiety is expected when practicing new behaviors. In fact, the goal is to perform the skills or steps *while feeling anxious*. If a child can perform the appropriate skills or steps under these conditions, then the skills are considered well established and are likely to persist in new situations, despite some anxiety. Children should be reminded that—just like everything else they have learned—the anxiety will decrease over time only with repeated practice.

WHAT'S THE EVIDENCE?

• Social skills training has been shown to significantly reduce anxiety in children with social phobia (Beidel et al., 2000; Miller et al., 1972; Spence et al., 2000).

WORKING WITH PARENTS: ACTIVE IGNORING

★ Objectives

The objective for this module is to introduce the skill of differential reinforcement to parents (or teachers). This technique involves the removal of reinforcement and attention for mild inappropriate behaviors (e.g., complaining, whining, reassurance seeking), paired with the increase of reinforcement and attention for more appropriate alternative behaviors. This module is often used when parents (or teachers) report responding frequently to mild inappropriate behavior or are (inadvertently) encouraging and rewarding avoidance.

⏱ If Pressed for Time

In most cases, this module should be covered completely, or nearly so, before its implementation. Partial application of this module may introduce new challenges. Thus, when time is a concern, one session should be devoted to covering the principles of differential reinforcement and a subsequent session should be dedicated to rehearsal of the strategy. In cases in which families seem especially prepared to implement this approach, it can be covered quickly but also should be rehearsed once together before assigning for home practice.

✉ Who Is Needed

Child
Parent(s) or teacher

✏ Materials

Active Ignoring Handout (parent, teacher, or both)
Observation Record (parent, teacher, or both)
Magazine or book for role play

Weekly Rating

Obtain the **Fear Ladder** ratings from both the child and parent(s). Inspect the Fear Ladder for unusually high or problematic items; these might need to be discussed during the meeting.

 Assignment Review

Review any practice assignments that were given in the previous session. Discuss what was learned, and consider rehearsing pieces of the homework together to consolidate the information. If the assignment was not completed, troubleshoot reasons why and consider the various options for handling whatever the obstacle might be. In all but the rarest of circumstances, do not proceed to new material if the assignment is not complete. It is better to take the planned session to perform the assignment together or to problem-solve how to accomplish it at home.

⌈1⌉ Set the Agenda

Meet with the parent(s) alone and talk about the various ideas and exercises you plan to cover in your meeting. Make sure these are spelled out in order, with approximate time limits given for how long each part might take. This information will add to the predictability of the meeting and minimize confusion. Ask the parent(s) if he or she has any issues to cover and put these on the agenda as well. It can be helpful to write these items on a dry erase board or easel pad to serve as a visual reminder. Finally, be sure to point out that there will be an opportunity for some positive time at the end of the meeting.

💬 Procedures

1. Continue meeting with the parent(s) alone and introduce the idea that behavior is strengthened or weakened by its consequences; that is, by what comes *after* the behavior. Explain that regardless of what a child is learning to do, his or her skills will be strengthened or weakened by the events that follow the learning activity.
2. Briefly discuss the idea of *reinforcement*. In order for a behavior to increase in strength, that behavior must be reinforced, or rewarded, after it occurs. Also, the reward cannot come at other times, only when the behavior occurs. Explain that if a child is rewarded regardless of whether he or she has performed the behavior or not (i.e., noncontingent reinforcement), then the reward will have no effect on the future performance of the behavior. However, if a child is rewarded *if, and only if,* the behavior is performed, the behavior will be more likely to occur again. Discuss the ways in which behaviors are increased in frequency and intensity of occurrence by

rewarding them, either with tangible objects (e.g., a sticker) or with attention from others.

✦ Example

If you cook a new recipe and you like how it tastes, you are likely to cook that meal again because it is rewarding.

If you do a favor for someone and he or she thanks you or gives you a gift, you are more likely to do another favor for that person later.

---

3. Point out that just as behaviors can be made to occur more often by the consequences that follow them, behaviors can also be lessened in strength or frequency by ignoring or *extinguishing* them. If a child continues to engage in a behavior but receives no reward for this behavior, the behavior should begin to lessen in frequency.

4. Introduce *active ignoring* as a tool for extinguishing mild problem behaviors. Explain that active ignoring means removing all attention from the child when the target behavior is being performed, so as not to reward undesirable behavior in any way. In children with anxiety, active ignoring is most often used in response to behaviors such as whining, crying, excessive reassurance seeking, or complaining (especially somatic complaints).

5. Discuss some examples of what usually happens when whining or complaining occurs. Be sure to point out how the parent's response is often rewarding for the child. Make clear how the parent's behavior is related to the consequences.

✦ Example

Therapist: What happens when your child complains about going to school?

Parent: We argue. I try to tell him why he has to go, but he just argues.

Therapist: So does your child end up going to school?

Parent: Sometimes. Usually we are just late from all the discussion and arguing.

Therapist: So, in a way, your child kind of gets his way—he gets to school late?

Parent: Uh-huh. That's how it usually goes.

Therapist: So there is kind of a reward in it for him if he keeps arguing.

Parent: There sure is.

---

6. Point out that the way to change this situation is not to respond. Responding can provide attention or relief in a way that ends up being a reward.

✦ Example

Therapist: What would happen if you just didn't argue? If you just set rules for bedtime and enforced them?

Parent: I guess my child would probably just give up arguing about bedtime eventually. Probably lose some rewards or privileges if she didn't get to bed on time.

Therapist: But the arguing would stop?

Parent: Probably, after a while.

7. Pick a behavior that the parent(s) would like to work on. Make sure the behavior is something mild or attention seeking. Good examples are whining, complaining, asking too many questions, pouting, or acting grumpy or upset.

8. For some parent(s) it is important to point out that sometimes the child's behavior is honest—even though it is rewarded by attention. For example, the child may actually have a stomachache on the way to school. The purpose of active ignoring is to get the child to develop a better way of coping when feeling bad in this way. We want the child to get rid of the habit of relying on Mom or Dad to help and to start using some of the new skills that he or she is learning in treatment.

9. Introduce the important features of "successful" ignoring:
   - Do not get drawn into arguing, scolding, or even talking. Many parents feel that they continually have to reexplain to their child why they are ignoring him or her during the behavior. The time to explain is *before* the behavior started.
   - Do not express anger or interest, either verbally or in your facial expression or movements.
   - Do not make eye contact with your child, and do not even glance at him or her more than briefly.
   - It helps to get absorbed in some other activity (e.g., going into another room, reading a book).

10. Explain to the parent(s) that the reason this technique is called *active* ignoring is because he or she should be working very hard to attend to and praise behaviors that are the opposite of the target behavior. Thus, when the child does not cry before school, the parent(s) should make extra efforts to provide praise and attention. If a child stops whining for even a minute, this is a good time to start attending and praising. If the child goes back to whining, the parent(s) must immediately begin ignoring the child again. It is this back and forth of attending to the good and ignoring the bad that makes this technique "active." Point out that the praise and attention for good behaviors are the most important part of active ignoring.

↳ Example

Therapist: The "active" part is the most important part of this technique. When do we usually notice children, when they are good, or when they are bad?

Parent: When they are bad.

Therapist: Right. What you have to try to do now is to notice when your child is good. The sooner the better. You can tell him things such as "That's really nice what you are doing," or you can answer a question or smile. That's how you can reward the right behaviors.

11. Some parents feel uncomfortable or even guilty using this technique. Point out that the parent(s) is not really being asked to ignore his or her *child*, but to ignore the unwanted *behavior*. The parent(s) should provide plenty of praise and attention when the child is doing well and not performing the unwanted behavior. Remind the parent(s) that this approach may feel very unnatural at first, because it does not always fit with one's "instincts," but assure the parent(s) that this technique is not harmful for the child. On the contrary, failure to use active ignoring could lead to bigger problems later, which is precisely why we would like the parent(s) to work so hard at active ignoring *now*.

12. Some parents may also feel guilty or angry because of the implication of this technique that parent behavior has caused child anxiety. These parents may conclude that they were responsible for their child's problems or that the therapist wishes to blame them in some way. Such parents should be reassured that child problems are typically the result of many factors that come together, such that it does not make sense to look for a single "cause." Also, attending to children when they are distressed is a natural parenting behavior that works well most of the time. It is the combination of this response with the child's existing anxiety and avoidance that can be trouble. Keep the parent(s) focused on the idea that therapy is present focused and that the idea is to use all the tools currently available to help. Active ignoring is one of those tools.

13. Tell the parent(s) that to review the concepts introduced above, you would like them to engage in a role play activity in which they can practice implementing these skills. Inform the parent(s) that you will act as their "child." Give the parent(s) the following directions:

🎭 Role Play

Start with something like this: "Let's practice what active ignoring will be like. I would like you to read a book or magazine while I play the part of your child. Try to use the techniques we have just discussed. When I am doing something bad, try to ignore me, and when I am good, try to praise me or pay attention."

You will need to alternate (about every minute) between engaging in appropriate (e.g., sitting quietly) versus inappropriate behavior (e.g., complaining or seeking reassurance). It is best to pick behaviors that the parent(s) often encounters with his or her child.

Praise the parent(s) for any successful parts of the role play. Point out what you liked most, and then repeat the role play if needed to address areas that could be improved (e.g., "That was great! Now we're going to try again, and we are just going to add one more thing").

14. Next, inform the parent(s) about the idea of an "extinction burst." Use examples (e.g., if you put money in a soda machine and nothing comes out, you might not just quit. You might put more money in, and you might even pound or shake the machine). Use these examples to express the idea that when we are used to getting

rewarded and then suddenly the reward stops, we often try harder or feel frustrated before giving up the behavior. The parent(s) should expect that active ignoring will be frustrating for the child at first and may cause a temporary increase in the behavior. Point out that this temporary increase *does not mean the parent(s) should give in*. On the contrary, it is a sign that the child has noticed the lack of reward and therefore the parent is doing the technique properly. The parent(s) should stick firmly to ignoring during extinction bursts and reassure him- or herself that these bursts are time limited.

15. Give the parent(s) the **Active Ignoring Handout** and answer any questions he or she has at this time.

16. Bring the child into the session and explain to the child that there will be some changes in communication in the family that are meant to be helpful for everyone. One thing we know makes it harder for children to use their new skills is *depending on parents at the wrong times*. As children begin to build their skills and get older, they will need to handle more situations on their own. You can tell the child that for the time being, the parent(s) is not allowed to respond to certain trouble behaviors. Use questions to make sure that the child understands that the parent(s) will not respond to, for example, complaints or crying for now.

 Example

Remember, if you are feeling sick before school, Mom is not allowed to talk to you about it. Sometimes you might forget and bring it up or try to talk with her, but she is not supposed to pay any attention. These rules are going to help everybody handle things better in the morning.

🎬 *In Vivo*

If possible, repeat the exercise you just role-played, now having the parent (or teacher) run through the strategy with the child. You may have to provide some prompts to the child as the *in vivo* progresses. In general, it is always best to rehearse a new skill at least once with the child in this way. The more, the better, and be sure to provide plenty of praise for everyone. Don't let them leave until it looks like they will get it right at home.

---

17. Remind the parent(s) to respond to the chosen undesirable behavior with active ignoring each time it occurs, and to praise the opposite or the absence of the behavior.

 Practice Assignment

Instruct the parent(s) in the use of the **Parent Observation Record** on which he or she will keep track of his or her response to each occasion of the child's unwanted behaviors. This monitoring will help the parent(s) track how well he or she is doing with this new technique.

☺ **End on a Positive**

If the child is present, end the session on a fun note with a game, activity, or other exercise that will leave the child feeling positive about the work you all have done together today. The parent(s) can be included in this activity as well. If the child is not present, take some time for supportive listening with the parent(s) if it appears to be pleasing.

☝ DON'T FORGET!

- Make sure that the parent takes home the **Parent Observation Record** (or **Teacher Observation Record** for a teacher).

✔ CHECKLIST

If two or more of the following items cannot be checked off, consider what problems may have arisen. Portions of the module might need to be repeated, or troubleshooting might be indicated to determine how to overcome or compensate for any challenges encountered.

_____ The parent(s) or teacher understood the concept of reinforcement.

_____ The parent(s) or teacher understood how attention—even negative attention—can be rewarding.

_____ The parent(s) or teacher understood that ignoring unwanted behaviors works hand-in-hand with praising good behaviors.

_____ The parent(s) or teacher was able to role-play successfully.

_____ The parent(s) or teacher was able to perform an *in vivo* exercise with the child successfully.

_____ A positive time together was shared at the end of the meeting, either with the child or in the form of supportive listening with the parent(s) or teacher.

ⓘ THINGS TO CONSIDER

- As noted, this module can also be used with teachers if the problem behaviors are happening in the classroom as well. Ideally, parents and teachers should be using the same program consistently. There is a separate **Active Ignoring Handout** and **Observation Record** for teachers.

❓ TROUBLESHOOTING

- **Intermittent attention**: If parents attend intermittently to unwanted behaviors, there is the possibility that the behaviors will get even worse. Thus it is important to inform parents, teachers, or caretakers who intend to use active ignoring of these risks. Those wishing to implement the technique should be told, in advance, that this is not a technique that can be used in a diluted fashion. A helpful analogy with parents or teachers is that of antibiotics. Patients are instructed to finish their entire dose of an antibiotic, because failure to do so could cause not only a return of the problem but even a more resistant version of the problem. The same is true with active ignoring. Partial application can lead to more treatment-resistant behaviors than were present before the treatment. In addition, it can be helpful to prepare parents for the possibility of an immediate worsening of the problem initially (i.e., "extinction burst"), which is common upon removal of a reinforcer. Parents should be prepared to watch for this phenomenon and to remain committed to the strategy despite the temporary challenges.

- **Too much explanation**: Sometimes parents engage in explanations of the technique while they are supposed to be ignoring the child. This misapplication is best noticed during the role play or *in vivo* exercise. It helps to warn parents of this tendency beforehand. In practice, families should be encouraged to provide only a single review of the rules of active ignoring with the child before the technique is implemented.

- **Ignoring the child**: Some parents ignore not only the unwanted behaviors but *all* behaviors. This problem, too, can be identified through role play and *in vivo* exercises, and it is best prevented rather than handled after the fact. It should be stated clearly to parents that they are never to try to ignore their children. In fact, with active ignoring, the overall amount of attention and praise to the child might actually increase rather than decrease. The strategy is all about the *timing* of attention, not the amount.

⊞ WHAT'S THE EVIDENCE?

- Differential attending to positive versus negative behaviors has been a successful strategy in dozens of studies of child behavior (e.g., Greene et al., 2004; Kazdin, Siegel, & Bass, 1992; Patterson, Chamberlain, & Reid, 1982; Wells & Egan, 1988).

- This technique has been used successfully to reduce complaints and other unwanted behaviors associated with childhood anxiety in several studies (e.g., Chorpita, Albano, Heimberg, & Barlow, 1996; King et al., 1998; Spence et al., 2000).

WORKING WITH PARENTS: REWARDS

★ Objectives

Objectives for this module are to review the concept of reinforcement with parents (or teachers) and to help establish a reward program for the home or classroom. This module is often used when there is a need to increase motivation to participate in exposure exercises, and possibly when the establishment of other behaviors is important to achieving the overall goals (e.g., going to bed on time).

⏲ If Pressed for Time

Cover the basic principles of how rewards work, set up a short list of rewards, and if time permits, connect these to the desired behaviors via a menu.

✉ Who Is Needed

Child
Parent(s) or teacher

✐ Materials

Rewards Handout (parent, teacher, or both)
Observation Record (parent, teacher, or both)
Fear Ladder (for reference, as needed)
Blank paper and a pen

🌡 Weekly Rating

Obtain the **Fear Ladder** ratings from both the child and parent(s). Inspect the Fear Ladder for unusually high or problematic items; these might need to be discussed during the meeting.

📄 Assignment Review

Review any practice assignments that were given in the previous session. Discuss what was learned, and consider rehearsing pieces of the homework together to consolidate the information. If the assignment was not completed, troubleshoot reasons why and consider the various options for handling whatever the obstacle might be. In all but the rarest of circumstances, do not proceed to new material if the assignment is not complete. It is better to take the planned session to perform the assignment together or to problem-solve how to accomplish it at home.

1 Set the Agenda

Meet with the parent(s) and child and talk about the various ideas and exercises you plan to cover in your meeting. Make sure these are spelled out in order, with approximate time limits given for how long each part might take. This information will add to the predictability of the meeting and minimize confusion. Ask the parent(s) if he or she has any issues to cover and put these on the agenda as well. It can be helpful to write these items on a dry erase board or easel pad to serve as a visual reminder. Finally, be sure to point out that there will be an opportunity for some positive time at the end of the meeting.

Procedures

1. Meet with the child alone and explain that you will be spending some time talking about the different kinds of activities that the child enjoys doing. Discuss the idea of rewards with the child. Elicit several types of items or activities that the child would find rewarding. Be sure to ask the child for smaller and larger items that would be reinforcing, reminding the child that rewards do not have to be large to make us feel good.
2. Meet with the parent(s) alone and discuss the idea of reinforcement and how it works with children. Remind the parent(s) that to be effective, reinforcement needs to occur very soon after the desired behavior has been exhibited. Indicate that giving rewards in the absence of the desired behavior or a long time after the behavior has occurred will not be very effective in increasing the likelihood of good behavior in the future.
3. Work with the parent(s) to add to the child's list of rewards. Be careful to ensure that the parent(s) only adds things that are truly enjoyable to the child. Encourage rewards that are small, can be given quickly, and do not cost much if at all. For example, it is best to use rewards such as praise, playing a game with a parent, going for a drive together, going to the mall together, watching a TV program, getting to stay up an extra half hour, picking a favorite meal for that night's dinner, or renting a movie. Rewards such as getting a bicycle or a new pet should be discouraged or saved for the completion of the treatment program altogether. It is much more important to work on a list of rewards that can be provided day to day.
4. Work with the parent(s) to create a list of desired behaviors. Current treatment goals and the child's **Fear Ladder** can be referenced to assist in the development of this list. One to three behaviors should be the maximum for now. More behaviors can be added later, after these first ones are well established.

5. Establish a schedule of reinforcement by selecting each behavior and deciding a reward (or allowing the child to choose among several rewards) that can be paired with it. For younger children, the rewards will need to be especially frequent, so that every time the behavior occurs, a small reward is given.

6. Indicate to the parent(s) that a child should be rewarded frequently in the beginning, so that he or she has the opportunity to experience success. However, it should become increasingly more challenging for the child to obtain rewards as treatment progresses. Explain to the parent(s) that if a child is getting too many rewards, then he or she is not being challenged and progress in treatment is not being made. Remind the parent(s) that the delivery of rewards must occur consistently and in a timely manner.

7. Meet with the child and parent(s) together to discuss the list and schedule of rewards. Work to resolve any discrepancies between child and parent(s) about how the system of rewards will work. The child should know that after meeting an agreed-upon goal (e.g., doing three exposure practices), he or she will get to pick something off the menu of rewards.

 In Vivo

If possible, have the parent(s) (or teacher) run through the strategy with the child. The child could pretend to engage in one of the behaviors, and the parent(s) could then mark down a reward on a piece of paper and announce to the child that a reward will be given. The parent(s) should provide lots of praise during this exercise.

You may have to provide some prompts to the child as the *in vivo* exercise progresses. In general, it is always best to rehearse a new skill at least once with the child in this way. The more, the better, and be sure to provide plenty of praise for child as well as parent(s). Don't let them leave until it looks like they will get it right at home.

8. Discuss with the child and parent(s) that these rewards are an ongoing part of working together. Consider posting the reward contract somewhere in the house (e.g., child's bedroom).

 Practice Assignment

Provide the parent(s) with the **Rewards Handout** and **Parent Observation Record** (or **Teacher Observation Record** for a teacher). Ask that the parent(s) record each time the desired behaviors occurred and what he or she did at that point. This record will be reviewed to see if the rewards are being given quickly and consistently, as well as to track whether the desired behaviors are occurring with the appropriate frequency.

☺ End on a Positive

If the child is present, end the session on a fun note with a game, activity, or other exercise that will leave the child feeling positive about the work you all have done together today. The parent(s) can be included in this activity as well. If the child is not present, take some time for supportive listening with the parent(s) if it appears to be pleasing.

 DON'T FORGET!

- Make sure that the parent(s) takes home the **Parent Observation Record** (or **Teacher Observation Record** for a teacher).

 CHECKLIST

If two or more of the following items cannot be checked off, consider what problems may have arisen. Portions of the module might need to be repeated, or troubleshooting might be indicated to determine how to overcome or compensate for any challenges encountered.

____ The parent(s) or teacher understood the concept of reinforcement.

____ The parent(s) or teacher understood how rewards increase behavior.

____ The child and parent(s) were able to develop an appropriate list of rewards.

____ The parent(s) or teacher was able to perform an *in vivo* exercise with the child successfully.

____ A positive time together was shared at the end of the meeting, either with the child or in the form of supportive listening with the parent(s).

 THINGS TO CONSIDER

- With younger children, the reward schedule should be as easy as possible at first, and the more immediate the better. The contract can always be made more challenging later. As a general rule, the child should get rewarded within a day or two of starting the rewards program. After he or she does well, the behaviors on the list can be changed to be more challenging, or they can be rewarded less frequently.
- With frequent behaviors (e.g., talking in class), it is not always possible to give out rewards each time the behavior occurs. It may be necessary to provide the child with a point system or sticker chart. Older children can simply earn points that are recorded on a score sheet. Younger children can get tokens (e.g., plastic game chips) or stickers to put up on a calendar. If this is the case, it will be helpful to make this calendar together in the session. Each time the child performs the desired behavior, a point or token or sticker is given. These points can be "cashed" in for things on the menu. With a point system, it is necessary to agree beforehand on a "price" for all items on the reward menu (i.e., how many points need to be cashed in for a reward). Set up the contract so that after a given length of time (e.g., 1 week), all points that don't get used up are taken away. The intent is to make sure that the child is actually experiencing the rewards and not just collecting points.
- The key to a successful rewards program is to keep the schedule from being too easy

or too hard. During each meeting, consider whether to adjust the reward or the points given for each behavior. If the child has not earned any rewards, the program should definitely be made easier (e.g., can the goal be approximated or done halfway at first?). If the child is getting frequent rewards, it is time to make the contract slightly more challenging. When discussing this rewards issue with a child, it is helpful to emphasize the similarity with someone "getting in shape." As you get better and stronger, you lift more weight or run farther each day, and that increase is a sign that you are really making progress. Over time, the rewards are faded out as the child learns to reward him- or herself with appreciation of his or her accomplishments (e.g., pride and self-praise).

- An important consideration with this module is the need for a sensitivity to class or the economic background of the family. With all families, it is important to emphasize that the best rewards do not cost money, but with economically disadvantaged families, it is especially important to be explicit about financial costs. Be sure that at least the first 10 items on the rewards menu are things that do not cost any money, and be especially reassuring that consistency, frequency, and immediacy of reward delivery are *always* more important than the material value of the reward.

- Continually remind the parent(s) that the best reward is praise. With enough praise from others, over time most children learn to self-praise and to take pride in their own accomplishments. These feelings are most likely to sustain the new behaviors in the long run.

- This module can also be used with teachers if the desired behaviors were supposed to appear in the classroom as well (e.g., asking questions in class). Ideally, the parent(s) and teachers should be using the same program consistently. There is a separate **Rewards Handout** and **Teacher Observation Record** for teachers.

? TROUBLESHOOTING

- **The rich baseline**: Some children already receive so many noncontingent "rewards" (i.e., for doing little or nothing positive) that it becomes a challenge to develop their interest in working for contingent rewards. In this scenario, it is important to discuss with the family the basic notion that although love for children is unconditional, most good things in life are not. Good things usually must be earned. Thus, much of what goes on the rewards menu should involve the behaviors in which the child already engages frequently (e.g., skateboarding, watching TV). If done hastily or improperly, however, this shift can come across as punishment or what is sometimes referred to as "response cost." For example, telling a child "Do your homework, or I will take away your video games for the night" does not reflect the proper application of a rewards program. Shifting the contingencies must be done within the framework of an open discussion about values related to effort and earning, with the idea that children do best in the long run if they learn how to get what they want through their own efforts. It is often helpful to have the child participate in some of this discussion as well. The child should know that he or she can have as many rewarding things as always, and that the overall level of rewards is under his or her control. It can be a subtle shift, but when done well ("Please finish your homework so you can still play your video game tonight"), it can increase the expected behaviors without creating resentment or withdrawal.

- **"I don't want anything"**: Some children will claim that they have no interest in anything and therefore will not nominate items for the reward menu. In such cases, look for behaviors that the child does often (e.g., watching TV, playing soccer). Ask the parent or child what he or she does with free time. Usually, the answer will provide some clue as to what is rewarding. For example, a child who "just hangs out in her room" has probably found something there that is reinforcing, such as books, toys, a puzzle, or just a resting place. Further discussion and a little detective work will usually turn up some ideas.

- **The distant future**: Sometimes parents or children will put rewards on the list that will take a long time to earn. Ironically, the best rewards are often those that cost little or no money and that can be delivered quickly. Examples include items such as trading cards (parents can buy a whole stack and give them out one at a time), stickers, or other little grab-bag objects from a "dollar store" or can include privileges such as picking what cereal to eat in the morning, getting to sit in the front seat of the car, or staying up an extra 15 minutes at bedtime. The therapist should make sure that most things on the rewards list can be delivered quickly and without great cost to the parents. If it is too difficult for children to wait or too difficult for parents to afford, the rewards program may break down.

- **Tangible dependency**: Sometimes parents express concern that their children will become dependent on treats and rewards or will become beggars. First, regarding begging, parents should be reminded that providing a reward in response to a child's request only rewards the request. Thus, in such cases, there should be ground rules that rewards are only delivered when the expected behavior (e.g., homework) is performed, and that the reward will be lost if a request is made. This means explaining to the child that to earn the reward, he or she must perform the appropriate behavior from the reward program *and* not ask for the reward. The best way to address the larger issue of dependency initially is to encourage the introduction of social reinforcers. Suggest the use of more praise, pats on the back, high-fives, victory dances, smiles, hugs, and thumbs-up whenever there is good behavior—even if the child also gets a tangible reward. This pairing ultimately makes it possible to fade out some of the tangible objects and treats while maintaining the social rewards. Eventually, children can maintain their behaviors on a leaner tangible rewards schedule, while still working for praise. Over time, the parent(s) should encourage the praise to become internalized by the child. That is, the parent(s) should progress from saying "You did a great job!" to asking "Didn't you do great?" to asking "How do you think you did?" Over time, the child should develop the capacity for self-praise, which can be applied even when there are no external rewards available. Finally, parents should take time to highlight the natural rewarding consequences of the child's good behavior (e.g., "Did you have fun with your friends at school today?"; "What did the teacher say when you got such a good grade?"). Ability to self-praise and to observe the natural rewards of one's behavior are the best insurance that those behaviors will become sustainable for the long run.

- **Bribery**: The parent(s) may express concern that he or she does not want to engage in "bribery" with their child. It can be helpful to point out here a major difference between bribery and rewards. Rewards are given *after* a behavior occurs, whereas bribes are given prior to the behavior. We never expect parents to give a reward first and then ask the child to perform a particular behavior as part of the deal. Another matter to highlight is that all people work for rewards, including adults. It might be less obvious, in that adults are capable of waiting a long time for a reward (e.g., a paycheck, a vacation), but everyone is motivated by rewards. It might be helpful to have this discussion with the parent(s) in the context of his or her own lives and behaviors first. Whether it be a cup of coffee, a few minutes of TV, a scented shampoo or soap in the shower, a glass of wine with dinner, or a favorite pair of jeans on the weekend, rewards are common for everyone. The major difference is that these rewards are often self-administered, not externally delivered. But they *are* rewards, in that they follow some event or achievement. Most adults don't start their day with the glass of wine or TV—they are rewards for a day of hard work. Coffee is a reward for getting out of bed, special soap for getting ready for the day, and comfy jeans a reward for working hard all week. Successful adults have multiple rewards throughout their day, and whether they know it or not, they have typically mastered the arrangement of their own routines (work, reward, work, reward) to maximize their performance and satisfaction. This is a lot to learn, and many children simply do not know how. Just like teaching children how to tie shoes and brush teeth, parents need to teach children how to self-reward so that they can be successful in the long run. The catch here is that for some children this training happens naturally, but for others the self-reward training starts with rewards delivered by parents. Children who need extra help first start out by learning the connection between their behavior and consequences—good behavior leads to good consequences. Over time, these children can be taught to self-administer rewards in the above manner. Parents can be reassured that their children will not become spoiled or unappreciative as a result of using a rewards program (unless, of course, spoiled or unappreciative behavior itself is unintentionally rewarded).

WHAT'S THE EVIDENCE?

- The use of rewards in therapy may be the most common practice in treatments supported by research, with dozens of successful studies across multiple areas (e.g., Henggeler et al., 1998; Kazdin et al., 1992; Patterson et al., 1982; Wells & Egan, 1988).
- This technique has been used widely in treatments for childhood anxiety, both to increase positive behaviors and to increase motivation to participate in practice exercises (e.g., Barrett, 1998; Barrett et al., 1996; Cobham et al., 1998; De Haan et al., 1998; Graziano & Mooney, 1980; Kendall, 1994; Kendall et al., 1997; King et al., 1998; King et al., 2000; Obler & Terwillinger, 1970; Pediatric OCD Treatment Study Team, 2004; Silverman, Kurtines, Ginsburg, Weems, Lumkin, et al., 1999; Spence et al., 2000).

WORKING WITH PARENTS: TIME-OUT

★ Objectives

The objective for this module is to introduce or review the procedure of time-out with the parent(s) (or teacher). This module is often used when moderately disruptive behaviors (e.g., throwing tantrums, hitting, being mean or disrespectful) prohibit working on other issues successfully. With some children, this is the first module covered after Learning about Anxiety, because they are too disruptive to do anything else, and the family may not be motivated to work on anything else first.

⏱ If Pressed for Time

Using the **Time-Out Handout**, go over the basic rules of time-out and pick at least one target behavior on which to practice at home before the next session.

✉ Who Is Needed

Child
Parent(s) or teacher

✏ Materials

Time-Out Handout (parent, teacher, or both)
Observation Record (parent, teacher, or both)

🌡 Weekly Rating

Obtain the **Fear Ladder** ratings from both the child and parent(s). Inspect the Fear Ladder for unusually high or problematic items; these might need to be discussed during the meeting.

📄 Assignment Review

Review any practice assignments that were given in the previous session. Discuss what was learned, and consider rehearsing pieces of the homework together to consolidate the information. If the assignment was not completed, troubleshoot reasons why and consider the various options for handling whatever the obstacle might be. In all but the rarest of circumstances, do not proceed to new material if the assignment is not complete. It is better to take the planned session to perform the assignment together or to problem-solve how to accomplish it at home.

1 Set the Agenda

Meet with the parent(s) alone and talk about the various ideas and exercises you plan to cover in your meeting. Make sure these are spelled out in order, with approximate time limits given for how long each part might take. This information will add to the predictability of the meeting and minimize confusion. Ask the parent(s) if he or she has any issues to cover and put these on the agenda as well. It can be helpful to write these items on a dry erase board or easel pad to serve as a visual reminder. Finally, be sure to point out that there will be an opportunity for some positive time at the end of the meeting.

Procedures

1. Continue to meet with the parent(s) alone and explain that, as a method of discipline, time-out means a brief interruption of activities for the child. The child is quickly removed from the situation in which the misbehavior occurred and placed in a quiet, boring place that is not fun at all.
2. Review with the parent(s) the reasons why children typically do not like time-out (e.g., they lose attention, temporary freedom, and more importantly, the power to upset and manipulate their parents). Because time-out is easy and convenient to use, children are unable get out of the punishment, as they often can with other parental threats.
3. Remind the parent(s) that children will do what works for them. If time-out is consistently applied for certain behaviors, the child will give up those behaviors and try other ways to get what he or she wants. Explain that the parent's job is to help the child find "good" ways to achieve desired ends by rewarding acceptable behaviors.
4. Inform the parent(s) of the short- and long-term benefits that can result from employing time-out:
   - Immediate benefit of reducing the occurrence of the problem behavior.
   - Immediate benefit of giving parents a chance to "cool off."
   - Long-term benefit of teaching children self-discipline; they learn to consider the consequences of their actions because the consequences are predictable.
5. Discuss with the parent(s) when it is best to use time-out. Explain that time-out should be used for stopping moderate-to-serious bad behavior (i.e., serious rudeness; aggressive, destructive, or nasty acts; behavior that might be dangerous to self or others, even if it wasn't intended to be). Remind the parent(s) that time-out is not effective for passive misbehavior (e.g., sulking) or for acts of omission, such as when the child fails to do something that the parent wanted him or her to do. Point out that when the goal is to get the child to start performing desired behaviors that are currently being avoided, rewards should be used instead.

6. Instruct the parent(s) to select only one to three target behaviors to begin with, explaining that other behaviors can be added once the family has had the chance to practice time-out for a while. Suggest that the parent(s) choose a behavior that occurs at least once a day, that is easily defined, and that can be observed at home.

7. Explain to the parent(s) that the place chosen for time-out should be a boring place (i.e., no other people available, away from toys, games, TV, books, pets, windows); it should *not* be a scary experience for the child. Parent(s) and child should be able to get to the time-out place within 10 seconds. Review the following guidelines for placing the child in time-out:
    - A separate room should be selected for older children (i.e., bathroom, laundry or utility room, hallway).
    - The child should be placed in the designated time-out place and left alone there for the duration of the time-out.
    - Other family members should be instructed not to talk to the child for the duration of the time-out.

8. Discuss with the parent(s) how to explain time-out to the child:
    - Suggest that the parent(s) choose a time when he or she and the child are relaxed and not upset. Both parents should be present for this discussion with the child, if possible, because the child needs to know that both parents have the same expectations of his or her behavior.
    - The parent(s) should tell the child that he or she is loved but that his or her behavior (indicate specific problematic behaviors) is causing problems for the parents and the family. The parent(s) should not ask for the child's agreement with this statement or argue with the child about it.

9. Discuss with the parent(s) what to do when misbehavior occurs, reviewing the steps that need to be taken to get the child to time-out quickly.

10. When a target behavior occurs, the parent(s) should get the child to time-out by using no more than 10 words in 10 seconds. The misbehavior should be labeled, and a command for time-out should be issued (e.g., "Because you pushed me, you have a time-out").

11. Instruct the parent(s) to use a portable timer because children learn quickly that they cannot argue with a timer. The timer should be placed within hearing distance of the child and set for 1 minute for each year of age. Tell the parent(s) that it is important to always use the same amount of time for time-out.

12. The timer should be reset for screaming or tantrums; all other attempts of the child to obtain parent(s) attention should be actively ignored.

13. Explain to the parent(s) the procedures to use following time-out. When the timer rings, the child should leave time-out and bring the timer to the parent(s). The child should then describe why he or she was sent to time-out. The parent(s) might say, "The timer rang, so you may come out now. Now, tell me why you had to go to time-out." If the child does not answer correctly why he or she was sent to time-out, tell him or her the reason and then ask again why he or she was sent to time-out.

14. The parent(s) should be told that, for all but the most serious misbehaviors, the inci-

dent should be dropped once the child has served a time-out. The parent(s) should be instructed to resist the temptation to scold the child further. When the time-out is completed, the child should be told that he or she may go play. If the child remains annoyed after the time-out, the parent(s) should be encouraged to ignore this behavior. The child has a right to these feelings, as long as the misbehavior does not continue.

15. Review with the parent(s) the common problems associated with implementing time-out:

   - **Talking back**: Each time the child talks back, he or she should earn another minute of time-out.
   - **Arguing**: If the talking back is substantial, the basic principle to apply is that the longer the child argues, the longer the duration of time-out. The parent(s) should be instructed to reset the timer once the child stops arguing.
   - **Refusing to go to time-out**: When the child refuses to go to time-out, he or she should lose 30 minutes of privileges (e.g., TV). If the child continues to refuse, he or she should lose privileges all day until the time-out is completed.
   - **Leaving time-out**: Whenever the child leaves time-out before the time is up, the timer should be reset.
   - **Making a mess**: If the child makes a mess in response to instructions to go to time-out, the child should clean the room and the timer should be reset.

16. It should be stressed to the parent(s) that time-out should never be used without rewarding the child for good behaviors at other times during the day.

🎭 Role Play

Start with something like this: "Let's practice what a time-out might look and sound like. I will play the part of your child. Try to use the techniques we have just discussed. When I am doing something bad, put me in time-out by using the steps we have discussed."

If it helps, you can have the parent(s) play the part of the child first, so that you can model the successful behavior and then have the parent(s) try it next.

Praise the parent(s) for any successful parts of the role play. Point out what you liked most and then repeat the role play, if needed, to address things that could be improved ("That was great! Now we're going to try again, and we are just going to add one more thing").

In Vivo

If possible, repeat the exercise you just role-played, now having the parent(s) (or teacher) run through the strategy with the child. You may have to provide some prompts to the child as the *in vivo* exercise progresses. In general, it is always best to rehearse a new skill at least once with the child in this way. The more, the better, and be sure to provide plenty of praise for everyone. Don't let them leave until it looks like they will get it right at home.

Practice Assignment

Provide the parent(s) with the **Time-Out Handout** and the **Parent Observation Record**. The parent(s) should be instructed to begin introducing time-out in the home and to monitor the child's behavior and his or her use of time-out on the **Parent Observation Record** during the next week.

☺ **End on a Positive**

If the child is present, end the session on a fun note with a game, activity, or other exercise that will leave the child feeling positive about the work you all have done together today. The parent(s) can be included in this activity as well. If the child is not present, take some time for supportive listening with the parent(s) if it appears to be pleasing.

☞ DON'T FORGET!

- Make sure that the parent takes home the **Parent Observation Record** and **Time-Out Handout** (or **Teacher Observation Record** and **Time-Out Handout** for a teacher).

✔ CHECKLIST

If two or more of the following items cannot be checked off, consider what problems may have arisen. Portions of the module might need to be repeated, or troubleshooting might be indicated to determine how to overcome or compensate for any challenges encountered.

____ The parent(s) or teacher understood that time-out involves the temporary removal of rewards.

____ The parent(s) or teacher understood the short- and long-term benefits of time-out.

____ The parent(s) or teacher understood which behaviors were appropriate for time-out.

____ The parent(s) or teacher was able to role-play successfully.

____ The parent(s) or teacher was able to perform an *in vivo* exercise with the child successfully.

____ A positive time together was shared at the end of the meeting, either with the child or in the form of supportive listening with the parent(s).

(i) THINGS TO CONSIDER

- Many parents will protest that "time-out does not work" for their child. Encourage them to consider that it is possible that what did not work before might work now, if given the chance. Most often, time-out fails because it is not used consistently or properly. If these problems can be fixed, it will probably work well with their child.
- Time-out can take a great deal of patience and effort at first. Assure the parent(s) that much of the success of time-out is in its "fine-tuning." If it is not successful right away, encourage the parent(s) not to give up; troubleshooting often reveals simple changes that will improve the success of using time-out.
- This module can also be used with teachers if the problem behaviors are happening in the classroom as well. Ideally, the parent(s) and teachers should be using the same program consistently. There is a separate **Time-Out Handout** and **Teacher Observation Record** for teachers.

? TROUBLESHOOTING

- **Slow starts**: Sometimes parents get involved in delaying, explaining, or negotiating when giving a time-out. This misapplication can be observed during the role play or *in vivo* exercise. Experts have suggested that the swiftness with which time-out is issued may be one of the best predictors of its effectiveness, and Russell Barkley has used the term "Swift Justice" to emphasize that aspect of the technique (e.g., Barkely et al., 2005). Parents and caretakers should therefore be prepared to identify and review the time-out behaviors with the child in advance, and then give an immediate time-out upon their occurrence.
- **Time-out is time in**: Sometimes parents implement a time-out in such a way as to allow the children to have time with rewards after all (such as in their room). Remind the parent(s) that the purpose of time-out is to remove all rewarding stimulation from the child for a brief period of time. This can be possible in a child's room, but it can take a considerable amount of work to remove all reinforcers from that environment. It is usually easier to pick a place to sit in some other part of the house, such as the kitchen or even the bathroom.
- **Fouling up the follow-up**: Parents sometimes engage in nagging, excessive discussion, or punitive remarks following a time-out. This misapplication can also be observed during the role play or *in vivo* exercise. The parent(s) should be instructed to keep the interaction following time-out brief. For example, a parent might ask, "Do you know why you got this time-out?" but once the reason was clear, would not pursue further discussion. If a demand was in place previously, now is the time to repeat it. And the follow-through should not only be short but also be sweet. That is, the tone should not be angry or aggressive, but calm and matter-of-fact.

WHAT'S THE EVIDENCE?

- The use of time-out to reduce unwanted negative behaviors has been supported in numerous studies of children with behavior problems (e.g., Kazdin et al., 1992; Patterson et al., 1982; Wells & Egan, 1988).
- This technique has been used successfully in treatments specifically designed for childhood anxiety (e.g., Barrett, 1998; Barrett et al., 1996; Chorpita et al., 2004; Cobham et al., 1998).
- Hamilton and MacQuiddy (1984) showed that a specific time-out procedure, used alone, resulted in clinically significant improvements in children with noncompliance problems relative to two control groups.

WORKSHEETS, RECORDS, AND HANDOUTS

Fear Ladder

Date: _____

Please give a rating for how scary each of these things is today. Remember to use the scale from 0 to 10.

Filled out by: ( ) child ( ) parent ( ) other _____

Feelings

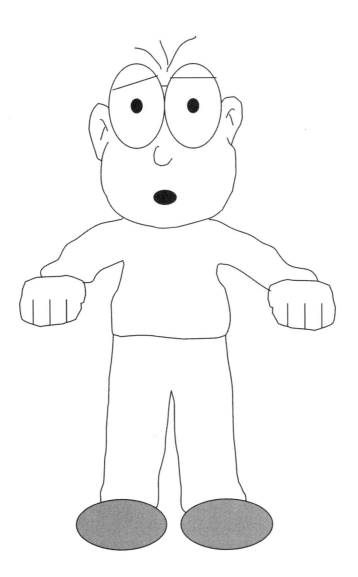

Feelings

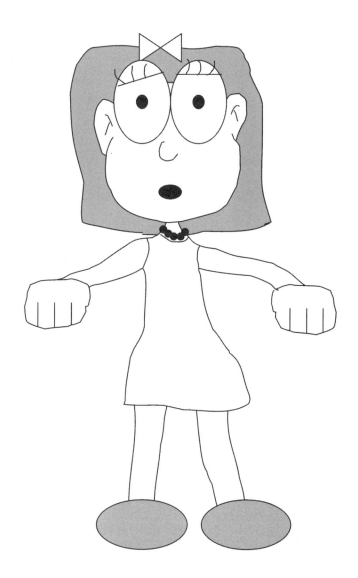

Thoughts

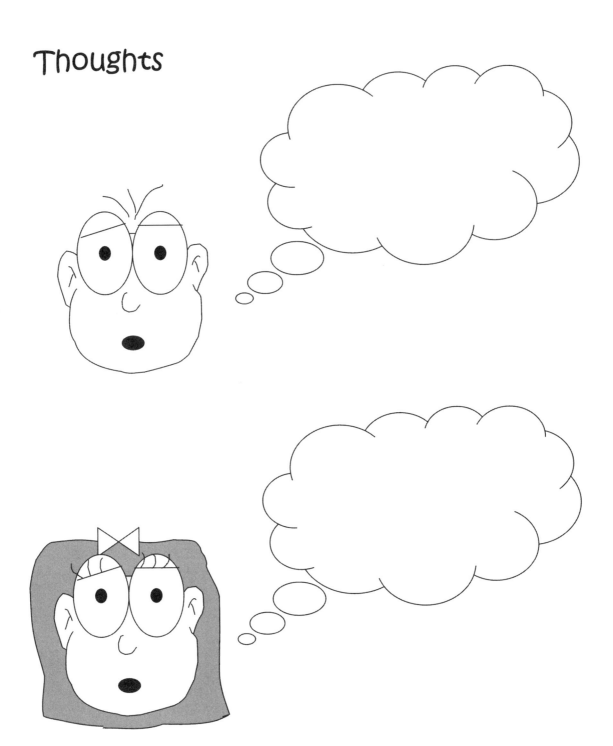

(page 3 of 3)

Anxiety and How It Works

WORKSHEET FOR CHILDREN

I learned a lot of new things about anxiety this week.

This worksheet will help me remember some of the most important things. Follow the numbers.

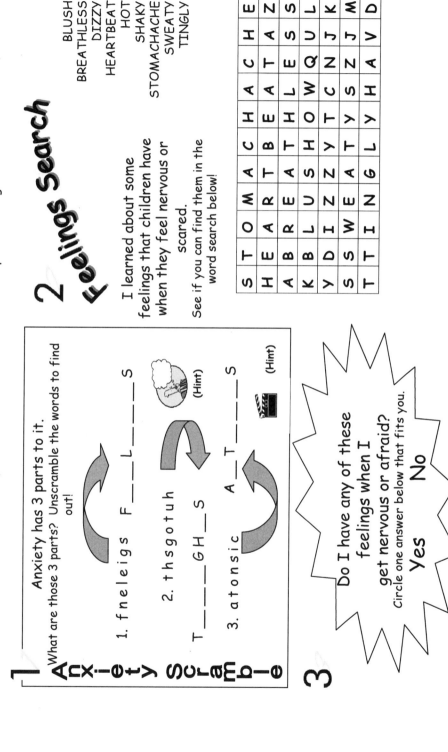

2 Feelings Search

BLUSH
BREATHLESS
DIZZY
HEARTBEAT
HOT
SHAKY
STOMACHACHE
SWEATY
TINGLY

I learned about some feelings that children have when they feel nervous or scared.

See if you can find them in the word search below!

S	T	O	M	A	C	H	A	C	H	E
H	E	A	R	T	B	E	A	T	A	Z
A	B	R	E	A	T	H	L	E	S	S
K	B	L	U	S	H	O	W	Q	U	L
Y	D	I	Z	Z	Y	T	C	N	J	K
S	S	W	E	A	T	Y	S	Z	J	M
T	T	I	N	G	L	Y	H	A	V	D

1 Anxiety Scramble

A. What are those 3 parts? Unscramble the words to find out!

1. fneleigs   F _ _ _ _ _ S

2. thsgotuh   T _ _ _ _ GH _ S   (Hint)

3. atonsic   A _ T _ _ _ S   (Hint)

3

Do I have any of these feelings when I get nervous or afraid?
Circle one answer below that fits you.

Yes   No

4 Remember all the feelings in the feelings search?
People get all sorts of feelings when they get scared.

Circle the feelings that you get.

BLUSHING   BUTTERFLIES
DIZZY   DRY MOUTH
FAST HEARTBEAT   FIDGETY
HEADACHE   HOT
SHAKY   SHORT OF BREATH
STOMACHACHE   SWEATY
TINGLY HANDS   UPSET TUMMY

6 When I feel nervous or scared, sometimes I act in certain ways.
List the things that these people are doing because they're nervous or scared.

This person is…

R _ N N _ _ _ G

This person is…

C _ Y _ N _ _

This person is…

Y _ L _ I _ G

5 When I feel nervous and scared, I often have certain thoughts.

List a thought that you have when you feel nervous or scared.

Thoughts Bubble

Example: When I go into a room, I think everyone will laugh at me.

_____
_____
_____
_____

226

7

When I get nervous or scared, I . . . .
(Circle what you do.)

CRY   STAY AWAY

YELL   RUN AWAY

WORRY   STAY BY MOM

CAN'T MOVE   GET MAD

anything else? _____

8

Anxiety is meant to be . . . .
Circle one

Good   Bad

Anxiety is the body's _____

(Hint)

Give an example of a
"Red Light" _____

_____
"Yellow Light"

9

Being scared can cause problems when we
feel really nervous or afraid but there is no
danger around us. Match the picture to the
word that best describes this.

False Alarm

True Alarm

10

How can you fix false alarms?
Fill in the letters below to find out!

(Hint: Remember, this is an important part of getting better with
nervous and scared feelings, just like it's an important part of getting
better at sports or playing an instrument.)

P _ _ _ _ _ _

17 By practicing things that make me nervous or scared, I can become braver when I'm in those situations (get rid of my false alarms.) When I practice, I should work from things that are less scary to those that are more scary.

Use what you know about practice and nervous and scared feelings to come up with exercises for people to try.

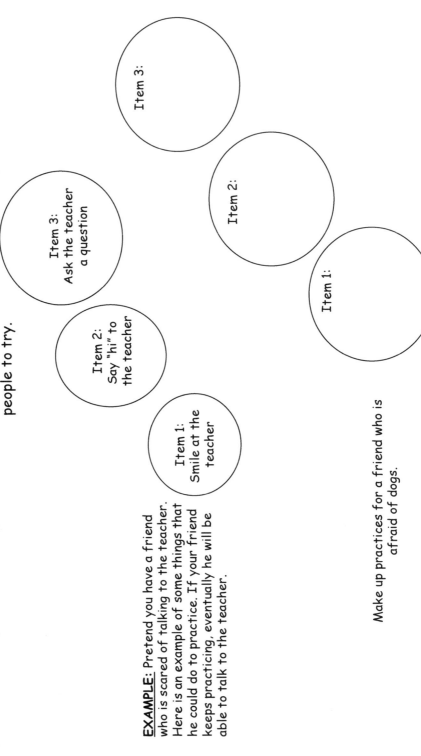

Item 1:
Smile at the teacher

Item 2:
Say "hi" to the teacher

Item 3:
Ask the teacher a question

Item 1:

Item 2:

Item 3:

EXAMPLE: Pretend you have a friend who is scared of talking to the teacher. Here is an example of some things that he could do to practice. If your friend keeps practicing, eventually he will be able to talk to the teacher.

Make up practices for a friend who is afraid of dogs.

228

12

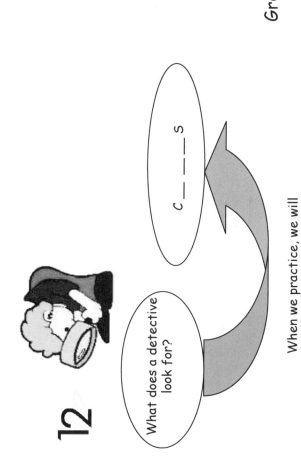

What does a detective look for?

c _ _ _ _ s

When we practice, we will be like detectives and gather clues.

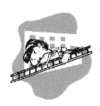
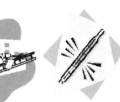

By using the fear thermometer and filling out the fear ladders, we will collect clues and track your nervous and scared feelings!

13

Great job! We're ready to get started! Now let's go and collect clues for you!

Anxiety and How It Works
WORKSHEET FOR TEENS

I learned a lot of new things about anxiety this week.

This worksheet will help me remember some of the most important things. Follow the numbers.

1 — Anxiety Scramble

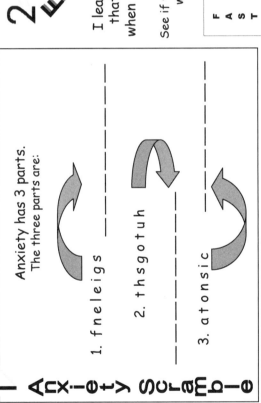

Anxiety has 3 parts.
The three parts are:

1. fneleigs _ _ _ _ _ _ _ _

2. thsgotuh _ _ _ _ _ _ _ _

3. atonsic _ _ _ _ _ _ _

2 — Feelings Search

I learned about feelings that some people have when they feel nervous or scared.

See if you can find them in the word search below!

- BLUSHING
- BUTTERFLIES
- DIZZY
- DRY MOUTH
- FAST BEATING HEART
- FIDGETY
- HEADACHE
- HOT
- SHAKY
- SHORT OF BREATH
- STOMACHACHE
- SWEATY
- TINGLY HANDS

```
F A D R Y M O U T H F L B
A M Z D A L E T K C A D D
S S H P S R T K M L Y Q T
T B U T T E R F L I E E S
B R C G W T O E B K E S W
E L C B N U H Y L S H X E
A Z Y I T C I T A D X C E
T K J G A J E L F Y I B A
I A P D H G L K W P D H T
N O A C D K A J Y R C Y
G E T I X H G M C X Z A D
H F F E S O O H A A Z M F
E O V Z B T P O I N G Y O N P
A S B L U A H Z H A N D S G
R Q H Z L A F N Z S Y A
T I N G L Y H A N D B E A T H
S H O R T O F B R E A T H
```

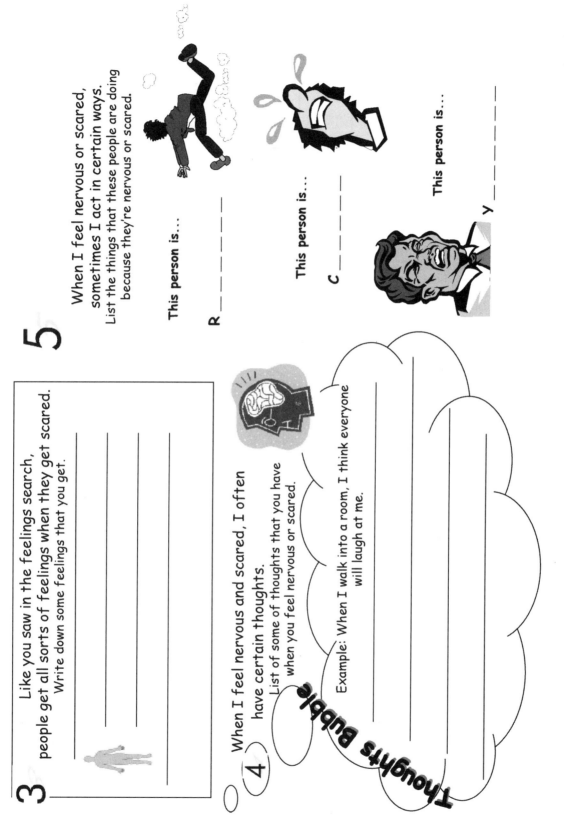

5

When I feel nervous or scared, sometimes I act in certain ways. List the things that these people are doing because they're nervous or scared.

This person is...

R _ _ _ _ _ _ _

This person is...

C _ _ _ _ _ _ _

This person is...

Y _ _ _ _ _ _ _

3

Like you saw in the feelings search, people get all sorts of feelings when they get scared. Write down some feelings that you get.

_ _ _ _ _ _ _ _ _ _
_ _ _ _ _ _ _ _ _ _
_ _ _ _ _ _ _ _ _ _

4

When I feel nervous and scared, I often have certain thoughts.

List of some of thoughts that you have when you feel nervous or scared.

Thoughts Bubble

Example: When I walk into a room, I think everyone will laugh at me.

_ _ _ _ _ _ _ _ _ _
_ _ _ _ _ _ _ _ _ _
_ _ _ _ _ _ _ _ _ _

7 Anxiety is meant to be . . .
Circle one

Good   **Bad**

Anxiety is the body's _____

(Hint)

Give an example of a
"Red Light" _____

"Yellow Light" _____

6

When I get nervous or scared, I . . . .
(Write in what you do.)

_____
_____
_____
_____
_____

8 We can get into trouble when we feel really nervous or afraid but there is no danger around us. Pretend an alarm is going off and match the picture to the word that best describes it.

False Alarm

True Alarm

9 How can you fix false alarms?
Fill in the letters below to find out! (Hint: Remember, this is an important part of getting better with nervous and scared feelings, just like it's an important part of getting better at sports or playing an instrument.)

P _ _ _ _ _ _

232

10 By practicing these things, I can become less nervous or scared when I'm in those situations (get rid of my false alarms.) When I practice, I should work from things that are less scary to those that are more scary.

Use what you know about practice and nervous and scared feelings to come up with exercises for people to try.

EXAMPLE: Pretend you have a friend who is scared of talking to the teacher. Here is an example of some things that he could do to practice. If your friend keeps practicing, eventually he will be able to talk to the teacher.

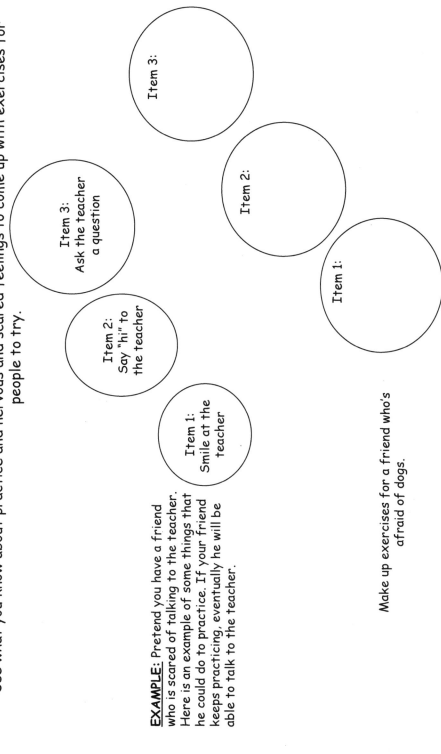

Item 1:
Smile at the teacher

Item 2:
Say "hi" to the teacher

Item 3:
Ask the teacher a question

Item 1:

Item 2:

Item 3:

Make up exercises for a friend who's afraid of dogs.

11

How do I know if my practice is helping me figure out if things are changing?

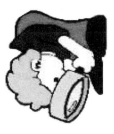

By using the fear ladder and taking ratings with the fear thermometer during practice, we can make sure that things keep getting better.

12

Good job! Now we are ready to work on getting rid of the extra anxiety in your life.

About Anxiety
PARENT HANDOUT

Anxiety Has Many Causes

Lots of things have been found to cause anxiety in children and adolescents, such as biological factors (things in your body), psychological factors (things you think and feel), and social factors (where you go to school, who your friends are). These factors most often come together as the combination of a child's

Children can have a "sensitive personality" that puts them at risk for anxiety problems.

"sensitive personality" with a variety of experiences that can intensify and focus anxiety problems. "Sensitive personality" in children involves an increased sensitivity to bad events or objects and information that may be threatening. In other words, these are children who get upset, worried, frightened, or sad more easily than others. This personality factor puts a child at risk to experience a variety of negative emotions throughout life and can lead to anxiety disorders and sometimes depression.

Feeling Out of Control

This "sensitive personality" can be intensified through a variety of experiences in a child's life. One of the most important influences appears to be related to a child's sense of control over things that happen in life. Some people have found that children who feel they cannot control certain things are likely to have a more negative reaction to bad experiences. This sense of things being out of one's control can be made worse through situations that limit a child's opportunity to experience the world, to master challenges, and to attract help at the appropriate times. Most importantly, a child needs to develop a sense that he or she can make bad things less bad by making them go away or by learning how to cope or deal with them.

The Role of Bad Experiences

In addition to these important feelings about control, certain bad experiences can occur in life that can lead a child's personality to express itself in a specific area. For example, a child at risk in this way who is bitten by a dog may develop a phobia of dogs; if the child is excessively teased, social phobia might develop; if the child has a bad experience with a stranger, separation anxiety may develop, and so forth. Thus, an anxiety disorder is usually the result of a lot of things that add up over time, including personality type, early feelings of being out of control, and specific bad experiences.

Effects on Thinking

Children with anxiety problems see the world in a slightly different way.

Children with anxiety problems are somewhat different from other children in the way that they think. In general, anxious children are better able to generate negative ideas. In other words, relative to other children, they can think of lots of ways

From Bruce F. Chorpita (2007). Copyright by The Guilford Press.

(page 1 of 3)

235

that things can go wrong. This tendency shows up in a number of specific ways, including problems with attention, interpretation, and "self-talk." For example, in a research study people presented children with pairs of words on a computer screen and found that anxious children were more likely to look at words that were threatening, such as "accident." In other studies, several researchers noticed that anxious children are more likely to interpret ambiguous situations as dangerous. For example, when asked a question such as "you hear a noise in the middle of the night—what do you think it is?" anxious children come up with a larger number of threatening possibilities, such as "a burglar." In yet another line of research, people observed that anxious children use more negative "self-talk" than nonanxious children, telling themselves such things as "I won't be able to handle this situation."

Effects on Feelings

When the world is seen in this way, the effects on the child are many, and this activates a number of important events in the brain and body. It is important to remember that anxiety is an emotion whose purpose is to prepare someone to handle danger. In its first stage, such as when a threat is still somewhat distant, anxiety shows up as worry, tension, increased attention to the

Anxiety is a natural human emotion that is meant to protect us from danger.

possible danger, and reduction of activities like running or playing. One researcher calls this first part the "stop, look, and listen" stage of anxiety. For example, a child who suddenly hears a dog barking as she walks to school might stop and listen, imagining the ways that the dog might be trouble and thinking about a safer way to get to school. This

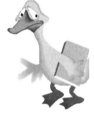

response is common in animals, such as when you first approach a bird, the way it will stop feeding and walking so that it can study you to see what you will do next. As you can see, the emotion of anxiety serves a useful purpose in looking out for danger and therefore helping to avoid it. In other words, **anxiety can be good**. It is only when people begin to experience anxiety when they are not supposed to—when there is no real threat or danger—that the emotion becomes a problem. Sometimes we call this kind of anxiety a "false alarm."

The emotion of anxiety has two "stages."

If the threat gets closer or more intense, the feelings escalate, and other parts of the body are called in and prepared to confront the danger. Again, this is all part of a natural and purposeful response to survive a threatening experience, such as an attack from an angry dog. In this situation, the body is wired to activate the second stage, often called fear or panic, also known as the "fight or flight" response. This response involves increased heartbeat, change in blood pressure, faster breathing, and a cascade of chemicals throughout the body to increase speed, strength, and alertness. Some of these chemicals, like adrenaline, can have side effects such as shakiness or nausea. In our example of the student, if the dog leaps at her, she moves on from stage one, worry and tension, to stage two: dry mouth, shaky hands, intense breathing, and pounding heart. All of this is to

(page 2 of 3)

help her run away or fight off the attacking dog. Similarly, if you continue to move toward the bird in the earlier example, it will fly away in a burst of energy—or, if that is not possible, it will try to defend itself. This is part of the body's design to handle danger. Again, the problem is that children with anxiety disorders can experience these emotions when there is no real danger, such as when children who always get good grades panic during a test. This is another example of a "false alarm."

Cognitive-Behavioral Therapy

The treatment approach that works best with anxiety is called *cognitive-behavioral therapy.* This approach is based on the idea that it is important to teach children the skills to identify when the danger is not real, when they are just having a "false alarm," and therefore when their anxiety is unnecessary. Giving children the ability to identify **accurately** when situations are safe helps reduce or eliminate the tension and worry as well as the feelings of fear and panic. Much of this happens through **practice exercises** designed to teach the children, using reasoning and experience, that their anxiety is not necessary—that what they feel is dangerous and scary is really safe. One of the main problems with anxious children is that by avoiding what they are afraid of, they limit the possibility for these helpful practice experiences. The therapist's role is to act as a guide to encourage and support the child to participate in these experiences so that things misperceived as threatening can eventually be seen as safe. As you will see, most of *cognitive-behavioral therapy* is about practice that will help your child think about things in a new and different way.

(page 3 of 3)

Principles of Success

IMPORTANT THINGS TO KEEP IN MIND
WHEN WORKING WITH YOUR CHILD'S ANXIETY

1. **Homework is more important than in-session work.** What happens at home and school is more important than what happens when your child is working with a therapist. Just like with music lessons, a therapist just reviews progress and assigns new things to practice. If the child does not practice in-between meetings with the therapist, little progress will be made.

2. **The therapist and parents are "coaches."** Things work best if parents take over an increasingly larger part of the coaching role as the program goes along.

3. **The program works best if it is a high priority to the child and parent(s).** If everyone in the family is not committed to the program, results will not be so good. For now, it might have to come first before other things, such as school plays, sports, weekend trips, etc.

4. **A minimum level of commitment is required.** When a child's enthusiasm is low, the parent's enthusiasm must be extra high; similarly, if a parent's enthusiasm is low, the enthusiasm of the child must be high. The best situation is when both the parent and child see practice and improvement as a high priority, just like in the picture below.

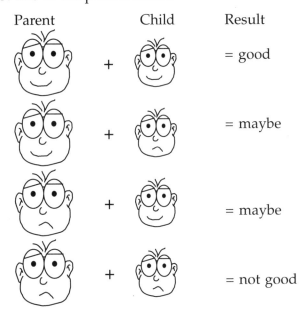

Parent		Child		Result
	+			= good
	+			= maybe
	+			= maybe
	+			= not good

5. **It is important to let some things be hard in the short term, so that your child's life can be easier in the long term.** For example, it is often easier to let your child just have fun by watching TV, playing video games, shopping, or hanging out with friends. This can put your child in a good mood, but the long-term anxiety problems won't go away. On the other hand, with some extra work now, anxiety problems can be much better for months or years.

(page 1 of 2)

6. **Things go better for parents who remember that practice is safe.** For example, sometimes your child might cry or complain during some of the practices. This is perfectly normal, and you should try to help your child stick it out in the tough situation and get used to whatever is difficult for him or her now. It is important to be supportive, but it is not a good idea to stop things for your child just because they are hard.

7. **You and your child's attendance or willingness to meet and speak on the phone with the therapist are extremely important.** Without that, there is little chance of success.

8. **When parents are anxious, treatment can often be more difficult.** Anxious parents often have a hard time letting their children practice challenging things. This is why the therapist is the coach in the beginning and decides what pace is best for your child. It is important to try to stay relaxed during the exercises your child will practice.

9. **Finally, it is common for many of these things to be difficult at first, and it is OK for you to talk about what is getting in the way of the program.** Parents who talk about what is not working for them and their family do better than families who don't tell anyone about the troubles they are having. Remember, someone is there now to help solve some of the problems for you, even with things like lack of time or doubts about your child's progress. If something feels like it is going wrong, bring it up.

About Anxiety

TEACHER HANDOUT

Anxiety Has Many Causes

Lots of things have been found to cause anxiety in children and adolescents, such as biological factors (things in your body), psychological factors (things you think and feel), and social factors (where you go to school, who your friends are). These factors most often come together as the combination of a child's

Children can have a "sensitive personality" that puts them at risk for anxiety problems.

"sensitive personality" with a variety of experiences that can intensify and focus anxiety problems. "Sensitive personality" in children involves an increased sensitivity to bad events or objects and information that may be threatening. In other words, these are children who get upset, worried, frightened, or sad more easily than others. This personality factor puts a child at risk to experience a variety of negative emotions throughout life and can lead to anxiety disorders and sometimes depression.

Feeling Out of Control

This "sensitive personality" can be intensified through a variety of experiences in a child's life. One of the most important influences appears to be related to a child's sense of control over things that happen in life. Some people have found that children who feel they cannot control certain things are likely to have a more negative reaction to bad experiences. This sense of things being out of one's control can be made worse through situations that limit a child's opportunity to experience the world, to master challenges, and to attract help at the appropriate times. Most importantly, a child needs to develop a sense that he or she can make bad things less bad by making them go away or by learning how to cope or deal with them.

The Role of Bad Experiences

In addition to these important feelings about control, certain bad experiences can occur in life that can lead a child's personality to express itself in a specific area. For example, a child at risk in this way who is bitten by a dog may develop a phobia of dogs; if the child is excessively teased, social phobia might develop; if the child has a bad experience with a stranger, separation anxiety may develop, and so forth. Thus, an anxiety disorder is usually the result of a lot of things that add up over time, including personality type, early feelings of being out of control, and specific bad experiences.

Effects on Thinking

Children with anxiety problems see the world in a slightly different way.

Children with anxiety problems are somewhat different from other children in the way that they think. In general, anxious children are better able to generate negative ideas. In other words, relative to other children, they can think of lots of ways that things can go wrong. This tendency shows up in a number of specific ways, including problems with attention, interpretation, and "self-talk." For example, in a research study people presented children with pairs of words on a computer screen and found that anxious children were more likely to look at words that were threatening, such as "accident." In other studies, several researchers noticed that anxious children are more likely to interpret ambiguous situations as dangerous. For example, when asked a question such as "you hear a noise in the middle of the night—what do you think it is?" anxious children come up with a larger number of threatening possibilities, such as "a burglar." In yet another line of research, people observed that anxious children use more negative "self-talk" than nonanxious children, telling themselves such things as "I won't be able to handle this situation."

Effects on Feelings

When the world is seen in this way, the effects on the child are many, and this activates a number of important events in the brain and body. It is important to remember that anxiety is an emotion whose purpose is to prepare someone to handle danger. In its first stage, such as when a threat is still somewhat distant, anxiety shows up as worry, tension, increased attention to the possible danger, and reduction of activities like running or playing. One researcher calls this first part the "stop, look, and listen" stage of anxiety. For example, a child who suddenly hears a dog barking as she walks to school might stop and listen, imagining the ways that the dog

Anxiety is a natural human emotion that is meant to protect us from danger.

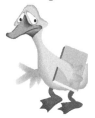
might be trouble and thinking about a safer way to get to school. This response is common in animals, such as when you first approach a bird, the way it will stop feeding and walking so that it can study you to see what you will do next. As you can see, the emotion of anxiety serves a useful purpose in looking out for danger and therefore helping to avoid it. In other words, **anxiety can be good**. It is only when people begin to experience anxiety when they are not supposed to—when there is no real threat or danger—that the emotion becomes a problem. Sometimes we call this kind of anxiety a "false alarm."

The emotion of anxiety has two "stages."

If the threat gets closer or more intense, the feelings escalate, and other parts of the body are called in and prepared to confront the danger. Again, this is all part of a natural and purposeful response to survive a threatening experience, such as an attack from an angry dog. In this situation, the body is wired to activate the second stage, often called fear or panic, also 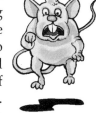 known as the "fight or flight" response. This response involves increased heart beat, change in blood pressure, faster breathing, and a cascade of chemicals throughout the body to increase speed, strength, and alertness. Some of these chemicals, like adrenaline, can have side effects such as shakiness or nausea. In our example of the student, if the dog leaps at her, she moves on from stage one, worry and tension, to stage two: dry mouth, shaky hands, intense breath-

(page 2 of 3)

ing, and pounding heart. All of this is to help her run away or fight off the attacking dog. Similarly, if you continue to move toward the bird in the earlier example, it will fly away in a burst of energy—or, if that is not possible, it will try to defend itself. This is part of the body's design to handle danger. Again, the problem is that children with anxiety disorders can experience these emotions when there is no real danger, such as when children who always get good grades panic during a test. This is another example of a "false alarm."

Cognitive-Behavioral Therapy

The treatment approach that works best with anxiety is called *cognitive-behavioral therapy*. This approach is based on the idea that it is important to teach children the skills to identify when the danger is not real, when they are just having a "false alarm," and therefore when their anxiety is unnecessary. Giving children the ability to identify **accurately** when situations are safe helps reduce or eliminate the tension and worry as well as the feelings of fear and panic. Much of this happens through **practice exercises** designed to teach the children, using reasoning and experience, that their anxiety is not necessary—that what they feel is dangerous and scary is really safe. One of the main problems with anxious children is that by avoiding what they are afraid of, they limit the possibility for these helpful practice experiences. The therapist's role is to act as a guide to encourage and support the child to participate in these experiences so that things misperceived as threatening can eventually be seen as safe. As you will see, most of *cognitive-behavioral therapy* is about practice that will help your student think about things in a new and different way.

(page 3 of 3)

Discrete Practice Record

Goal: Each time you practice, repeat _____ times or until your rating comes down to _____. You can do it!

Start Date: _____

Day _____ _____ _____ _____ _____ _____ _____
Item _____ _____ _____ _____ _____ _____ _____

Before / After thermometer scales (0–10)

Day _____ _____ _____ _____ _____ _____ _____
Item _____ _____ _____ _____ _____ _____ _____

Before / After thermometer scales (0–10)

From Bruce F. Chorpita (2007). Copyright by The Guilford Press.

Continuous Practice Record

Goal: Each time you practice, take ratings every _____ minutes. Stop after _____ minutes or when your rating comes down to a _____.

Start Date: _____

Day _____
Item _____

Day _____
Item _____

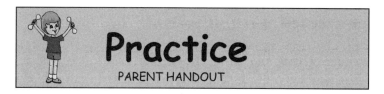

Practice
PARENT HANDOUT

"What is practice?"

Practice for fear or anxiety means doing things that are hard in order to get used to them. It works a lot like practicing a musical instrument or a sport. You can get better at playing the trumpet or soccer if you practice. You can get less nervous about dogs or about what other people think if you practice. Practice leads to improvement. Of course, practice is not always easy. Practicing things that cause anxiety does not always feel good at the time, just like music practice or exercise drills might not always seem fun. This is why your child really needs your help and support.

"When should my child practice?"

Practice is a lot like exercise. It is important to start small and start slowly, and then as your child "gets in shape," she or he can take on bigger challenges and practice more often. We will work together with your child to make sure he or she is practicing the right amount.

Practice can decrease anxiety about: animals, high places, riding the bus, going to school, being teased, being embarrassed, swimming, being in the dark, being away from parents, talking to other people, trying to be perfect, feeling out of breath, feeling out of control, getting a shot, being around adults, being around other children, and lots and lots of other things.

"What are the benefits of practice?"

✓ It is the best possible way to overcome fear.

✓ It is an easy way for me to help your child.

✓ Your child will quickly learn to do things that were too hard before.

(page 1 of 4)

"How do I get started with practice?"

(1) **First, pick something** that your child is afraid of. It is best to start with something that is not too hard. One way to make something easier is to break it down into steps. Remember, once your child starts practicing more, he or she can move on to harder things. "A fear I would like to see go away is:

_____."

(2) **Next, pick a time** that you can help your child with practice. It should be a time when everything is calm, and no one feels rushed. Sometimes practice can take a while, so remember to leave plenty of time. "An example of a good time to help my child practice is:

_____."

(3) **Have a fear thermometer** to take ratings. These ratings range from 0 to 8, and higher numbers mean higher amounts of fear or anxiety. The goal is to get these numbers to go down over time.

(4) **Have a practice form** to keep track of the ratings. This is the best way to know how well the practice is working, and you will need these ratings to know what to practice next.

(5) **Remember** that your child will need plenty of praise and support from as many people as possible. Sometimes practice can feel like a chore, but is the only way to get over feeling nervous or afraid. Help keep your child interested and encouraged.

"What are the steps?"

(1) **When your child is ready,** begin the practice. It can be standing near a dog, sleeping over at a friend's house, talking to an adult, whatever.

(2) **Take ratings.** Use the practice form to take ratings. You will probably take them every few minutes or so. We can show you how to do this.

(3) **Wait as long as you need to.** Sometimes it takes a while for your child to get used to something. Small children might protest or even cry during practice. The best thing to do is to keep going and tell your child he or she is doing well. It may take a little longer, but your child will soon get used to what he or she is practicing.

(4) **Practice, practice, and more practice.** Once things are going pretty well, you can repeat a practice as much as you want. Just like exercise, the more your child does, the better your child will feel. This is the best way to help your child with anxiety or fears. Just make sure there is time left over for fun things, too.

(5) **As your child does better, make things a little harder.** When your child gets good at doing a certain practice, you can move onto something harder. Again, this is just like exercise. Once you can run 5 laps well, then you can try running 6 or 7 laps next time. Be careful not to make it too hard too fast or your child will get frustrated. We can help you with knowing what to practice and knowing how fast to advance your child. This can take some time and patience.

(6) **Keep a regular routine.** Even after something gets better, it is always good to go back to it every now and then to make sure it stays easy. It is important to "stay in shape."

"Help! Practice isn't working!"

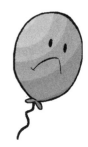

"My child's ratings won't go down." This could be because the practices are too short, or the things you are practicing are too hard for right now. If you are sure you have not picked something that is too hard, try making the practice go longer—eventually your child's fear will decrease and the ratings will come down.

"My child's ratings go down, but the next time we practice they are right back up where they started." When this happens, it usually means there has been too much time between practice. If you are practicing only once or twice a week, try four or five times. Sometimes it can take practicing every day to see improvement.

"My child is too scared to get started." This means it is time to break things down into smaller steps. Think of ways you can make the practice easier (without making it shorter). There are other solutions to this problem, too, and we can usually can help with it.

"My child is getting more scared instead of less." This can happen if you quit in the middle of a practice or if the practices are too short. If you are having problems, you can always go back to practicing something easier for now. Make sure not to stop in the middle—keep it going until the ratings really come down.

"My child says he or she doesn't need to practice anymore." Remember to explain that practice is about building a skill. If you don't keep using it, it will go away. Even when things are not hard anymore, it is important to show you can do them every now and then. This can keep the anxiety from coming back.

(page 4 of 4)

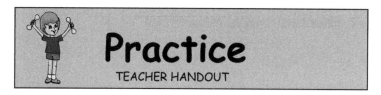

Practice
TEACHER HANDOUT

"What is practice?"

Practice for fear or anxiety means doing things that are hard in order to get used to them. It works a lot like practicing a musical instrument or a sport. You can get better at playing the trumpet or soccer if you practice. You can get less nervous about dogs or about what other people think if you practice. Practice leads to improvement. Of course, practice is not always easy. Practicing things that cause anxiety does not always feel good at the time, just like music practice or exercise drills might not always seem fun. This is why your student really needs your help and support.

"When should my student practice?"

Practice is a lot like exercise. It is important to start small and start slowly, and then as your student "gets in shape," he or she can take on bigger challenges and practice more often. We will work together with your student to make sure he or she is practicing the right amount.

Practice can decrease anxiety about: talking in class, class trips, riding the bus, going to school, being teased, being embarrassed, swimming, doing sports, being away from parents, talking to other people, trying to be perfect, feeling out of breath, feeling out of control, being around adults, being around other children, taking tests, and lots and lots of other things.

"What are the benefits of practice?"

✓ It is the best possible way to overcome fear.

✓ It is an easy way for you to help your student.

✓ Your student will quickly learn to do things that were too hard before.

(page 1 of 4)

"How do I get started with practice?"

(1) **First, pick something** that your student is afraid of. It is best to start with something that is not too hard. One way to make something easier is to break it down into steps. Remember, once your student starts practicing more, he or she can move on to harder things. "A fear at school I would like to see go away is:

_____."

(2) **Next, pick a time** that you can help your student with practice. It often can involve practice talking in class or to teachers. Sometimes practice can take a while, so remember to leave plenty of time if you think you will need it. "An example of a good time to help my student practice is:

_____."

(3) **Remind the child beforehand** to take ratings. These ratings range from 0 to 8, and higher numbers mean higher amounts of fear or anxiety. The goal is to get these numbers to go down over time.

(4) **You can use a practice form** to keep track of the ratings. This is the best way to know how well the practice is working, and you can use these ratings to know what to practice next.

(5) **Remember** that your student will need plenty of praise and support from as many people as possible. Sometimes practice can feel like a chore, but is the only way to get over feeling nervous or afraid. Help keep your student interested and encouraged.

(page 2 of 4)

"What are the steps?"

(1) When your student is ready, begin the practice. It can be raising a hand, writing on the board, talking to an adult, or whatever.

(2) Take ratings. The child should use the practice form to take ratings, probably every few minutes or so. We can show your student to do this.

(3) Wait as long as you need to. Sometimes it takes a while for your student to get used to something. The best thing to do is to keep going with it and tell your student he or she is doing well. It may take a little while, but your student will soon get used to what he or she is practicing.

(4) Practice, practice, and more practice. Once things are going pretty well, a child can repeat a practice as much as needed. Just like exercise, the more your student does, the better he or she will feel. If your student is practicing talking in class, make sure to call on him or her a lot as you see improvement.

(5) As your student does better, make things a little harder. When your student gets good at doing a certain practice, you can move onto something harder. Again, this is just like exercise. Once you can run 5 laps well, then you can try running 6 or 7 laps next time. Be careful not to make it too hard too fast, or your student will get frustrated. We can help you with knowing what to practice and knowing how fast to advance your student. This can take some time and patience.

(6) Keep a regular routine. Even after something gets better, it is always good to go back to it every now and then to make sure it stays easy. It is important to "stay in shape."

"Help! Practice isn't working!"

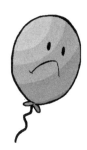

"My student's ratings won't go down." This can be because the practices are too short, or the things you are practicing are too hard for right now. If you are sure you have not picked something that is too hard, try making the practice go longer— eventually your student's fear will decrease and the ratings will come down.

"My student's ratings go down, but the next time we practice they are right back up where they started." When this happens, it usually means there has been too much time between practice. If you are practicing only once or twice a week, try four or five times if possible. Sometimes it can take practicing every day to see improvement.

"My student is too scared to get started." This means it is time to break things down into smaller steps. Think of ways you can make the practice easier (without making it shorter).

"My student is getting more scared instead of less." This can happen if you quit in the middle of a practice, or if the practices are too short. If you are having problems, you can always go back to practicing something easier for now. Make sure not to stop in the middle—keep it going until the ratings really come down.

"My student says he or she doesn't need to practice anymore." Remember to explain that practice is about building a skill. If you don't keep using it, it will go away. Even when things are not hard anymore, it is important to show you can do them every now and then. This can keep the anxiety from coming back.

(page 4 of 4)

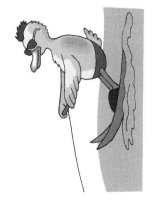

What I Took Back from Anxiety

Maintaining the gains

Your child has probably completed quite a bit of practice and has made some real progress with anxiety. As you know, this progress usually comes from a lot of hard work. Learning to be brave and to overcome anxiety is not easy, and your child and family deserve a lot of credit. Congratulations!

"What happens now?"

You will gradually be decreasing the number of meetings. There will probably be some progress review and question-and-answer time every couple of weeks, and possibly less frequently before finishing. The pace is a little different for each child. What is important to remember is that it won't be long before your family takes over the program and your child continues to face fears and practice on his or her own. Now is the time to ask questions you might have about doing it on your own. The last meeting will probably be a good time to celebrate and plan something fun together.

(page 1 of 4)

"How do we keep things going well?"

Learning to be brave and to handle anxiety is a lot like getting in shape with exercise. At first, there is a lot of effort, and the work can be tiring. After a while, it gets to be more of a regular routine, and the new skills become more and more natural. It is important to remember that just like with exercise, people can get out of shape again without regular practice.

The practice does not need to be as challenging as it was at first, but a little bit now and then will probably help to keep things going well. Just like running and stretching a few times a week will keep someone fit.

This is the time for your child to think of ways to continue to challenge him- or herself a few times a week with "mini-practice" exercises. And remember to keep using any skills or new things that you have learned, too.

"Some ways I can help my child keep practicing":

_____

_____

_____

Remember to praise

As always, praise is one of the best ways to keep things going. Remember to let your child know how proud you are and how hard he or she worked to get things going better. Once in a while, it is a good idea to point out how well things are going—even little things—to keep up your child's courage and enthusiasm.

"Things I can look for to praise":

_____

_____

_____

"What if we feel that there are still some problems?"

Usually there are still a few little things left to work on when the program comes to an end. This is actually part of the plan. The point is to leave some things for your child and family to work on together with the new skills that you have learned. As your child and family work successfully on your own, you will probably find that your child's confidence for handling anxiety increases. It is common for children to continue to improve for 6 months or more after finishing this program, just by working on their own.

(page 3 of 4)

"What if things get bad again?"

It is important to know the difference between a "lapse" and a "relapse." Lapses are natural, and involve minor steps backward. It is normal for children with anxiety to have lapses their whole life, and it just means that a few things need to be practiced again. Lapses are more common during stressful times, and it is perfectly normal for some anxiety to return now and then or for some new thing to become the focus of anxiety.

Remember what we learned in the beginning: A little bit of anxiety is normal and even helpful. Don't jump to the conclusion that you are having a "relapse" or a full return of the problem. Relapses almost never happen, and if they do, it is only because children stop practicing or someone panics when there is a lapse. If you have some trouble, do not jump to the conclusion that you are "back at square one." Stay calm and remember that all of the skills that your child learned will always be there, ready for him or her to use when they are needed. All your child needs to do is use them again when anxiety starts to be a problem.

If things ever get to the point where you feel that even the new skills and tools are not working, you can always seek some assistance again to get things back on track. Sometimes just a few simple suggestions can get things going well again.

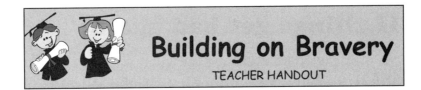

Maintaining the gains

Your student has probably completed quite a bit of practice and has made some real progress with anxiety. As you know, this progress usually comes from a lot of hard work. Learning to be brave and to overcome anxiety is not easy, and you and your student deserve a lot of credit. Congratulations!

"What happens now?"

Your student will gradually be decreasing the number of therapy sessions. There will probably be some progress review and question-and-answer time every couple of weeks, and possibly less frequently before finishing. The pace is a little different for each child. What is important to remember is that it won't be long before the child and family take over the program and your student continues to face fears and practice on his or her own. Now is the time to ask questions you might have about how the program will keep running in your class. The goal is for your student to work as independently as possible, with support from you when he or she needs it. For example, it might be helpful to try to continue to guide the child to practice from time to time.

"How do we keep things going well?"

Learning to be brave and to handle anxiety is a lot like getting in shape with exercise. At first, there is a lot of effort, and the work can be tiring. After a while, it gets to be more of a regular routine, and the new skills become more and more natural. It is important to remember that just like with exercise, people can get out of shape again without regular practice.

The practice does not need to be as challenging as it was at first, but a little bit now and then will probably help to keep things going well. Just like running and stretching a few times a week will keep someone fit.

This is the time for your student to think of ways to continue to challenge him- or herself a few times a week at school with "mini-practice" exercises. And remember to keep using any new programs that you have started, too, like time out or rewards.

"Some ways I can help my student keep practicing":

_____

_____

_____

Remember to praise

As always, praise is one of the best ways to keep things going. Remember to let your student know how proud you are and how hard he or she worked to get things going better. Once in a while, it is a good idea to point out how well things are going—even little things—to keep up your student's courage and enthusiasm.

"Things I can look for to praise":

_____

_____

_____

"What if I feel that there are still some problems?"

Usually there are still a few little things left to work on when the therapy comes to an end. This is actually part of the plan. The point is to leave some things for the child, family, and teacher to work on together with the new skills that they have learned. As your student and his or her family work successfully on their own, you will probably find that your student's confidence increases. It is common for children to continue to improve for 6 months or more after finishing this program, just by working on their own.

(page 3 of 4)

"What if things get bad again?"

It is important to know the difference between a "lapse" and a "relapse." Lapses are natural, and involve minor steps backward. It is normal for children with anxiety to have lapses their whole life, and it just means that a few things need to be practiced again. Lapses are more common during stressful times, and it is perfectly normal for some anxiety to return now and then or for some new thing to become the focus of anxiety.

Remember: A little bit of anxiety is normal and even helpful. Don't jump to the conclusion that your student is having a "relapse" or a full return of the problem. Relapses almost never happen, and if they do, it is only because children stop practicing or someone panics when there is a lapse. If you have some trouble, do not jump to the conclusion that your student is "back at square one." Remember that all of the skills that your student learned will always be there, ready for him or her to use when they are needed. All your student needs to do is use them again when anxiety starts to be a problem.

If things ever get to the point where you feel that the child's new skills and tools are not working, you can always seek some assistance again to get things back on track. It may be helpful to have a meeting with parents to discuss these issues.

Two-Column Thought Record

When you have a nervous thought, write it in the column on the left, and then rate how likely you think it is to come true. Remember to write your thought as a **prediction** or a guess about what will happen in the future.

Thought?	How likely is it? (0 to 100%)

Five-Column Thought Record

When you have a nervous thought, write it in the column on the left, and then rate how likely you think it is to come true. Next, write down an alternative thought and proof that you think it is true. Finally, rerate how likely you think your <u>original</u> nervous thought is, considering the proof you came up with.

Thought?	How likely does it feel? (0 to 100%)	Alternative Thought?	Proof?	How likely is it really? (0 to 100%)

Seven-Column Thought Record

When you have a nervous thought, write it in down and rate how likely you think it is to come true. Next, write down an alternative thought and proof that you think it is true. Then rerate how likely you think your <u>original</u> nervous thought is. Finally, write whether you can handle the situation if it comes true, and the evidence that you can do it.

Thought?	How likely does it feel? (0 to 100%)	Alternative Thought?	Proof?	How likely is it really? (0 to 100%)	If it happens, can I handle it?	Evidence I can handle it?

From Bruce F. Chorpita (2007). Copyright by The Guilford Press.

STOP Worksheet

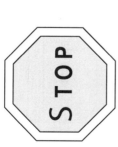

S is the first letter in the word "scared." Let's learn more about feeling scared. What are some other words for feeling scared?

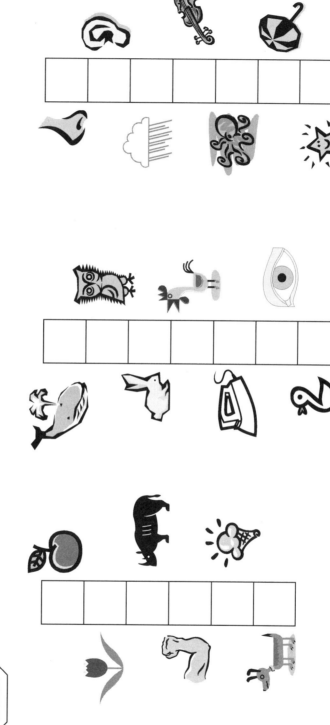

How do we know what someone is feeling?

STOP

See if you can figure out how they are feeling.

Write why you think they are feeling that way.

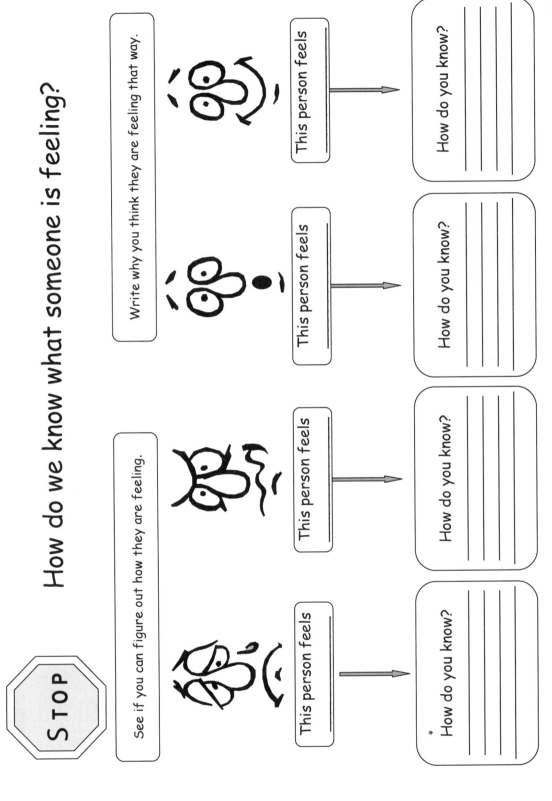

This person feels ___

This person feels ___

This person feels ___

This person feels ___

How do you know? _____

How do you know? _____

How do you know? _____

How do you know? _____

266

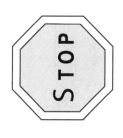

Here are things you can feel when you are scared. Draw a line to match the word with the feeling in the picture

STOP

blushing

sweaty

butterflies

racing heart

shaky

out of breath

dizzy

It is important to know when you feel scared, nervous, or worried so that you can practice feeling better.

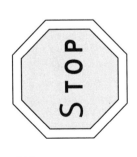

STOP

What are
some times
that you feel
like this?

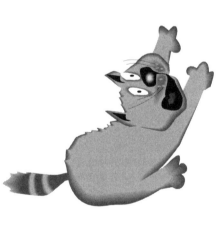

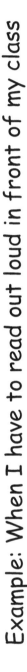

Example: When I have to read out loud in front of my class

1. _____

2. _____

3. _____

T stands for "thoughts." Fill in the thoughts below.

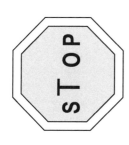

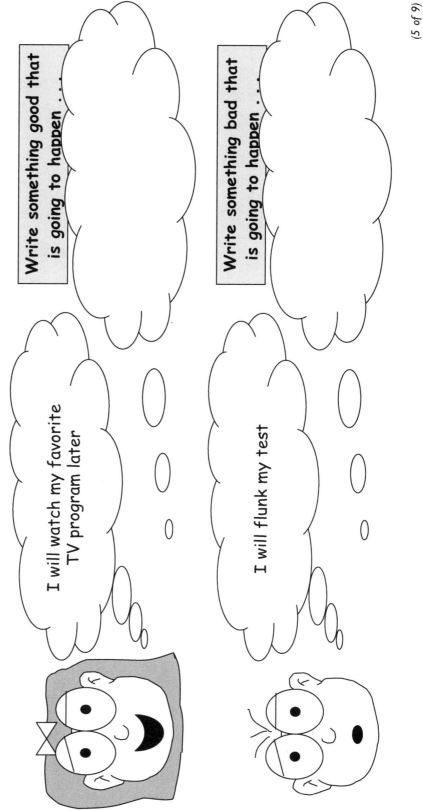

I will watch my favorite TV program later

Write something good that is going to happen . . .

I will flunk my test

Write something bad that is going to happen . . .

269

Remember: The thoughts you have can change how you feel. What thoughts do these people have about the dog? Who feels better?

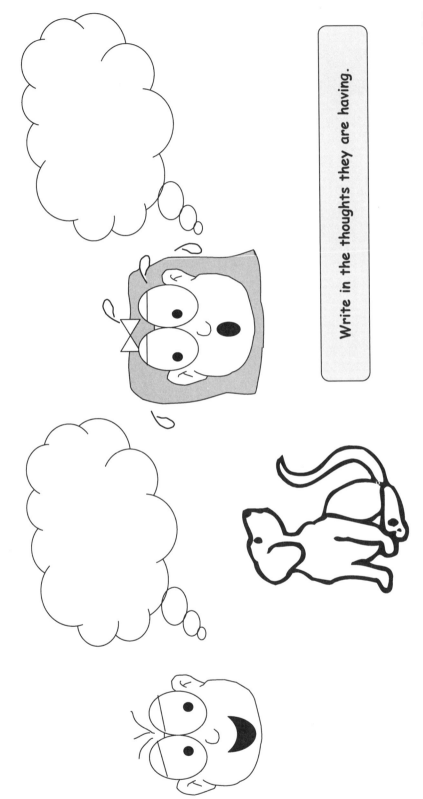

Write in the thoughts they are having.

STOP

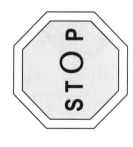

STOP

O stands for "other thoughts." We can learn to have other thoughts about things, so that we don't feel scared or nervous. Write some other thoughts below.

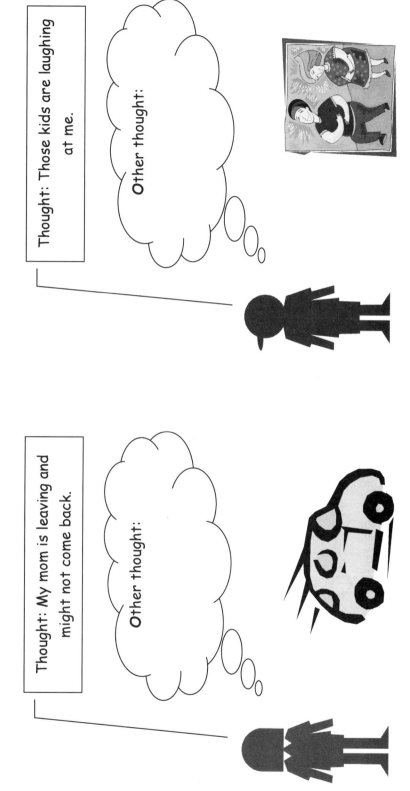

Thought: Those kids are laughing at me.

Other thought:

Thought: My mom is leaving and might not come back.

Other thought:

What are some scary or nervous thoughts you have sometimes? Write those down and see if you can think of **O**ther thoughts that are not so scary.

STOP

Nervous Thought:

Other:

Nervous Thought:

Other:

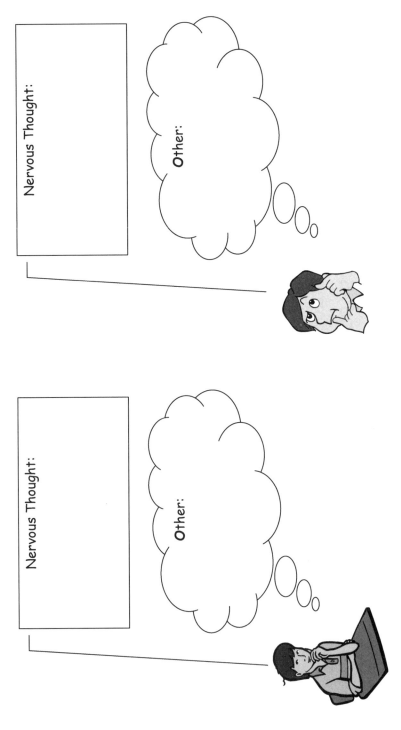

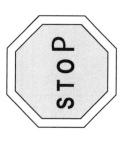

S = Scared
T = Thoughts
O = Other thoughts
P stands for "praise!" It is the last part of STOP.

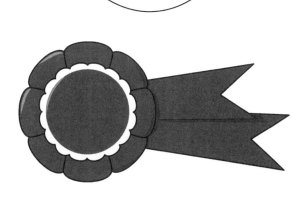

Remember to tell yourself that you are
DOING A GREAT JOB
when you use STOP to make yourself feel
less scared or nervous!!!

Things you can say to praise yourself:

_____

_____

STOP Record

If you feel **S**cared, write down where and when it happened over on the left. Then write any scary **T**houghts that you had. In the next column, put any **O**ther thoughts you could have that are less scary. Remember to **P**raise yourself at the end!

Scared? (where and when)	**T**houghts?	**O**ther Thoughts?	Did you **P**raise yourself?

Meeting and Greeting Worksheet

This week I'm going to learn some things about how to talk to people.

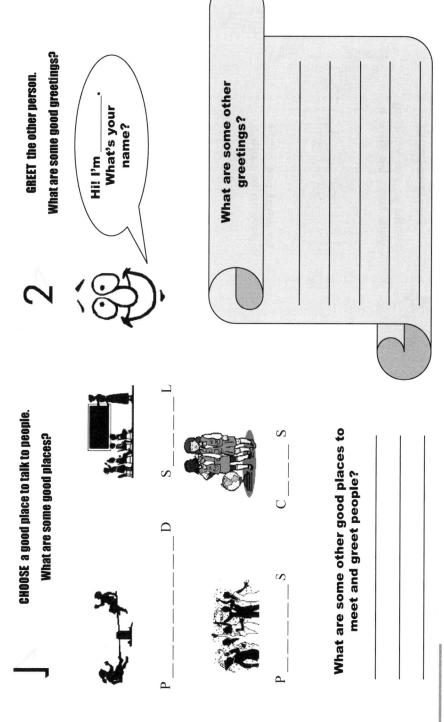

1 CHOOSE a good place to talk to people.

What are some good places?

P _ _ _ _ _ _ D

S _ _ _ _ _ L

P _ _ _ _ _ S

C _ _ _ _ S

What are some other good places to meet and greet people?

_____

_____

2 GREET the other person.

What are some good greetings?

Hi! I'm _____. What's your name?

What are some other greetings?

4

Take Turns Talking.

While you're waiting your turn, be sure t‹

Listen

to what the other person is saying

5

What do I do when it's my turn to talk?

Ask
a question.

Tell
how you feel.

Say
something about what the other person was talking about.

3

But what do I talk about after I greet someone?

Good things to talk about:

P _ _ _ _ S

M _ _ _ _ _ S

S _ _ _ _ _ L

THE END

What are some other good things to talk about?

_____

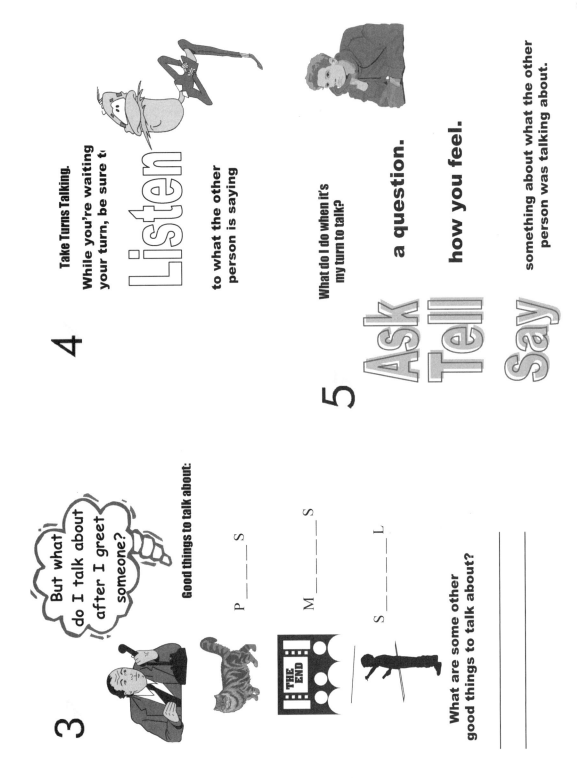

276

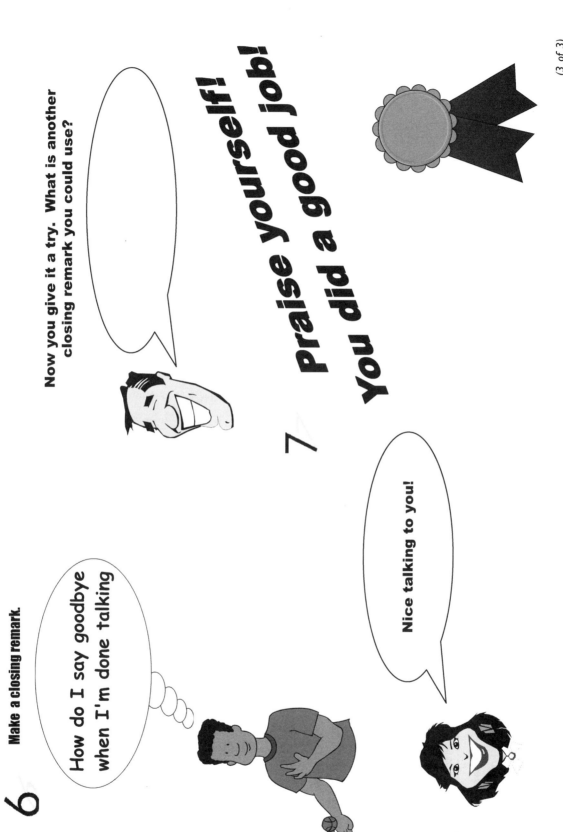

7   **Praise yourself!**
    You did a good job!

6   Make a closing remark.

How do I say goodbye when I'm done talking

Nice talking to you!

Now you give it a try. What is another closing remark you could use?

277

Meeting and Greeting Record

For each time that **you have a conversation with someone else**, rate how it went below. For this week, **practice having conversations with _____ people.**

Date	Where were you?	Who did you talk to?	What did you talk about?	What went well?	What was tough?

Don't Forget

Choose a place → Greet person → Take turns (Listen, Ask, Tell, or Say Something) → Make a closing remark

From Bruce F. Chorpita (2007). Copyright by The Guilford Press.

Nonverbal Skills Worksheet

When talking with people, it's important to also pay attention to the things that you do with your body and the messages that those things convey.

Some things are important to do
to help everyone feel more comfortable during a conversation.

Let's try some exercises to show you how the things that you do affect how comfortable you feel talking with someone.

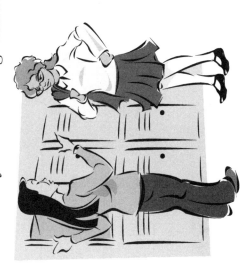

Remember: When practicing, you don't want to do TOO MUCH of something but you don't want to do TOO LITTLE. We're going to try to do things at the JUST RIGHT amount!

Taking Distance

Activity 1

❶ You stand about **4 feet** away from the other person.

❷ Face each other and have a short conversation.

After Activity 1

How comfortable did you feel?

Pick an answer based on your feelings.

I felt that the other person was:

T o o f a r
a w a y   Just the right   **Too close**
                 distance away

Ask the other person how he/she felt.

The other person felt that I was:

T o o f a r
a w a y   Just the right   **Too close**
                 distance away

What did you learn from Activity 1?

_____

_____

Activity 2

❶ Now stand about **1 foot** away from the other person.

❷ Face each other and have a short conversation.

After Activity 2

How comfortable did you feel?

Pick an answer based on your feelings.

I felt that the other person was:

T o o f a r
a w a y   Just the right   **Too close**
                 distance away

Ask the other person how he/she felt.

The other person felt that I was:

T o o f a r
a w a y   Just the right   **Too close**
                 distance away

What did you learn from Activity 2?

_____

_____

Talking Distance, Page 2

(3 of 6)

Now let's figure out how to look at people when you're talking with them.

What did you learn from Activity 3?

_____

_____

The distance would get . . .

L a r g e r   Stay the same   Smaller

Activity 3

❶ Stand at a distance from the other person that you feel is comfortable.
❷ Ask the other person if it is also comfortable for him/her.
❸ Adjust the distance until both people can agree on a comfortable distance.
❹ Face each other and have a short conversation.

After Activity 3

About how large was that distance?

_____ feet or inches

What do you think would happen to the talking distance if the other person was a good friend or close family member?

Sometimes those distances are different depending on the different type of relationships that you have with people that you know.

What you just did was the comfortable distance for talking to friends, people whom you just met, or relatives whom you don't know so well.

281

Eye Contact

Activity 1

❶ The other person will not look at you while talking or listening.

❷ Face each other and have a short conversation.

After Activity 1

How did you feel?

Pick an answer based on your feelings.

I felt that the other person was:

Very interested in what I had to say

Not interested in what I had to say

I felt:

Comfortable talking to Person B

Uncomfortable talking to Person B

What did you learn from Activity 1?

_____

_____

Activity 2

❶ The other person will look at you the whole time while talking or listening.

❷ Face each other and have a short conversation.

After Activity 2

How did you feel?

Pick an answer based on your feelings.

I felt that the other person was:

Very interested in what I had to say

Not interested in what I had to say

I felt:

Comfortable talking to Person B

Uncomfortable talking to Person B

What did you learn from Activity 2?

_____

_____

What happens when you talk with someone who always talks in the same tone the whole time and talks so softly that it's hard to hear that person? Let's find out!

Activity 1

❶ Person B will talk with Person A in a voice that is too quiet and has a low, unchanging tone.
❷ Face each other and have a short conversation.

After Activity 1

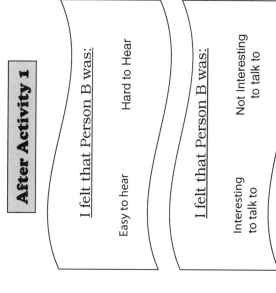

I felt that Person B was:

Easy to hear   Hard to Hear

I felt that Person B was:

Interesting   Not Interesting
to talk to   to talk to

S p e a k i n g   V o i c e

Eye Contact
Page 2

Activity 3

❶ You and the other person will make eye contact with each other about half the time while listening and talking.
❷ Face each other and have a short conversation.

After Activity 3

How did you feel?
Pick an answer based on your feelings.

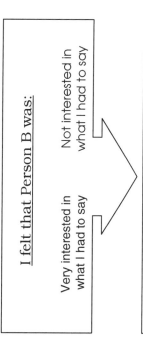

I felt that Person B was:

Very interested in   Not interested in
what I had to say   what I had to say

I felt:

Comfortable   Uncomfortable talking
talking to   to Person B
Person B

What did you learn from Activity 3?

_____

283

Speaking Voice, Page 2

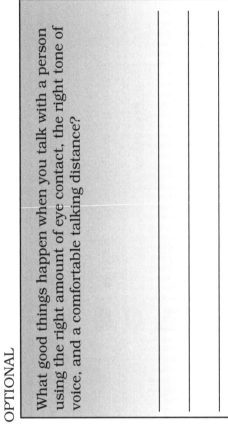

I felt that Person B was:

Easy to hear   Hard to hear

I felt that Person B was:

Interesting   Not interesting
to talk to   to talk to

After Activity 2

**What did you learn
from Activities 1 and 2?**

_____

OPTIONAL

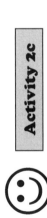

What good things happen when you talk with a person
using the right amount of eye contact, the right tone of
voice, and a comfortable talking distance?

_____

_____

_____

Activity 2a

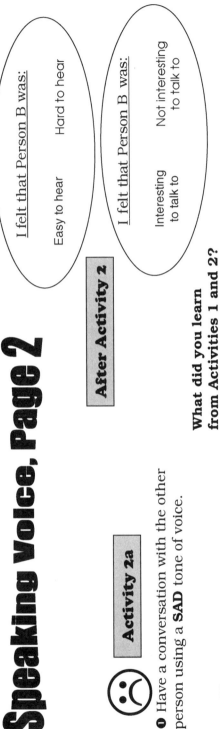

❶ Have a conversation with the other
person using a **SAD** tone of voice.

Activity 2b

❶ Have a conversation with the other
person using an **ANGRY** tone of voice.

Activity 2c

❶ Have a conversation with the other
person using an **EXCITED or HAPPY**
tone of voice.

284

Nonverbal Skills Record

For each time that you have a conversation or see a conversation, rate it below. For this week, practice having
_____ conversations. Practice watching _____ conversations.

Date	Place Where were the people talking?	Relationship How do the people know each other? (e.g., friends, strangers, parent and child)	Talking Distance How far apart did each person stand from each other? (pick 1)	Eye Contact How much eye contact did the persons have with each other? (pick 1)	Speaking Voice Did people talk in a loud enough voice while using a normal tone? (pick all that apply)
			☐ Too far ☐ Too close ☐ Just right distance	☐ Not enough ☐ Too much ☐ Just right	☐ Not loud enough ☐ Didn't use normal tone ☐ Loud enough to be heard ☐ Used a normal tone
			☐ Too far ☐ Too close ☐ Just right distance	☐ Not enough ☐ Too much ☐ Just right	☐ Not loud enough ☐ Didn't use normal tone ☐ Loud enough to be heard ☐ Used a normal tone
			☐ Too far ☐ Too close ☐ Just right distance	☐ Not enough ☐ Too much ☐ Just right	☐ Not loud enough ☐ Didn't use normal tone ☐ Loud enough to be heard ☐ Used a normal tone
			☐ Too far ☐ Too close ☐ Just right distance	☐ Not enough ☐ Too much ☐ Just right	☐ Not loud enough ☐ Didn't use normal tone ☐ Loud enough to be heard ☐ Used a normal tone
			☐ Too far ☐ Too close ☐ Just right distance	☐ Not enough ☐ Too much ☐ Just right	☐ Not loud enough ☐ Didn't use normal tone ☐ Loud enough to be heard ☐ Used a normal tone

Parent Observation Record

Each time you notice your child _____, please put a checkmark (√) in the second column. Please also record what you did in the next column, and the results in the last column.

Day	Behaviors (√)	What did you do?	Did it work? circle one
Monday			yes no unsure
Tuesday			yes no unsure
Wednesday			yes no unsure
Thursday			yes no unsure
Friday			yes no unsure
Saturday			yes no unsure
Sunday			yes no unsure
Monday			yes no unsure
Tuesday			yes no unsure
Wednesday			yes no unsure
Thursday			yes no unsure
Friday			yes no unsure
Saturday			yes no unsure
Sunday			yes no unsure

From Bruce F. Chorpita (2007). Copyright by The Guilford Press.

Teacher Observation Record

Each time you notice your student _____, please put a checkmark (√) in the second column. Please also record what you did in the next column, and the results in the last column.

Day	Behaviors (√)	What did you do?	Did it work? circle one
Monday			yes no unsure
Tuesday			yes no unsure
Wednesday			yes no unsure
Thursday			yes no unsure
Friday			yes no unsure
Monday			yes no unsure
Tuesday			yes no unsure
Wednesday			yes no unsure
Thursday			yes no unsure
Friday			yes no unsure

From Bruce F. Chorpita (2007). Copyright by The Guilford Press.

287

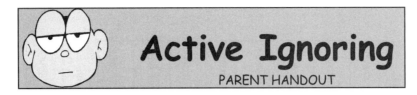

Active Ignoring
PARENT HANDOUT

"What is active ignoring?"

Active ignoring means not paying any attention to your child when a problem behavior is happening. Sometimes kids do things to get out of doing something they don't like, to get attention from their parents, or just to get their parents upset. Ignoring your child when she or he behaves this way is one way to get your child to stop doing this behavior.

"When do I use active ignoring?"

Active ignoring is meant for children between the ages of 2 and 12. It is useful for times when your child is being fussy or complaining.

Use active ignoring for behaviors like these: pouting, being grumpy, complaining, whining, mild arguing, talking back, making noises, asking the same question over and over, repeating things, or doing things to get your attention.

Do not use active ignoring for behaviors like these: hitting, slapping, pinching, throwing or breaking things, being mean to animals or people, doing dangerous things, disobeying a command, cursing, swearing, or threatening others, getting a bad grade, forgetting to do chores or homework, being afraid or shy, or wanting to be alone.

"What are the benefits of active ignoring?"

✓ It quickly stops many types of problem behaviors.

✓ It is easy to learn and with practice it is easy to use.

✓ It does not harm your child emotionally.

✓ Parents feel less angry and upset when they use active ignoring.

"How do I start using active ignoring?"

(1) First, pick a behavior you want to see go away. You can write it in the space that follows. Make sure it is the right kind of behavior for active ignoring. "From now on, I will ignore my child when":

_____

(2) Next, pick some behaviors you want to see instead. These are things like asking politely, being quiet, accepting a decision, playing nicely. "Some behaviors I will pay attention to are":

_____

(3) Next, think of ways to praise your child. These will be helpful to think about beforehand. There are many nice things you could do or say to let your child know you like what he or she is doing. "One way to praise my child is":

_____

(4) Next, pick a time to tell your child and family about active ignoring. The best time to talk about it is when everything is going well and everyone is calm. Your child should know that using active ignoring still means that you care as a parent, but that some behaviors will not get your attention and others will. This is not something that your child can argue about. It is part of the new rules for living in your home, and it is meant to make everyone feel better when they are together. "I will explain active ignoring to my family":

_____

"What are the steps?"

(1) **When the behavior happens,** look the other way or do something that will make it easy for you to ignore it. Sometimes it is best to leave the room.

(2) **Don't explain,** argue, scold, or even talk with your child. Many parents feel that they have to explain to their children why they are ignoring them while they are misbehaving. You already explained this before.

(3) **Don't look** angry or upset, if you can help it. Again, it is sometimes easier if you can busy yourself with something like TV or a book to hide your reaction.

(4) **Remember the active part** of active ignoring. For this to work, you have to catch your child being good and ignore your child being bad. Pay attention to your child as soon as the bad behavior stops. Make it obvious that you are interested by looking at your child, talking, and praising. If the behavior starts again, go back to ignoring.

(5) **Hang in there** if things get worse at first. This is actually a sign that things are going just as they are supposed to. It means your child is aware of what you are doing, and active ignoring is starting to have an effect. Children often try harder to get your attention before they give up, and with active ignoring, things sometimes get a little worse before they get better. This is the time to keep your cool.

"Help! Active ignoring isn't working!"

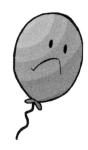

"The problem is getting worse instead of better."

Are you sure that you have been ignoring the *whole* time? The problem can get worse if you ignore only some of the time and then give in or get angry after a while. Once you decide to ignore a behavior, you have to go all the way with it. This is hard work, but it will be worth it.

"My child cries and screams."

This is also something that you can ignore, as long as your child doesn't do anything harmful to him- or herself or to others. It takes a lot of patience, but it will stop.

"My child is getting aggressive."

If your child is going to hurt you or someone else or starts hitting, slapping, or throwing things, active ignoring may not be enough. It is probably time to use some other tools, like "time-out." If you don't use "time-out," this might be a good time to start.

"My child is always angry at me now that we started active ignoring."

Sometimes this will happen when parents ignore their child all the time, instead of just ignoring the problem behaviors. Your child needs lots of attention, so when he or she is good, be sure to share and do fun things together. Only ignore the problem behaviors that you decided were important to make go away.

"Sometimes others in my home are not helpful."

Everyone has to work together. The same rules have to be used by everyone. Talk to your family about this when things are quiet and explain how important this is that you all work together.

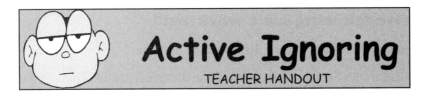

Active Ignoring
TEACHER HANDOUT

"What is active ignoring?"

Active ignoring means not paying any attention to a child when a problem behavior is happening. Sometimes kids do things to get out of doing something they don't like, to get attention from their peers, or just to get their teacher upset. Ignoring your student when he or she behaves this way is one way to stop this behavior.

"When do I use active ignoring?"

Active ignoring is best for children between the ages of 2 and 12. It is useful for times when your student is being fussy or complaining.

Use active ignoring for behaviors like these: pouting, being grumpy, complaining, whining, tapping pencils, mumbling, making noises, asking the same question over and over, repeating things, or doing things to get your attention.

Do not use active ignoring for behaviors like these: hitting, slapping, pinching, throwing or breaking things, being mean to animals or people, doing dangerous things, disobeying a command, cursing, swearing, or threatening others, getting a bad grade, forgetting to do class work or homework, being afraid or shy, or wanting to be alone.

"What are the benefits of active ignoring?"

✓ It quickly stops many types of problem behaviors.

✓ It is easy to learn and with practice it is easy to use.

✓ It does not harm your student emotionally.

✓ Teachers feel less angry and upset when they use active ignoring.

From Bruce F. Chorpita (2007). Copyright by The Guilford Press.

"How do I start using active ignoring?"

(1) **First, pick a behavior** you want to see go away. You can write it in the space that follows. Make sure it is the right kind of behavior for active ignoring. "From now on, I will ignore my student when":

_____

(2) **Next, pick some behaviors** you want to see instead. These are things like asking politely, being quiet, accepting a decision, playing nicely. "Some behaviors I will pay attention to are":

_____

(3) **Next, think of ways to praise** your student. These will be helpful to think about beforehand. There are many nice things you could do or say to let your student know you like what he or she is doing. "One way to praise my student is":

_____

(4) **Next, pick a time** to tell your student about active ignoring. The best time to talk about it is when everything is going well and things are calm. Your student should know that using active ignoring still means that you respect him or her, but that some behaviors will not get your attention and others will. This is not something that your student can argue about. It is part of the new rules for working in your class, and it is meant to make everyone feel better when they are together. "I will explain active ignoring to my student":

_____

"What are the steps?"

(1) **When the behavior happens,** look the other way or do something that will make it easy for you to ignore it. Sometimes it is best to attend to another child.

(2) **Don't explain,** argue, scold, or even talk with your student. Many teachers feel that they have to explain to their student why they are ignoring him or her while they are misbehaving. You will have already explained this before.

(3) **Don't look** angry or upset, if you can help it. Again, it is sometimes easier if you can busy yourself with other students to hide your reaction.

(4) **Remember the active part** of active ignoring. For this to work, you have to catch your student being good and ignore your student being bad. Pay attention to the child as soon as the bad behavior stops. Make it obvious that you are interested by looking at your student, talking, or praising. If the behavior starts again, go back to ignoring.

(5) **Hang in there** if things get worse at first. This is actually a sign that things are going just as they are supposed to. It means your student is aware of what you are doing, and active ignoring is starting to have an effect. Children often try harder to get your attention before they give up, and with active ignoring, things sometimes get a little worse before they get better. This is the time to keep your cool.

(page 3 of 4)

"Help! Active ignoring isn't working!"

"The problem is getting worse instead of better."

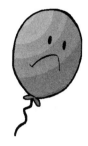

Are you sure that you have been ignoring the *whole* time? The problem can get worse if you ignore only some of the time and then give in or get angry after a while. Once you decide to ignore a behavior, you have to go all the way with it. This is hard work, but it will be worth it.

"My student cries when I ignore the behavior."

This is also something that you can ignore, as long as your student doesn't do anything harmful to him- or herself or to others. If the crying gets too disruptive, you might need to move your student to another room. This takes a lot of patience, but it will stop.

"My student is getting aggressive."

If your student is going to hurt you or someone else or starts hitting, slapping, or throwing things, active ignoring may not be enough. It is probably time to use some other tools, like "time-out." If you don't use "time-out," this might be a good time to start. It also means that a meeting with parents would be a good idea at this point.

"My student is always angry at me now that we started active ignoring."

Sometimes this will happen when teachers ignore a student all the time, instead of just ignoring the problem behaviors. Your student needs lots of attention, so when he or she is good, be sure to share and praise. Only ignore the problem behaviors that you decided were important to make go away.

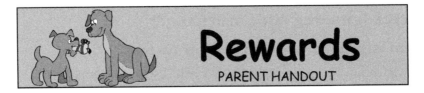

Rewards
PARENT HANDOUT

"What are rewards?"

Rewards are those things you give to your child when he or she is good. They can be anything, like time with a toy, attention from a loved one, a gift, a smile, or a hug. Rewards are often the most important tools that parents have to encourage good behavior and discourage bad behavior. When things are not going well at home, using rewards can often help.

"When do I use rewards?"

Rewards can be used with children as young as 1. When parents smile at their baby for doing something nice, they are already using rewards. Rewards can also be used with teenagers and even adults. Different kinds of rewards are important, depending on the age of your child.

Rewards can increase behaviors like these: being on time, being polite, sharing, doing homework, coming home on time, remembering important things, doing chores, going to bed on time, or anything else you think is important for your child to learn. Although it might not seem possible, using rewards is also one of the best ways to get rid of problem behaviors. You see, if your child is always trying to be good, there is less time to get into trouble.

"What are the benefits of using rewards?"

✓ They quickly increase good behaviors.

✓ They are easy to learn about and easy to use.

✓ They teach your child about the value of working hard.

✓ Parents and children feel less angry and upset when they use rewards.

(page 1 of 4)

"How do I start using rewards?"

(1) **First, pick a behavior** you want to see increase. It should be very specific, like "finish homework before 6 o'clock." Rewards work best when everyone knows exactly what the behavior is and can agree when it happens. "A behavior I would like to see increase is":

_____

(2) **Next, make a list** of rewards you think you can use. Sometimes it helps to talk with your child about this. They don't have to be big things or things that cost money—they can be things like spending time playing a favorite game together, or staying up an extra 15 minutes, things like that. Think of as many as you can. "An example of a small reward my child would like is":

_____

(3) **Next, come up with a <u>contract</u>** for what your child has to do to get the rewards. Use an "IF–THEN" sentence. For example, "If my child can finish his homework by dinnertime, then he can have TV time that night." Write an example here:

If _____

Then _____

(4) **Next, pick a way** to keep track of the contract. For young children, you can use a chart with stickers. Each time your child does the good behavior, you can give a sticker. When enough stickers are earned, they can be used to get a reward. For older children, a point system can be used, with a card to keep track of points.

"What are the steps?"

(1) **When the behavior happens,** give the sticker or point right away. The sooner you do this, the better the rewards will work.

(2) **Have your child spend the points.** Some children save up their stickers or points and don't want to spend them. After a while, they can have so many points that they don't want to work any more. One way to prevent this is to have children spend all their points by the end of the weekend, and have the points start back at 0 each week.

(3) **As your child does better, make things a little harder.** When your child gets good at doing the behavior, you can "raise the price of rewards." For example, if something cost 3 points or stickers, it can now cost 4 points or stickers. Be careful not to make it too hard too fast, or your child can get frustrated. Progress can take time.

(4) **Don't give rewards when your child asks for them.** Children who ask for rewards should not get them at that time (this just rewards them for asking). The reward should only come after the behavior you have decided to increase.

(5) **Don't make the rewards too hard to earn in the beginning.** If it takes too long or too much effort at first, children will lose interest in a reward program, even when the rewards are big. Instead of promising a bicycle if your child gets good grades, give small rewards each time your child does homework. Small rewards given often work best. The younger the child, the more often you will have to give rewards.

(6) **Remember to praise.** Praise is always a good thing to give along with a reward. It helps build a sense of accomplishment that will motivate your child.

(page 3 of 4)

"Help! Rewards aren't working!"

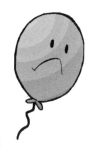

"I feel like I am bribing my child." Some parents feel like they are bribing their child to be good, and that children shouldn't need rewards. That may be true when children grow up, but many children need extra help learning to do things at first. Rewards get them started. Later, the rewards can be made smaller, so that children will eventually behave and work hard just because it makes them feel good.

"My child is not following through." Make sure you are giving the rewards *after* the behavior, not before. If you say, "You can watch TV now if you promise to do your homework later," your child may not honor the promise. Remember to use IF–THEN sentences when talking about rewards, and give the rewards only after the behavior.

"My child already has everything he [or she] wants." Often children get rewards even when they don't earn them. Think about many of the fun things your child gets, and see if you can have your child earn them with good behavior.

"My child is trying, but rewards are not working." The three biggest problems with rewards not working are that (1) the behavior is too hard; (2) the rewards are not being given right away; or (3) the rewards are not interesting. Make sure the behavior can be done at first. If not, break it into small steps and reward for each one. Remember to reward right away, and be sure to reward with something your child really likes.

"Sometimes others in my home are not helpful." Everyone has to work together, and it really helps if all caretakers in the home give out the points or stickers. Talk to your family about this when things are quiet, and explain how important this is that you all work together.

Rewards
TEACHER HANDOUT

"What are rewards?"

Rewards are those things you give to a child when he or she is good. They can be anything, like time with a toy, attention from a teacher, a smile, or special privileges. Rewards are often the most important tools that teachers have to encourage good behavior and discourage bad behavior. When things are not going well at school, using rewards can often help.

"When do I use rewards?"

Rewards can be used with children as young as 1. When parents smile at their baby for doing something nice, they are already using rewards. Rewards can also be used with teenagers and even adults. Different kinds of rewards are important, depending on the age of your student.

Rewards can increase behaviors like these: being on time, being polite, sharing, doing homework, coming to class on time, remembering important things, doing class work, paying attention, or anything else you think is important for your student to learn. Although it might not seem possible, using rewards is also one of the best ways to get rid of problem behaviors. You see, if your student is always trying to be good, there is less time to get into trouble.

"What are the benefits of using rewards?"

✓ They quickly increase good behaviors.

✓ They are easy to learn about and easy to use.

✓ They teach your student the value of working hard.

✓ Teachers and children feel less angry and upset when they use rewards.

(page 1 of 4)

"How do I start using rewards?"

(1) **First, pick a behavior** you want to see increase. It should be very specific, like "finish work before lunch time." Rewards work best when everyone knows exactly what the behavior is and can agree when it happens. "A behavior I would like to see increase is":

_____

(2) **Next, make a list** of rewards you think you can use. Sometimes it helps to talk with your student and his or her parents about this. Rewards don't have to be big things or things that cost money—they can be things like taking a break, playing a game together, or working on the computer, things like that. Think of as many as you can. "A small reward my student might like is":

_____

(3) **Next, come up with a <u>contract</u>** for what your student has to do to get the rewards. Use an "IF–THEN" sentence. For example, "If my student can finish her work by lunch time, then she can play on the computer later." Write an example here:

If _____

Then _____

(4) **Next, pick a way** to keep track of the contract. For young children, you can use a chart with stickers. Each time your student does the good behavior, you can give a sticker. When enough stickers are earned, they can be used to get a reward. For older children, a point system can be used, with a card to keep track of points.

"What are the steps?"

(1) **When the behavior happens,** give the sticker or point right away. The sooner you do this, the better the rewards will work.

(2) **Have your student spend the points.** Some children save up their stickers or points and don't want to spend them. After a while, they can have so many points that they don't want to work any more. One way to prevent this is to have children spend all their points by Friday, and have the points start back at 0 each week.

(3) **As your student does better, make things a little harder.** When your student gets good at doing the behavior, you can "raise the price of rewards." For example, if something cost 3 points or stickers, it can now cost 4 points or stickers. Be careful not to make it too hard too fast, or the child can get frustrated. Progress can take time.

(4) **Don' t give rewards when your student asks for them.** Children who ask for rewards should not get them at that time (this just rewards them for asking). The reward should only come after the behavior you have decided to increase.

(5) **Don't make the rewards too hard to earn in the beginning.** If it takes too long or too much effort at first, children will lose interest in a reward program, even when the rewards are big. Instead of promising a bicycle if your child gets good grades, give small rewards each time your child does homework. Small rewards given often work best. The younger the child, the more often you will have to give rewards.

(6) **Remember to praise.** Praise is always a good thing to give along with a reward. It helps build a sense of accomplishment that will motivate your student.

(page 3 of 4)

"Help! Rewards aren't working!"

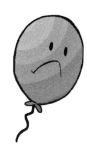

"I feel like I am bribing my student." Some teachers feel like they are bribing their student to be good, and that children shouldn't need rewards. That may be true when children grow up, but many children need extra help learning to do things at first. Rewards get them started. Later the rewards can be made smaller, and eventually children will behave and work hard just because it makes them feel good.

"My student is not following through." Make sure you are giving the rewards *after* the behavior, not before. If you say, "You can take a break now if you promise to do your assignment later," the child may not honor the promise. Remember to use IF–THEN sentences when talking about rewards, and give the rewards only after the behavior.

"My student already has everything he or she wants." Often children get rewards even when they don't earn them. Think about many of the fun things your student gets during the day, and see if you can have him or her earn some of them with good behavior. Sometimes it helps to talk to parents about making sure that the child does not bring toys or games to school.

"My student is trying, but rewards are not working." The three biggest problems with rewards not working are that (1) the behavior is too hard; (2) the rewards are not being given right away; or (3) the rewards are not interesting. Make sure the behavior can be done at first. If not, break it into small steps and reward for each one. Remember to reward right away, and be sure to reward with something your student really likes.

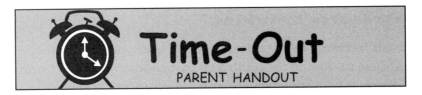

"What is time-out?"

"Time-out," like in sports, is a short break in activities for your child. It means that your child has a "time-out" from rewards, attention, and interesting things. Time-out prevents your child from being rewarded for behaviors that are a problem.

"When do I use time-out?"

Time-out is meant for children between the ages of 2 and 12. It is useful for times when your child is being mean or aggressive or is acting without thinking.

Use time-out for behaviors like these: hitting, slapping, pinching, talking back to parents, throwing or breaking things, being mean to animals or people, doing dangerous things, disobeying a command to stop a problem behavior, cursing, swearing, or threatening others.

Do not use time-out for behaviors like these: pouting or grumpiness, getting a bad grade, forgetting to do chores or homework, being afraid or shy, or wanting to be alone. Also, do not use time-out unless you have seen the problem behavior happen.

"What are the benefits of time-out?"

✓ It quickly stops many types of problem behaviors.

✓ It is easy to learn and, with practice, it is easy to use.

✓ It does not harm your child emotionally.

✓ Parents feel less upset when they use time-out.

(page 1 of 4)

"How do I start using time-out?"

(1) **First, pick a behavior** you want to work on. You can write it in the space that follows. Make sure it is the right kind of behavior for time-out. "From now on, my child will get a time-out for":

_____

(2) **Next, pick a place** for time-out. It should be as boring as possible. If your child is younger than 4, pick a chair that you can keep in view. For older children, choose a place that does not have TV, toys, or other distractions, such as the bathroom or a hallway. "The place I will use for time-out is":

_____

(3) **Next, pick a time** to tell your child and family about time-out. The best time to talk about it is when everything is going well and everyone is calm. Your child should know that using time-out still means that you care as a parent, but that some behaviors are not allowed. Time-out is not something that your child can argue about. It is part of the new rules for living in your home. If your child does not agree to do time-out, some fun things like TV time will be taken away. "I will explain time-out to my family":

_____

(4) **Get a timer** to use for time-out. Put it near the time-out place so that it will be ready.

(5) **Remember** to use plenty of praise and rewards when things are going well.

"What are the steps?"

(1) **When the behavior happens,** tell your child "You need to go to time-out." Do this right away, and do it every time the behavior happens.

(2) **Don' t explain.** You already explained time-out before. If your child argues or asks why, just say "We will talk about this after you do your time-out." This is no time for discussion. Don't repeat this more than once or twice. If your child tries to argue too much, add a minute to the time-out by saying, "I just added a minute, please start your time-out." Continue adding a minute until the arguing stops and time-out starts.

(3) **Set the timer** for 1 minute for every year of age for your child.

(4) **Place the timer** out of your child's reach but close enough to be seen. Do not let your child touch the timer.

(5) **Reset the timer** if your child is not quiet and still. Time-out starts when your child is quiet. Remember, no one should talk to your child during time-out.

(6) **Talk with your child calmly** after time-out. Ask your child why you gave the time-out. If your child can't remember, now is the time to explain. Remember, this is not a time to yell or punish—time-out was the punishment.

"Help! Time-out isn't working!"

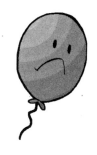

"My child makes a mess during time-out." Require your child to clean the mess before leaving time-out. If anything is damaged, your child will have to pay by doing extra chores.

"My child cries and screams during time-out." Ignore your child and stay away from the time-out place. Wait until your child is quiet to reset the timer. This can be hard at first, but it will get easier.

"What if we are not at home?" If problems often happen when you are out, bring the timer with you. You can sometimes do time-out by having your child sit some quiet place outside. Other times, you can have your child sit in a boring place right where you are. Make sure the place is safe and that you can see your child at all times.

"My child doesn't believe that I will give a time-out." Never give more than one warning for time-out. If the behavior happens again, you must always send your child to time-out right away. If you do not follow through, your child will not respond to your warnings.

"Sometimes others in my home are not helpful." Everyone has to work together. The same rules have to be used by everyone. Talk to your family about this when things are quiet, and explain how important this is that you work together.

"My child escapes from time-out." You can pick up young children and put them back in time-out and reset the timer. For older children, take away an activity (like TV) until the time-out is finished.

(page 4 of 4)

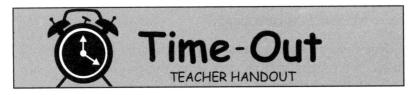

"What is time-out?"

"Time-out," like in sports, is a short break in activities for a child. It means that your student has a "time-out" from rewards, attention, and interesting things. Time-out prevents your student from being rewarded for behaviors that are a problem.

"When do I use time-out?"

Time-out is meant for children between the ages of 2 and 12. It is useful for times when your student is being mean or aggressive or is acting without thinking.

Use time-out for behaviors like these: hitting, slapping, pinching, talking back to teachers, throwing or breaking things, being mean to other children, doing dangerous things, disobeying a command to stop a problem behavior, cursing, swearing, or threatening others.

Do not use time-out for behaviors like these: pouting or grumpiness, getting a bad grade, forgetting to do class work or homework, being afraid or shy, or wanting to be alone. Also, do not use time-out unless you have seen the problem behavior happen.

"What are the benefits of time-out?"

✓ It quickly stops many types of problem behaviors.

✓ It is easy to learn and, with practice, it is easy to use.

✓ It does not harm your student emotionally.

✓ Teachers feel less upset when they use time-out.

From Bruce F. Chorpita (2007). Copyright by The Guilford Press.

(page 1 of 4)

"How do I start using time-out?"

(1) **First, pick a behavior** you want to work on. You can write it in the space that follows. Make sure it is the right kind of behavior for time-out. "From now on, my student will get a time-out for":

_____

(2) **Next, pick a place** for time-out. It should be as boring as possible. If your student is younger than 4, pick a chair that you can keep in view. For older children, choose a place that does not have games, toys, or other distractions, such as the back of the room or the hallway. "The place I will use for time-out is":

_____

(3) **Next, pick a time** to tell your student about time-out. The best time to talk about it is when everything is going well and the child is calm. Your student should know that using time-out still means that you respect him or her, but that some behaviors are not allowed. Time-out is not something that your student can argue about. It is part of the new rules for the classroom. If your student does not agree to do time-out, the family can be notified, and some privileges can be taken away. "I will explain time-out to my student":

_____

(4) **Get a timer** to use for time-out. Put it near the time-out place so that it will be ready.

(5) **Remember** to use plenty of praise and rewards when things are going well.

"What are the steps?"

(1) **When the behavior happens,** tell your student "You need to go to time-out." Do this right away, and do it every time the behavior happens.

(2) **Don't explain.** You already explained time-out before. If your student argues or asks why, just say, "We will talk about this after you do your time-out." This is no time for discussion. Don't repeat this more than once or twice. If your student tries to argue too much, add a minute to the time-out by saying, "I just added a minute, please start your time-out." Continue adding a minute until the arguing stops and time-out starts.

(3) **Set the timer** for 1 minute for every year of age for your student.

(4) **Place the timer** out of your student's reach but close enough to be seen. Do not let the child touch the timer.

(5) **Reset the timer** if your student is not quiet and still. Time-out starts when the child is quiet. Remember, no one should talk to your student during time-out, including other students or teachers.

(6) **Talk with your student calmly** after time-out. Ask your student why you gave the time-out. If he or she can't remember, now is the time to explain. Remember, this is not a time to yell or punish—the time-out was the punishment.

(page 3 of 4)

"Help! Time-out isn't working!"

"My student makes a mess during time-out." Require your student to clean the mess before leaving time-out. If anything is damaged, this can be discussed with the family.

"My student cries or whines during time-out." Ignore your student and stay away from the time-out place. Wait until the child is quiet to reset the timer. This can be hard at first, but it will get easier. You may have to use the office or some other place, so the other students are not disrupted.

"My student doesn't believe that I will give a time-out." Never give more than one warning for time-out. If the behavior happens again, you must always send your student to time-out right away. If you do not follow through, the child (and other children) will not respond to your warnings.

"My student thinks the program is not fair." Time-out programs work best when they apply to all children in the classroom. Talk to your class about this when things are calm and quiet, and explain how important this is that all children follow the same rules together.

"My student escapes from time-out." If your student runs out of the class, more serious measures might need to be taken. If it is possible to have time-out supervised in another location (e.g., principal's office), that can sometimes help. Otherwise, a meeting with the family may be required to talk about a more intensive plan.

(page 4 of 4)

References

Addis, M. E., & Krasnow, A. D. (2000). A national survey of practicing psychologists' attitudes toward psychotherapy treatment manuals. *Journal of Consulting and Clinical Psychology, 68,* 331–339.

Albano, A. M., Chorpita, B. F., & Barlow, D. H. (1996). Childhood anxiety disorders. In E. J. Mash & R. A. Barkley (Eds.), *Child psychopathology* (pp. 196–241). New York: Guilford Press.

Albano, A. M., Chorpita, B. F., & Barlow, D. H. (2003). Childhood anxiety disorders. In E. J. Mash & R. A. Barkley (Eds.), *Child psychopathology* (2nd ed., pp. 279–329). New York: Guilford Press.

Alloy, L. B., Kelly, K. A., Mineka, S., & Clements, C. M. (1990). Comorbidity of anxiety and depressive disorders: A helplessness–hopelessness perspective. In J. D. Maser & C. R. Cloninger (Eds.), *Comorbidity of mood and anxiety disorders* (pp. 499–543). Washington, DC: American Psychiatric Press.

American Psychiatric Association. (2000). *Diagnostic and statistical manual of mental disorders* (4th ed., text rev.). Washington, DC: Author.

Anderson, D. J., Williams, S., McGee, R., & Silva, P. A. (1987). DSM-III disorders in preadolescent children: Prevalence in a large sample from the general population. *Archives of General Psychiatry, 44,* 69–76.

Annon, J. S. (1975). *The behavioral treatment of sexual problems. I: Brief therapy.* Oxford, UK: Enabling Systems.

Armbruster, P., & Fallon, T. (1994). Clinical, sociodemographic, and systems risk factors for attrition in a children's mental health clinic. *American Journal of Orthopsychiatry, 64,* 577–585.

Armbruster, P., & Kazdin, A. E. (1994). Attrition in child psychotherapy. *Advances in Clinical Child Psychology, 16,* 81–108.

Bandura, A. (1969). *Principles of behavior modification.* New York: Holt, Rinehart & Winston.

Bandura, A., Blanchard, E. B., & Ritter, B. (1969). Relative efficacy of desensitization and modeling approaches for inducing behavioral, affective, and attitudinal changes. *Journal of Personality and Social Psychology, 13,* 173–199.

Bandura, A., Grusec, J. E., & Menlove, F. L. (1967). Vicarious extinction of avoidance behavior. *Journal of Personality and Social Psychology, 5,* 16–23.

Barabasz, A. F. (1973). Group desensitization of test anxiety in elementary school. *Journal of Psychology, 83,* 295–301.

Barlow, D. H. (1988). *Anxiety and its disorders: The nature and treatment of anxiety and panic.* New York: Guilford Press.

Barlow, D. H. (2000). Unraveling the mysteries of anxiety and its disorders from the perspective of emotion theory. *American Psychologist, 55,* 1247–1263.

Barlow, D. H. (2002). *Anxiety and its disorders: The nature and treatment of anxiety and panic* (2nd ed.). New York: Guilford Press.

Barlow, D. H., Chorpita, B. F., & Turovsky, J. (1996). Fear, panic, anxiety, and the disorders of emotion. In D. A. Hope (Ed.), *Perspectives on anxiety, panic, and fear* (Vol. 43, pp. 251–328). Lincoln, NE: University of Nebraska Press.

Barrett, P. M. (1998). Evaluation of cognitive-behavioral group treatments for childhood anxiety disorders. *Journal of Clinical Child Psychology, 27,* 459–468.

Barrett, P. M., Dadds, M. R., & Rapee, R. M. (1996). Family treatment of childhood anxiety: A controlled trial. *Journal of Consulting and Clinical Psychology, 64,* 333–342.

Barrett, P. M., Rapee, R. M., Dadds, M. M., & Ryan, S. M. (1996). Family enhancement of cognitive style in anxious and aggressive children. *Journal of Abnormal Child Psychology, 24,* 187–203.

Barrios, B. A., & Hartmann, D. P. (1997). Fears and anxieties. In E. J. Mash & L. G. Terdal (Eds.), *Assessment of childhood disorders* (3rd ed., pp. 230–327). New York: Guilford Press.

Barrios, B. A., & O'Dell, S. L. (1998). Fears and anxieties. In E. J. Mash & R. A. Barkley (Eds.), *Treatment of childhood disorders* (2nd ed., pp. 249–337). New York: Guilford Press.

Beck, A. T., Rush, A. J., Shaw, B. F., & Emery, G. (1979). *Cognitive therapy of depression.* New York: Guilford Press.

Beidel, D. C. (1991). Social phobia and overanxious disorder in school-age children. *Journal of the American Academy of Child and Adolescent Psychiatry, 30,* 545–552.

Beidel, D. C., Turner, S. M., & Morris, T. L. (2000). Behavioral treatment of childhood social phobia. *Journal of Consulting of Clinical Psychology, 68,* 1072–1080.

Bell-Dolan, D. J. (1995). Social cue interpretation of anxious children. *Journal of Clinical Child Psychology, 24,* 2–10.

Berg, C. J., Rapoport, J. L., & Flament, M. (1986). The Leyton Obsessional Inventory—Child Version. *Journal of the American Academy of Child and Adolescent Psychiatry, 25,* 84–91.

Bernstein, G. A., & Borchardt, C. M. (1991). Anxiety disorders of childhood and adolescence: A critical review. *Journal of the American Academy of Child and Adolescent Psychiatry, 30,* 519–532.

Beutler, L. E., & Harwood, T. M. (2000). *Prescriptive psychotherapy: A practical guide to systematic treatment selection.* New York: Oxford University Press.

Bickman, L., Lambert, E. W., Karver, M., & Andrade, A. R. (1998). Two low-cost measures of child and adolescent functioning for services research. *Evaluation and Program Planning, 21,* 263–275.

Blanchard, E. B. (1970). Relative contributions of modeling, informational influences, and physical contact in extinction of phobic behavior. *Journal of Abnormal Psychology, 76,* 55–61.

Bornstein, P. H., & Knapp, M. (1981). Self-control desensitization with a multi-phobic boy: A multiple baseline design. *Journal of Behavior Therapy and Experimental Psychiatry, 12,* 281–285.

Bronfenbrenner, U. (1986). Ecology of the family as a context for human development: Research perspectives. *Developmental Psychology, 22,* 723–742.

Burke, A. E., & Silverman, W. K. (1987). The prescriptive treatment of school refusal. *Clinical Psychology Review, 7,* 353–362.

Cacioppo, J. T., Petty, R. E., & Stoltenberg, C. D. (1985). Processes of social influence: The Elaboration Likelihood model of persuasion. In P. C. Kendall (Ed.), *Advances in cognitive-behavioral research and therapy* (Vol. 4, pp. 215–274). San Diego: Academic Press.

Cannon, W. B. (1929). *Bodily changes in pain, hunger, fear and rage* (2nd ed.). Oxford, UK: Appleton.

Chorpita, B. F. (2001). Control and the development of negative emotions. In M. W. Vasey & M. R. Dadds (Eds.), *The developmental psychopathology of anxiety* (pp. 112–142). New York: Oxford University Press.

Chorpita, B. F. (2003). The frontier of evidence-based practice. In A. E. Kazdin & J. R. Weisz (Eds.), *Evidence-based psychotherapies for children and adolescents* (pp. 42–59). New York: Guilford Press.

Chorpita, B. F., Albano, A. M., & Barlow, D. H. (1996). Cognitive processing in children: Relationship to anxiety and family influences. *Journal of Clinical Child Psychology, 25,* 170–176.

Chorpita, B. F., Albano, A. M., & Barlow, D. H. (1998). The structure of negative emotions in a clinical sample of children and adolescents. *Journal of Abnormal Psychology, 107,* 74–85.

Chorpita, B. F., Albano, A. M., Heimberg, R. G., & Barlow, D. H. (1996). A systematic replication of the prescriptive treatment of school refusal behavior in a single subject. *Journal of Behavior Therapy and Experimental Psychiatry, 27*, 281–290.

Chorpita, B. F., & Barlow, D. H. (1998). The development of anxiety: The role of control in the early environment. *Psychological Bulletin, 117*, 3–19.

Chorpita, B. F., & Daleiden, E. L. (2002). Tripartite dimensions of emotion in a child clinical sample: Measurement strategies and implications for clinical utility. *Journal of Consulting and Clinical Psychology, 70*, 1150–1160.

Chorpita, B. F., Daleiden, E. L., Moffitt, C. E., Yim, L. M., & Umemoto L. A. (2000). Assessment of tripartite factors of emotion in children and adolescents. I: Structural validity and normative data of an Affect and Arousal Scale. *Journal of Psychopathology and Behavioral Assessment, 22*, 141–160.

Chorpita, B. F., Daleiden, E., & Weisz, J. R. (2005a). Identifying and selecting the common elements of evidence based interventions: A distillation and matching model. *Mental Health Services Research, 7*, 5–20.

Chorpita, B. F., Daleiden, E., & Weisz, J. R. (2005b). Modularity in the design and application of therapeutic interventions. *Applied and Preventive Psychology, 11*, 141–156.

Chorpita, B. F., & Donkervoet, C. M. (2005). Implementation of the Felix Consent Decree in Hawaii: The impact of policy and practice development efforts on service delivery. In R. G. Steele & M. C. Roberts (Eds.), *Handbook of mental health services for children, adolescents, and families* (pp. 317–332). New York: Kluwer.

Chorpita, B. F., Moffitt, C. E., & Gray, J. A. (2005). Psychometric properties of the Revised Child Anxiety and Depression Scale in a clinical sample. *Behaviour Research and Therapy, 43*, 309–322.

Chorpita, B. F., & Nakamura, B. J. (2006). *Dynamic structure in diagnostic structured interviewing: A comparative test of accuracy and efficiency.* Manuscript submitted for publication.

Chorpita, B. F., Plummer, C. M., & Moffitt, C. E. (2000). Relations of tripartite dimensions of emotion to childhood anxiety and mood disorders. *Journal of Abnormal Child Psychology, 28*, 299–310.

Chorpita, B. F., & Southam-Gerow, M. (2006). Fears and anxieties. In E. J. Mash & R. A. Barkley (Eds.), *Treatment of child disorders* (3rd ed., pp. 271–335). New York: Guilford Press.

Chorpita, B. F., Taylor, A. A., Francis, S. E., Moffitt, C. E., & Austin, A. A. (2004). Efficacy of modular cognitive behavior therapy for childhood anxiety disorders. *Behavior Therapy, 35*, 263–287.

Chorpita, B. F., Tracey, S., Brown, T. A., Collica, T. J., & Barlow, D. H. (1997). Assessment of worry in children and adolescents: An adaptation of the Penn State Worry Questionnaire. *Behaviour Research and Therapy, 35*, 569–581.

Chorpita, B. F., Vitali, A. E., & Barlow, D. H. (1997). Behavioral treatment of choking phobia in an adolescent: An experimental analysis. *Journal of Behavior Therapy and Experimental Psychiatry, 28*, 307–315.

Chorpita, B. F., Yim, L. M., Moffitt, C. E., Umemoto L. A., & Francis, S. E. (2000). Assessment of symptoms of DSM-IV anxiety and depression in children: A Revised Child Anxiety and Depression Scale. *Behaviour Research and Therapy, 38*, 835–855.

Chorpita, B. F., Yim, L. M., & Tracey, S. A. (2002). Feasibility of a simplified and dynamic Bayesian system for use in structured diagnostic interviews. *Journal of Psychopathology and Behavioral Assessment, 24*, 13–23.

Clark, L. A., & Watson, D. (1991). A tripartite model of anxiety and depression: Psychometric evidence and taxonomic implications. *Journal of Abnormal Psychology, 100*, 316–336.

Clark, L. A., Watson, D., & Mineka, S. (1994). Temperament, personality, and the mood and anxiety disorders. *Journal of Abnormal Psychology, 103*, 103–116.

Cobham, V. E., Dadds, Mark R., & Spence, S. H. (1998). The role of parental anxiety in the treatment of childhood anxiety. *Journal of Consulting and Clinical Psychology, 66*, 893–905.

Cohen, J. A., Deblinger, E., Mannarino, A. P., & Steer, R. A. (2004). A multisite, randomized controlled trial for children with sexual abuse-related PTSD symptoms. *Journal of the American Academy of Child and Adolescent Psychiatry, 43*(4), 393–402.

Costello, E. J., Angold, A., Burns, B. J., Erkanli, A., Stangl, D. K., & Tweed, D. L. (1996). The Great

Smoky Mountains study of youth: Functional impairment and serious emotional disturbance. *Archives of General Psychiatry, 53,* 1137–1143.

Crano, W. D., & Prislin, R. (2006). Attitudes and persuasion. *Annual Review of Psychology, 57,* 345–374.

Cuffe, S. P., Addy, C. L., Garrison, C. Z., Waller, J. L., Jackson, K., McKeown, R. E., & Chilappagari, S. (1998). Prevalence of PTSD in a community sample of older adolescents. *Journal of the American Academy of Child and Adolescent Psychiatry, 37,* 147–154.

Cunningham, P. B., & Henggeler, S. W. (1999). Engaging multiproblem families in treatment: Lessons learned throughout the development of multisystemic therapy. *Family Process, 38,* 265–286.

Daleiden, E. L., & Chorpita, B. F. (2005). From data to wisdom: Quality improvement strategies supporting large-scale implementation of evidence based services. In B. J. Burns & K. E. Hoagwood (Eds.), *Child and adolescent psychiatric clinics of North America* (pp. 329–349). Philadelphia: Saunders.

Daleiden, E. L., Chorpita, B. F., & Lu, W. (2000). Assessment of tripartite factors of emotion in children and adolescents II: Construct validity and reliability of an Affect and Arousal Scale. *Journal of Psychopathology and Behavioral Assessment, 22,* 161–177.

Dawes, R. M., Faust, D., & Meehl, P. E. (1989). Clinical versus actuarial judgment. *Science, 243,* 1668–1674.

Deffenbacher, J. L., & Kemper, C. C. (1974). Counseling test-anxious sixth graders. *Elementary School Guidance and Counseling, 21,* 23–29.

De Haan, E., Hoogduin, K., Buitelaar, J. K., & Keijsers, G. P. J. (1998). Behavior therapy versus clomipramine for the treatment of obsessive–compulsive disorder in children and adolescents. *Journal of the American Academy of Child and Adolescent Psychiatry, 37,* 1022–1029.

deRoss, R., Chorpita, B. F., & Gullone, E. (2002). The Revised Child Anxiety and Depression Scale: A psychometric investigation with Australian youth. *Behaviour Change, 19,* 90–101.

DiNardo, P. A., O'Brien, G. T., Barlow, D. H., Waddell, M. T., & Blanchard, E. B. (1983). Reliability of DSM-III anxiety disorders using a new structured interview. *Archives of General Psychiatry, 22,* 1070–1078.

Doucette, A., & Bickman, L. (2001). *Therapeutic Alliance Scale (TAS).* Nashville, TN: Authors.

Durand, V. M. (1990). *Severe behavior problems: A functional approach to communication training.* New York: Guilford Press.

Dweck, C., & Wortman, C. (1982). Learned helplessness, anxiety, and achievement. In H. Krone & L. Laux (Eds.), *Achievement, stress and anxiety* (pp. 93–125). New York: Hemisphere.

Edelbrock, C., & Costello, A. J. (1990). Structured interviews for children and adolescents. In G. Goldstein & M. Hersen (Eds.), *Handbook of Psychological Assessment* (2nd ed., pp. 308–323). New York: Pergamon.

Eisen, A. R., & Silverman, W. K. (1991). Treatment of an adolescent with bowel movement phobia using self-control therapy. *Journal of Behavior Therapy and Experimental Psychiatry, 22,* 45–51.

Eisen, A. R., & Silverman, W. K. (1998). Prescriptive treatment for generalized anxiety disorder in children. *Behavior Therapy, 29,* 105–121.

Essau, C. A., Conradt, J., & Petermann, F. (2000). Frequency, comorbidity, and psychosocial impairment of specific phobia in adolescents. *Journal of Clinical Child Psychology, 29,* 221–231.

Evans, P. D., & Harmon, G. (1981). Children's self-initiated approach to spiders. *Behaviour Research and Therapy, 19,* 543–546.

Eysenck, H. J. (1979). The conditioning model of neurosis. *Behavioral and Brain Sciences, 2*(2), 155–199.

Falloon, I. R. H. (Ed.). (1988). *Handbook of behavioral family therapy.* New York: Guilford Press.

Flament, M. F., Whitaker, A., Rapoport, J. L., Davies, M., Zeremba-Berg, C., Kalikow, K. S., et al. (1988). Obsessive compulsive disorder in adolescence: An epidemiological study. *Journal of the American Academy of Child and Adolescent Psychiatry, 27,* 764–771.

Foa, E. B., & Kozak, M. J. (1986). Emotional processing of fear: Exposure to corrective information. *Psychological Bulletin, 99,* 20–35.

Giebenhain, J., & Barrios, B. A. (1986, November). *Multichannel assessment of children's fears.* Paper presented at the meeting of the Association for Advancement of Behavior Therapy, Chicago.

Ginsburg, G. S., La Greca, A. M., & Silverman, W. K. (1998). Social anxiety in children with anxiety disorders: Relation with social and emotional functioning. *Journal of Abnormal Child Psychology, 26,* 175–185.

Goenjian, A. K., Karayan, I., Pynoos, R. S., Minassian, D., Najarian, L. M., Steinberg, A. M., et al. (1997). Outcome of psychotherapy among early adolescents after trauma. *American Journal of Psychiatry, 154,* 536–542.

Goldberg, L. R. (1968). Simple models or simple processes? Some research on clinical judgments. *American Psychologist, 23,* 483–496.

Gray, J. A. (1987). *The psychology of fear and stress* (2nd ed.). Cambridge, UK: Cambridge University Press.

Gray, J. A., & McNaughton, N. (1996). The neuropsychology of anxiety: Reprise. In D. A. Hope (Ed.), *Nebraska Symposium on Motivation, 1995: Perspectives on anxiety, panic, and fear* (pp. 61–134). Lincoln, NE: University of Nebraska Press.

Graziano, A. M., & Mooney, K. C. (1980). Family self-control instruction for children's nighttime fear reduction. *Journal of Consulting and Clinical Psychology, 48,* 206–213.

Greene, R. W., Ablon, J. S., Monuteaux, M. C., Goring, J. C., Henin, A., Raezer-Blakely, L., et al. (2004). Effectiveness of collaborative problem solving in affectively dysregulated children with oppositional defiant disorder. *Journal of Consulting and Clinical Psychology, 72,* 1157–1164.

Hamilton, S. B., & MacQuiddy, S. L. (1984). Self-administered behavioral parenting training: Enhancement of treatment efficacy using a time-out signal seat. *Journal of Clinical Child Psychology, 13,* 61–69.

Handwerk, M. L., Larzelere, R. E., Soper, S. H., & Friman, P. C. (1999). Parent and child discrepancies in reporting severity of problem behaviors in three out-of-home settings. *Psychological Assessment, 11,* 14–23.

Hatch, M. L., Friedman, S., & Paradis, C. M. (1996). Behavioral treatment of obsessive–compulsive disorder in African Americans [Special issue]. *Cognitive and Behavioral Practice, 3,* 303–315.

Heesacker, M. (1986). Counseling pretreatment and the Elaboration Likelihood Model of attitude change. *Journal of Counseling Psychology, 33,* 107–114.

Henggeler, S. W., Rodick, J. D., Bourdin, C. M., Hanson, C. L., Watson, S. M., & Urey, J. R. (1986). Multisystemic treatment of juvenile offenders: Effects on adolescent behavior and family interaction. *Developmental Psychology, 22,* 132–141.

Henggeler, S. W., Schoenwald, S. K., Borduin, C. M., Rowland, M. D., & Cunningham, P. B. (1998). *Multisystemic treatment of antisocial behavior in children and adolescents.* New York: Guilford Press.

Heyne, D., King, N. J., Tonge, B. J., Rollings, S., Young, D., Pritchard, M., & Ollendick, T. H. (2002). Evaluation of child therapy and caregiver training in the treatment of school refusal. *Journal of the American Academy of Child and Adolescent Psychiatry, 41,* 687–695.

Hodges, K. (1998). *Child and Adolescent Functional Assessment Scale.* Ann Arbor, MI: Functional Assessment Systems.

Hodges, K., & Wong, M. M. (1996). Psychometric characteristics of a multidimensional measure to assess impairment: The Child and Adolescent Functional Assessment Scale. *Journal of Child and Family Studies, 5,* 445–467.

Hodges, K., & Wong, M. M. (1997). Use of the Child and Adolescent Functional Assessment Scale to predict service utilization and cost. *Journal of Mental Health Administration, 24,* 278–290.

Jacobson, N. S., Schmaling, K. B., Holtzworth-Munroe, A., Katt, J. L., Wood, L. F., & Follette, V. M. (1989). Research-structured vs. clinically flexible versions of social learning-based marital therapy. *Behaviour Research and Therapy, 27,* 173–180.

Johnson, T., Tyler, V., Thompson, R., & Jones, E. (1971). Systematic desensitization and assertive training in the treatment of speech anxiety in middle-school students. *Psychology in the Schools, 8,* 263–267.

Joiner, T. E., Catanzaro, S. J., & Laurent, J. (1996). Tripartite structure of positive and negative affect, depression, and anxiety in child and adolescent psychiatric inpatients. *Journal of Abnormal Psychology, 105,* 401–409.

Jones, M. C. (1924). The elimination of children's fears. *Journal of Experimental Psychology, 1,* 383–390.

Kandel, H. J., Ayllon, T., & Rosenbaum, M. S. (1977). Flooding or systematic exposure in the treatment of extreme social withdrawal in children. *Journal of Behavior Therapy and Experimental Psychiatry, 8,* 75–81.

Kanfer, F. H., Karoly, P., & Newman, A. (1975). Reduction of children's fear of the dark by competence-related and situational threat-related verbal cues. *Journal of Consulting and Clinical Psychology, 43,* 251–258.

Kashani, J. H., & Orvaschel, H. (1988). Anxiety disorders in midadolescence: A community sample. *American Journal of Psychiatry, 145,* 960–964.

Kashani, J. H., Orvaschel, H., Rosenberg, T. K., & Reid, J. C. (1989). Psychopathology in a community sample of children and adolescents: A developmental perspective. *Journal of the American Academy of Child and Adolescent Psychiatry, 28,* 701–706.

Kazdin, A. E., Holland, L., & Crowley, M. (1997). Family experience of barriers to treatment and premature termination from child therapy. *Journal of Consulting and Clinical Psychology, 65,* 453–463.

Kazdin, A. E., Siegel, T. C., & Bass, D. (1992). Cognitive problem-solving skills training and parent management training in the treatment of antisocial behavior in children. *Journal of Consulting and Clinical Psychology, 60,* 733–747.

Kearney, C. A. (2001). *School refusal behavior in youth: A functional approach to assessment and treatment.* Washington, DC: American Psychological Association.

Kearney, C. A., & Silverman, W. K. (1990). A preliminary analysis of a functional model of assessment and treatment for school refusal behavior. *Behavior Modification, 14,* 340–366.

Keller, M. B., Lavori, P., Wunder, J., Beardslee, W. R., Schwartz, C. E., & Roth, J. (1992). Chronic course of anxiety disorders in children and adolescents. *Journal of the American Academy of Child and Adolescent Psychiatry, 31,* 595–599.

Kendall, P. C. (1992). Childhood coping: Avoiding a lifetime of anxiety. *Behavioural Change, 9,* 1–8.

Kendall, P. C. (1994). Treating anxiety disorders in children: Results of a randomized clinical trial. *Journal of Consulting and Clinical Psychology, 62,* 100–110.

Kendall, P. C. (2002). *Coping Cat Therapist Manual.* Ardmore, PA: Workbook Publishing.

Kendall, P. C., & Flannery-Schroeder, E. (1998). Methodological issues in treatment research for anxiety disorders in youth [Special issue]. *Journal of Abnormal Child Psychology, 26,* 27–38.

Kendall, P. C., Flannery-Schroeder, E., Panichelli-Mindel, S. M., Southam-Gerow, M., Henin, A., & Warman, M. (1997). Therapy for youths with anxiety disorders: A second randomized clinical trial. *Journal of Consulting and clinical Psychology, 65,* 366–380.

Kendall, P. C., Kane, M., Howard, B., & Siqueland, L. (1990). *Cognitive-behavioral treatment of anxious children: Treatment manual.* Ardmore, PA: Workbook Publishing.

Kendall, P. C., & Sugarman, A. (1997). Attrition in the treatment of childhood anxiety disorders. *Journal of Consulting and Clinical Psychology, 65,* 883–888.

Kendall, P. C., & Treadwell, K. R. H. (1996). Cognitive-behavioral treatment for childhood anxiety disorders. In E. D. Hibbs & P. S. Jensen (Eds.), *Psychosocial treatments for child and adolescent disorders: Empirically based strategies* (pp. 23–41). Washington, DC: American Psychological Association.

King, N. J., Tonge, B. J., Heyne, D., Pritchard, M., Rollings, S., Young, D., et al. (1998). Cognitive-behavioral treatment of school-refusing children: A controlled evaluation. *Journal of the American Academy of Child and Adolescent Psychiatry, 37,* 395–403.

King, N. J., Tonge, B. J., Mullen, P., Myerson, N., Heyne, D., Rollings, S., et al. (2000). Treating sexually abused children with posttraumatic stress symptoms: A randomized clinical trial. *Journal of the American Academy of Child and Adolescent Psychiatry, 39,* 1347–1355.

Klein, R. G. (1991). Parent–child agreement in clinical assessment of anxiety and other psychopathology: A review [Special issue]. *Journal of Anxiety Disorders, 5,* 187–198.

Knox, L. S., Albano, A. M., & Barlow, D. H. (1996). Parental involvement in the treatment of childhood obsessive compulsive disorder: A multiple-baseline examination incorporating parents. *Behavior Therapy, 27,* 93–115.

La Greca, A. M., & Stone, N. (1993). Social Anxiety Scale for Children—Revised: Factor structure and concurrent validity. *Journal of Clinical Child Psychology, 22,* 17–27.

Lang, P. J., & Lazovic, A. D. (1963). Experimental desensitization of a phobia. *Journal of Abnormal and Social Psychology, 66,* 519–525.

Last, C. G., Perrin, S., Hersen, M., & Kazdin, A. E. (1992). DSM-III-R anxiety disorders in children: Sociodemographic and clinical characteristics. *Journal of the American Academy of Child and Adolescent Psychiatry, 31*, 1070–1076.

Last, C. G., Strauss, C. C., & Francis, G. (1987). Comorbidity among childhood anxiety disorders. *Journal of Nervous and Mental Disease, 175*, 726–730.

Laurent, J., Catanzaro, S. J., Joiner, T. E., Rudolph, K. D., Potter, K. I., Lambert, S., et al. (1999). A measure of positive and negative affect for children: Scale development and preliminary validation. *Psychological Assessment, 11*, 326–338.

Laxer, M., & Walker, K. (1970). Counterconditioning versus relaxation in the desensitization of test anxiety. *Journal of Counseling Psychology, 17*, 431–436.

Lazarus, A. A. (1974). Multimodal behavioral treatment of depression. *Behavior Therapy, 5*, 549–554.

Lewis, S. (1974). A comparison of behavior therapy techniques in the reduction of fearful avoidance behavior. *Behavior Therapy, 5*, 648–655.

Liberman, R. P., Mueser, K., & Glynn, S. (1988). Modular behavioral strategies. In I. R. H. Falloon (Ed.), *Handbook of behavioral family therapy* (pp. 27–50). New York: Guilford Press.

Lonigan, C. J., Carey, M. P., & Finch, A. J. (1994). Anxiety and depression in children and adolescents: Negative affectivity and the utility of self-report. *Journal of Consulting and Clinical Psychology, 62*, 1000–1008.

Lonigan, C. J., Hooe, E. S., David, C. F., & Kistner, J. A. (1999). Positive and negative affectivity in children: Confirmatory factor analysis of a two-factor model and its relation to symptoms of anxiety and depression. *Journal of Consulting and Clinical Psychology, 67*, 374–386.

Lonigan, C. J., & Phillips, B. M. (2001). Temperamental influences on the development of anxiety disorders. In M. W. Vasey & M. R. Dadds (Eds.), *The developmental psychopathology of anxiety* (pp. 60–91). New York: Oxford University Press.

Maggini, C., Ampollini, P., Gariboldi, S., Cella, P. L., Peqlizza, L., & Marchesi, C. (2001). The Parma High School epidemiological survey: Obsessive compulsive symptoms. *Acta Psychiatrica Scandinavica, 103*, 441–446.

Mann, J., & Rosenthal, T. L. (1969). Vicarious and direct counter-conditioning of test anxiety through individual and group desensitization. *Behaviour Research and Therapy, 31*, 9–15.

March, J. S., Amaya-Jackson, L., Murray, M. C., & Schulte, A. (1998). Cognitive-behavioral psychotherapy for children and adolescents with posttraumatic stress disorder after a single-incident stressor. *Journal of the American Academy of Child and Adolescent Psychiatry, 37*, 585–593.

March, J. S., Parker, J. D. A., Sullivan, K., Stallings, P., & Conners, K. (1997). The Multidimensional Anxiety Scale for Children (MASC): Factor structure, reliability, and validity. *Journal of the American Academy of Child and Adolescent Psychiatry, 36*, 554–565.

March, J. S., Sullivan, K., & Parker, J. D. A. (1999). Test–retest reliability of the multidimensional anxiety scale for children. *Journal of Anxiety Disorders, 13*, 349–358.

Marks, I. M. (1969). *Fears and phobias.* New York: Academic Press.

Matarazzo, J. D. (1983). The reliability of psychiatric and psychological diagnosis. *Clinical Psychology Review, 3*, 103–145.

McGee, R., Fehan, M., Williams, S., Partridge, F., Silva, P. A., & Kelly, J. (1990). DSM-III disorders in a large sample of adolescents. *Journal of the American Academy of Child and Adolescent Psychiatry, 29*, 611–619.

Meehl, P. E. (1954). *Clinical versus statistical prediction: A theoretical analysis and a review of the evidence.* Lanham, MD: Aronson.

Melamed, B. G., Hawes, R., Heiby, E., & Glick, J. (1975). Use of filmed modeling to reduce uncooperative behavior of children during dental treatment. *Journal of Dental Research, 54*, 757–801.

Melamed, B. G., & Siegel, L. J. (1975). Reduction of anxiety in children facing hospitalization and surgery by use of filmed modeling. *Journal of Consulting and Clinical Psychology, 43*, 511–521.

Menzies, R. G., & Clarke, J. C. (1993). A comparison of *in vivo* and vicarious exposure in the treatment of childhood water phobia. *Behaviour Research and Therapy, 31*, 9–15.

Miller, L. C., Barrett, C. L., Hampe, E., & Noble, H. (1972). Comparison of reciprocal inhibition, psychotherapy, and waiting list control for phobic children. *Journal of Abnormal Psychology, 79*, 269–279.

Minuchin, S., & Fishman, H. (1981). *Family therapy techniques.* Cambridge, MA: Harvard University Press.

Moreau, D., & Weissman, M. M. (1992). Panic disorder in children and adolescents: A review. *American Journal of Psychiatry, 149,* 1306–1314.

Mowrer, O. H. (1939). A stimulus–response analysis of anxiety and its role as a reinforcing agent. *Psychological Review, 46,* 553–565.

Muris, P., Merckelbach, H., Holdrinet, I., & Sijsenaar, M. (1998). Treating phobic children: Effects of EMDR verus exposure. *Journal of Consulting and Clinical Psychology, 66,* 193–198.

Murphy, C. M., & Bootzin, R. R. (1973). Active and passive participation in the contact desensitization of snake fear in children. *Behavior Therapy, 4,* 203–211.

Neal, A. M., & Turner, S. M. (1991). Anxiety disorders research with African Americans: Current status. *Psychological Bulletin, 109,* 400–410.

Nelles, W. B., & Barlow, D. H. (1988). Do children panic? *Clinical Psychology Review, 8,* 359–372.

Nock, M. K., & Kazdin, A. E. (2001). Parent expectancies for child therapy: Assessment and relation to participation in treatment. *Journal of Child and Family Studies, 10,* 155–180.

Nock, M. K., & Kazdin, A. E. (2005). Randomized controlled trial of a brief intervention for increasing participation in parent management training. *Journal of Consulting and Clinical Psychology, 73,* 872–879.

Norcross, J. C. (Ed.). (2002). *Psychotherapy relationships that work: Therapist contributions and responsiveness to patients.* Oxford, UK: Oxford University Press.

Obler, M., & Terwilliger, R. F. (1970). Pilot study on the effectiveness of systematic desensitization with neurologically impaired children with phobic disorders. *Journal of Consulting and Clinical Psychology, 34,* 314–318.

Ollendick, T. H. (1995). Cognitive behavioral treatment of panic disorder with agoraphobia in adolescents: A multiple baseline design analysis. *Behavior Therapy, 26,* 517–531.

Ollendick, T. H., & Francis, G. (1988). Behavioral assessment and treatment of childhood phobias [Special issue]. *Behavior Modification, 12,* 165–204.

Ollendick, T. H., Hagopian, L. P., & Huntzinger, R. M. (1991). Cognitive-behavior therapy with nighttime fearful children. *Journal of Behavior Therapy and Experimental Psychiatry, 22,* 113–121.

Ollendick, T. H., & King, N. J. (1994a). Diagnosis, assessment, and treatment of internalizing problems in children: The role of longitudinal data. *Journal of Consulting and Clinical Psychology, 62,* 918–927.

Ollendick, T. H., & King, N. J. (1994b). Fears and their level of interference in adolescents. *Behaviour Research and Therapy, 32,* 635–638.

Ollendick, T. H., & King, N. J. (1998). Empirically supported treatments for children with phobic and anxiety disorders. *Journal of Clinical Child Psychology, 27,* 156–167.

Ollendick, T. H., King, N. J., & Yule, W. (Eds.). (1994). *International handbook of phobic and anxiety disorders in children and adolescents: Issues in clinical child psychology.* New York: Plenum Press.

Ollendick, T. H., Vasey, M. W., & King, N. J. (2001). Operant conditioning influences in childhood anxiety. In M. W. Vasey & M. R. Dadds (Eds.), *The developmental psychopathology of anxiety* (pp. 231–252). New York: Oxford University Press.

Ollendick, T. H., Yang, B., King, N. J., Dong, Q., & Akande, A. (1996). Fears in American, Australian, Chinese, and Nigerian children and adolescents: A cross-cultural study. *Journal of Child Psychology and Psychiatry, 37,* 213–220.

Oskamp, S. (1962). The relation of clinical experience and training methods to several criteria of clinical prediction. *Psychological Monographs 76,* 27.

Öst, L. G., Svensson, L., Hellström, K., & Lindwall, R. (2001). One-session treatment of specific phobias in youths: A randomized clinical trial. *Journal of Consulting and Clinical Psychology, 69,* 814–824.

Parish, T. S., Buntman, A. D., & Buntman, S. R. (1976). Effect of counterconditioning on test anxiety as indicated by digit span performance. *Journal of Educational Psychology, 68,* 297–299.

Patterson, G. R., Chamberlain, P., & Reid, J. B. (1982). A comparative evaluation of a parent-training program. *Behavior Therapy, 13,* 638–650.

Pavlov, I. (1927). *Conditioned reflexes.* New York: Oxford University Press.

Pediatric OCD Treatment Study Team. (2004). Cognitive behavior therapy, sertraline, and their combination for children and adolescents with obsessive compulsive disorder: The Pediatric OCD Treatment Study (POTS) randomized controlled trial. *Journal of the American Medical Association, 292*, 1969–1976.

Persons, J. B. (1989). *Cognitive therapy in practice: A case formulation approach.* New York: Norton.

Persons, J. B. (1991). Psychotherapy outcome studies do not accurately represent current models of psychotherapy: A proposed remedy. *American Psychologist, 46*, 99–106.

Persons, J. B., & Tompkins, M. A. (1997). Cognitive-behavioral case formulation. In T. D. Eells (Ed.), *Handbook of psychotherapy case formulation* (pp. 314–339). New York: Guilford Press.

Petty, R. E., & Cacioppo, J. T. (1984). The effects of involvement on responses to argument quantity and quality: Central and peripheral routes to persuasion. *Journal of Personality and Social Psychology, 46*, 69–81.

Pfiffner, L., Barkley, R. A., & DuPaul G. J. (2006). Treatment of ADHD in school settings. In R. A. Barkley (Ed.) *Attention-Deficit Hyperactivity Disorder: A Handbook for Diagnosis and Treatment* (3rd ed., pp. 547–589). New York: Guilford Press.

Phillips, N. K., Hammen, C. L., Brennan, P. A., Najman, J. M., & Bor, W. (2005). Early adversity and the prospective prediction of depressive and anxiety disorders in adolescents. *Journal of Abnormal Child Psychology, 33*, 13–24.

Pina, A. A., Silverman, W. K., Fuentes, R. M., Kurtines, W. M., & Weems, C. F. (2003). Exposure-based cognitive-behavioral treatment for phobic and anxiety disorders: Treatment effects and maintenance for Hispanic/Latino relative to European-American youths. *Journal of the American Academy of Child and Adolescent Psychiatry, 42*, 1179–1187.

Pine, D. S. (1994). Child–adult anxiety disorders. *Journal of the American Academy of Child and Adolescent Psychiatry, 33*, 2280.

Rachman, S. (1977). The conditioning theory of fear-acquisition: A critical examination. *Behaviour Research and Therapy, 15*, 375–387.

Reid, J. B., Patterson, G. R., & Snyder, J. (Eds.). (2002). *Antisocial behavior in children and adolescents: A developmental analysis and model for intervention.* Washington, DC: American Psychological Association.

Ritter, B. (1968). The group desensitization of children's snake phobias using vicarious and contact desensitization procedures. *Behaviour Research and Therapy, 6*, 1–6.

Rogers, E. M. (1995). *Diffusion of innovations* (4th ed.). New York: Free Press.

Rutter, M., Tizard, J., & Whitmore, K. (Eds.). (1970). *Education, health and behaviour.* London: Longmans.

Saigh, P. A. (1986). *In vitro* flooding in the treatment of a six-year-old boy's posttraumatic stress disorder. *Behaviour Research and Therapy, 24*, 685–688.

Saigh, P. A. (1987). *In vitro* flooding of a posttraumatic stress disorder. *School Psychology Review, 16*, 203–211.

Santisteban, D. A., Sazpocznik, J., Perez-Vidal, A., Kurtines, W. M., Murray, E. J., & LaPerriere, A. (1996). Efficacy of intervention for engaging youth and families into treatment and some variables that may contribute to differential effectiveness. *Journal of Family Psychology, 10*, 35–44.

Schoenwald, S. K., & Henggeler, S. W. (2003). Current strategies for moving evidence-based interventions into clinical practice: Introductory comments. *Cognitive and Behavioral Practice, 10*, 275–277.

Schulte, D., Kuenzel, R., Pepping, G., & Schulte-Bahrenberg, T. (1992). Tailor-made versus standardized therapy of phobic patients. *Advances in Behaviour Research and Therapy, 14*, 67–92.

Seligman, M. E. (1970). On the generality of the laws of learning. *Psychological Review, 77*, 406–418.

Seligman, M. E. (1971). Phobias and preparedness. *Behavior Therapy, 2*, 307–320.

Shirk, S. R., & Saiz, C. C. (1992). Clinical, empirical, and developmental perspectives on the therapeutic relationship in child psychotherapy [Special issue]. *Development and Psychopathology, 4*, 713–728.

Silverman, W. K., & Albano, A. M. (1996). *Anxiety Disorders Interview Schedule for Children–IV, Child and Parent Versions.* San Antonio, TX: Psychological Corporation.

Silverman, W. K., Kurtines, W. M., Ginsburg, G. S., Weems, C. F., Lumpkin, P. W., & Carmichael, D. H. (1999). Treating anxiety disorders in children with group cognitive-behavioral therapy: A randomized clinical trial. *Journal of Consulting and Clinical Psychology, 67*(6), 995–1003.

Silverman, W. K., Kurtines, W. M., Ginsburg, G. S., Weems, C. F., Rabian, B., & Serafini, L. T. (1999) Contingency management, self-control, and education support in the treatment of childhood phobic disorders: A randomized clinical trial. *Journal of Consulting and Clinical Psychology, 67*(5), 675–687.

Silverman, W. K., Saavedra, L. M., & Pina, A. A. (2001). Test–retest reliability of anxiety symptoms and diagnoses with Anxiety Disorders Interview Schedule for DSM-IV: Child and Parent Versions. *Journal of the American Academy of Child and Adolescent Psychiatry, 40*, 937–944.

Southam-Gerow, M. A., Chorpita, B. F., Miller, L. M., & Taylor, A. A. (2006). *Private and public referrals in a child anxiety disorders clinic: Similarities and differences.* Manuscript submitted for publication.

Southam-Gerow, M. A., Weisz, J. R., & Kendall, P. C. (2003). Youth with anxiety disorders in research and service clinics: Examining client differences and similarities. *Journal of Clinical Child and Adolescent Psychology, 32*, 375–385.

Spence, S. H., Donovan, C., & Brechman-Toussaint, M. (2000). The treatment of childhood social phobia: The effectiveness of a social skills training-based, cognitive-behavioural intervention, with and without parental involvement. *Journal of Child Psychology and Psychiatry, 41*, 713–726.

Stavrakaki, C., Vargo, B., Roberts, N., & Boodoosingh, L. (1987). Concordance among sources of information for ratings of anxiety and depression in children. *Journal of the American Academy of Child and Adolescent Psychiatry, 26*, 733–737.

Strauss, C. C. (1993). Anxiety disorders. In T. H. Ollendick & M. Hersen (Eds.), *Handbook of child and adolescent assessment* (pp. 239–250). Needham Heights, MA: Allyn & Bacon.

Strauss, C. C., Last, C. G., Hersen, M., & Kazdin, A. E. (1988). Association between anxiety and depression in children and adolescents with anxiety disorders. *Journal of Abnormal Child Psychology, 16*, 57–68.

Strauss, C. C., Lease, C. A., Last, C. G., & Francis, G. (1988). Overanxious disorder: An examination of developmental differences. *Journal of Abnormal Child Psychology, 16*, 433–443.

Substance Abuse and Mental Health Services Administration. (1993). Final notice establishing definitions for (1) children with a serious emotional disturbance, and (2) adults with a serious mental illness. *Federal Register, 58*, 422–429.

Swedo, S. E., Rapoport, J. L., Leonard, H., Lenane, M., & Cheslow, D. (1989). Obsessive–compulsive disorder in children and adolescents: Clinical phenomenology of 70 consecutive cases. *Archives of General Psychiatry, 46*, 335–341.

Treadwell, K. R. H., Flannery-Schroeder, E. C., & Kendall, P. C. (1995). Ethnicity and gender in relation to adaptive functioning, diagnostic status, and treatment outcome in children from an anxiety clinic. *Journal of Anxiety Disorders, 9*, 373–384.

Treadwell, K. R. H., & Kendall, P. C. (1996). Self-talk in youth with anxiety disorders: States of mind, content specificity, and treatment outcome. *Journal of Consulting and Clinical Psychology, 64*, 941–950.

Ultee, C. A., Griffioen, D., & Schellekens, J. (1982). The reduction of anxiety in children: A comparison of the effects of "systematic desensitization *in vitro*" and "systematic desensitization *in vivo*." *Behaviour Research and Therapy, 20*, 61–67.

Van Hasselt, V. B., Hersen, M., Bellack, A. S., Rosenblum, N. D., & Lamparski, D. (1979). Tripartite assessment to the effects of systematic desensitization in a multi-phobic child: An experimental analysis. *Journal of Behavior Therapy and Experimental Psychiatry, 10*, 51–55.

Vasey, M. W., & Daleiden, E. L. (1994). Worry in children. In G. C. L. Davey & F. Tallis (Eds.), *Worrying: Perspectives on theory, assessment and treatment* (pp. 185–207). Oxford, UK: Wiley.

Vasey, M. W., Daleiden, E. L., Williams, L. L., & Brown, L. M. (1995). Biased attention in childhood anxiety disorders: A preliminary study. *Journal of Abnormal Child Psychology, 23*, 267–279.

Verhulst, F. C., van der Ende, J., Ferdinand, R. F., & Kasius, M. C. (1997). The prevalence of DSM-III-R diagnoses in a national sample of Dutch adolescents. *Archives of General Psychiatry, 54*, 329–336.

Warren, R., & Zgourides, G. (1988). Panic attacks in high school students: Implications for prevention and intervention. *Phobia Practice and Research Journal, 1*, 97–113.

Watson, D., & Clark, L. A. (1984). Negative affectivity: The disposition to experience negative emotional states. *Psychological Bulletin, 96*, 465–490.

Watson, J. B., & Morgan, J. J. B. (1917). Emotional reactions and psychological experimentation. *American Journal of Psychology, 28*, 163–174.

Watson, J. B., & Rayner, R. (1920). Conditioned and emotional reactions. *Journal of Experimental Psychology, 3,* 1–14.

Weissbrod, C. W., & Bryan, J. H. (1973). Filmed treatment as an effective fear-reduction technique. *Journal of Abnormal Child Psychology, 1,* 196–201.

Weisz, J. R., Donenberg, G. R., Han, S. S., & Kauneckis, D. (1995). Child and adolescent psychotherapy outcomes in experiments versus clinics: Why the disparity? [Special issue]. *Journal of Abnormal Child Psychology, 23,* 83–106.

Weisz, J. R., Donenberg, G. R., Han, S. S., & Weiss, B. (1995). Bridging the gap between laboratory and clinic in child and adolescent psychotherapy. *Journal of Consulting and Clinical Psychology, 63,* 688–701.

Weisz, J. R., Weersing, V. R., Valeri, S. M., & McCarty, C. A. (1999). *Therapist's Manual PASCET: Primary and secondary control enhancement training program.* Los Angeles: University of California.

Wells, K. C., & Egan, J. (1988). Social learning and systems family therapy for childhood oppositional disorder: Comparative treatment outcome. *Comprehensive Psychiatry, 29,* 138–146.

Wilson, G. T. (1996). Manual-based treatments: The clinical application of research findings. *Behaviour Research and Therapy, 34,* 295–314.

Wilson, G. T. (1998). Manual-based treatment and clinical practice. *Clinical Psychology: Science and Practice, 5,* 363–375.

Wilson, G. T. (2000, November). *Manual-based treatment in clinical practice: Future directions.* Paper presented at the AABT annual convention, New Orleans.

Wolpe, J. (1989). The derailment of behavior therapy: A tale of conceptual misdirection. *Journal of Behaviour Therapy and Experimental Psychiatry, 20,* 3–15.

Wolpe, J., & Lazarus, A. A. (1966). *Behavior therapy techniques: A guide to the treatment of neuroses.* Elmsford, NY: Pergamon Press.

Wolpe, J., & Rowan, V. C. (1988). Panic disorder: A product of classical conditioning. *Behaviour Research and Therapy, 26,* 441–450.

Zohar, A. H., Ratzoni, G., Pauls, D. L., Apter, A., Bleich, A., Kron, S., et al. (1992). An epidemiological study of obsessive–compulsive disorder and related disorders in Israeli adolescents. *Journal of the American Academy of Child and Adolescent Psychiatry, 31,* 1057–1061.

Index

Items in **bold** indicate reproducible worksheets and handouts.
t indicates table; *f* indicates figure

Cognitive-behavioral therapy, 44–45
Cognitive procedures
    overview, 94–95, 95f
    troubleshooting, 105–106
Cognitive restructuring
    Cognitive Restructuring: Catastrophic
        Thinking module, 174–180
    Cognitive Restructuring: Probability
        Overestimation module, 168–173
    Cognitive Restructuring: STOP module,
        181–187
    overview, 44–45
    troubleshooting, 106
Cognitive Restructuring: Catastrophic
    Thinking module, 174–180
Cognitive Restructuring modules, 125, 168–
    173, 174–180, 181–187
Cognitive Restructuring: Probability
    Overestimation module, 168–173
Cognitive Restructuring: STOP module, 181–
    187
Cognitive techniques, 43t
Collaboration, impaired. See Impaired
    collaboration
Collaborative strategies
    engagement and, 115–117
    intensity strategies and, 117–119
Commitment to treatment, 148, 149. See also
    Engagement
Complaining behaviors, 197–204
Comprehensive assessment. See Assessment,
    comprehensive
Compulsions, 18
Concentration difficulties, 17
Consent, informed, 116
Consequences of exposure, 156
Continuous Practice Record
    complete, 244
    Practice: In Vivo module, 151–156
Control, perception of, 20–21
Coping self-talk, 44
Core treatment plan. See Treatment plan
Cost–benefit ratio
    collaborative strategies and, 115
    engagement and, 114, 114t
Course of anxiety disorders, 15

Covert modeling, 45
Creativity in designing exposures, 74–77, 78t
Crying
    Active Ignoring module and, 96
    social phobia and, 17
Cultural considerations
    attrition risk and, 113
    overview, 68

D

Decision-making, clinical, 41–42
Delinquency, 117–118
Demographics, 113
Dependency, tangible, 103–104, 210
Depression, 35t
Diagnosis
    anxiety syndromes, 16–19, 16t
    assessment and, 34, 35t, 36, 36t, 39
    exposure and, 69–74
    multiple, 15
    overview, 15
Direct confrontation exposure. See In vivo
    exposure
Discrete Practice Record
    complete, 243
    Practice: Imaginal module, 157–162
    Practice: In Vivo module, 151–156
Disruptive behavior disorders, 35t
Dizziness, panic attacks and, 19
Drawings Worksheet, 137
DSM-IV-TR
    anxiety syndromes, 16–19, 16t
    negative affectivity, 20

E

Educational implications of anxiety, 15
"80/20" approach to termination, 111
Emotional processing theory
    exposure and, 54
    overview, 66
Emotions, confusing with thoughts, 106, 173,
    179–180, 187

Therapist behavior
    before, during and after exposure, 58–60,
        67–68
    rapport and, 63–64
Thought records
    five-column, 168–173, 263
    seven-column, 174–180, 264
    two-column, 168–173, 262
Thoughts. *See also* Cognitive restructuring
    anxious thinking, 22–23
    cognitive procedures and, 95*f*
    Cognitive Restructuring: Catastrophic
        Thinking module, 174–180
    Cognitive Restructuring: Probability
        Overestimation module, 168–173
    Cognitive Restructuring: STOP module,
        181–187
    confusing with emotions, 106, 173, 179–180,
        187
    during a panic attack, 19
Thoughts Record, 224
Threats, reactions to, 23–24
Tic disorders, assessment and, 35*t*
Time-Out Handout
    for parents, 304–307
    for teachers, 308–311
    Working With Parents: Time-Out module,
        212–218
Time-Out module
    overview, 96–97
    troubleshooting, 109–110
    Working With Parents: Time-Out module,
        212–218
Toolbox approach, 124–125
Treatment flexibility
    how the modules support, 82–83, 83*f*
    individualizing treatment, 81–82
    modular treatment and, 83–88, 85*f*, 86*f*, 87*f*
    pace of interventions and, 124
Treatment manuals, 10–11
Treatment plan. *See also* Exposure
    assessment and, 48–50, 49*f*, 50*f*
    "core four" procedures, 47–48, 48*f*
    how the modules support, 82–83, 83*f*, 89*t*
    importance of exposure in, 45–47, 46*f*
    individualizing treatment, 81–82
    overview, 41–42

treatment options, 42, 43*t*, 44–45
Treatment planning, 84–88, 85*f*, 86*f*, 87*f*, 91–92,
    91*f*
Treatments for anxiety, 42, 43*t*, 44–45. *See also*
    Exposure
Troubleshooting
    Active Ignoring module, 106–108, 203–204
    cognitive procedures and, 105–106
    Cognitive Restructuring: Catastrophic
        Thinking module, 179–180
    Cognitive Restructuring: Probability
        Overestimation module, 173
    Cognitive Restructuring: STOP module,
        186–187
    Fear Ladder module, 100–101
    fundamentals of treatment and, 99
    Learning about Anxiety module, 143
    Learning about Anxiety—Parent module,
        150
    Maintenance and Relapse Prevention
        module, 166–167
    Maintenance module, 110–111
    Making a Fear Ladder module, 134–135
    overview, 9, 91*f*, 97–98
    Practice: Imaginal module, 161–162
    Practice: *In Vivo* module, 155–156
    Psychoeducation module, 101–102
    Rewards module, 102–105, 209–211
    Social Skills: Meeting New People module,
        191
    Social Skills: Nonverbal Communication
        module, 196
    social skills training, 108–109
    Time-Out module, 109–110, 217
    Working With Parents: Active Ignoring
        module, 203–204
    Working With Parents: Rewards module,
        102–105, 209–211
    Working With Parents: Time-Out module,
        109–110, 217
Trust, posttraumatic stress disorder and, 73
Turning-point phenomenon, 66–67
Two-Column Thought Record
    Cognitive Restructuring: Probability
        Overestimation module, 168–173
    complete, 262
Two-stage model of anxiety, 23–24